Progress in Drug Research
Fortschritte der Arzneimittelforschung
Progrès des recherches pharmaceutiques
Vol. 45

Progress in Drug Research
Fortschritte der Arzneimittelforschung
Progrès des recherches pharmaceutiques
Vol. 45

Edited by / Herausgegeben von / Rédigé par
Ernst Jucker, Basel

Authors / Autoren / Auteurs
Vijendra K. Singh · Margaret E. Gnegy · S.P. Gupta · R. Leurs, R.C. Vollinga and H. Timmerman · Ray W. Fuller · Nissim Claude Cohen and Vincenzo Tschinke · Elaine J. Benaksas, E. David Murray, Jr. and William J. Wechter · Indra Dwivedy and Suprabhat Ray

1995

Birkhäuser Verlag
Basel · Boston · Berlin

Editor:

Dr. E. Jucker
Steinweg 28
CH-4107 Ettingen
Switzerland

Softcover reprint of the hardcover 1st edition 1995

Printed on acid-free paper produced from chlorine-free pulp. TCF ∞

ISBN-13: 978-3-0348-7166-2 e-ISBN-13: 978-3-0348-7164-8
DOI: 10.1007/978-3-0348-7164-8

9 8 7 6 5 4 3 2 1

Contents · Inhalt · Sommaire

Foreword

Volume 45 of "Progress in Drug Research" contains eight reviews and the various indexes which facilitate its use and establish the connection with the previous volumes. The articles in this volume deal with neuropeptides as native immune modulators, with Calmodulin and with effects of cell stimuli and drugs on cellular activation, with recent advances in benzodiazepine receptor binding studies, with the medicinal chemistry and therapeutic potentials of ligands of the histamine H_3 receptor, with Serotonin uptake inhibitors, with computer-aided drug design, with natriuretic hormones and with the recent developments in the chemotherapy of osteoporosis.

In the 36 years that PDR has existed, the Editor has enjoyed the valuable help and advice of many colleagues. Readers, the authors of the reviews and, last but not least, the reviewers have all contributed greatly to the success of this series. Although the comments received so far have generally been favorable, it is nevertheless necessary to analyze and to reassess the current position and the future direction of such a series of monographs.

So far, it has been the Editor's intention to help disseminate information on the vast domain of drug research, and to provide the reader with a tool with which to keep abreast of the latest developments and trends. The reviews in PDR are useful to the nonspecialist, who can obtain an overview of a particular field of drug research in a relatively short time. The specialist readers of PDR will appreciate the reviews' comprehensive bibliographies, and, in addition, they may even get fresh impulses for their own research. Finally, the readers can use the 45 volumes of PDR as an encyclopedic source of information.

It gives me great pleasure to present this new volume to our readers. At the same time I would like to extend my gratitude to the authors who willingly accepted the task of preparing extensive reviews. My sincere thanks also go to Birkhäuser Verlag, and in particular to Mrs. L. Koechlin and Mssrs. H.-P. Thür, E. Mazenauer and G. Messmer. Without their personal commitment and assistance, editing PDR would be a nearly impossible task.

Basel, October 1995 DR. E. JUCKER

Vorwort

Der vorliegende 45. Band der Reihe «Fortschritte der Arzneimittelforschung» enthält acht Beiträge sowie die verschiedenen Register, welche das Arbeiten mit diesem Band erleichtern und den Zugriff auf die vorhergehenden Bände ermöglichen.

Die Artikel des 45. Bandes behandeln wiederum verschiedene aktuelle Themen des komplexen Gebietes der Arzneimittelforschung. Neuropeptide und ihre Rolle als Modulatoren des Immunsystems werden behandelt und Calmodulin und seine Wirkungen beschrieben. Ein Beitrag befasst sich mit dem Benzodiazepinrezeptor, und die Übersicht über Liganden des Histamin H_3 Rezeptors beleuchtet seine potentiellen therapeutischen Möglichkeiten. Die Verwendung von Serotonin-Aufnahme Inhibitoren in der Therapie wird zusammengefasst und die Möglichkeiten des Einsatzes von Computern in der Entwerfung neuer Strukturen dargestellt. In einem weiteren Beitrag werden die neuesten Ergebnisse der Untersuchungen an Natriuretischen Hormonen behandelt, und der letzte Beitrag fasst schliesslich das Neueste in der Chemotherapie der Osteoporose zusammen.

Seit der Gründung der Reihe sind 36 Jahre vergangen. In dieser langen Zeitspanne konnte der Herausgeber immer auf den Rat der Fachkollegen, der Leser und der Autoren zählen. Manche Anregungen empfing ich auch von den Rezensenten. Obwohl die grosse Mehrzahl der Besprechungen positiv war, stellt sich doch immer wieder die Frage nach dem Sinn und Zweck der «Fortschritte». Nach wie vor ist es unser Ziel, neueste Forschungen in Form von Übersichtsreferaten darzustellen und dem Leser auf diese Weise zu ermöglichen, sich verhältnismässig rasch und mühelos über bestimmte aktuelle Richtungen der Arzneimittelforschung zu informieren. Er erhält damit die Möglichkeit, sich in diesem komplexen und rasant sich entwickelnden Fachgebiet auf dem Laufenden zu halten. Dem Spezialisten hingegen bieten die «Fortschritte» eine wertvolle Quelle der Originalliteratur dar, erlauben ihm Vergleichsmöglichkeiten und können u.U. seine eigenen Untersuchungen befruchten. Für alle Leser stellen die «Fortschritte» mit ihren umfangreichen Registern eine nützliche Quelle von enzyklopädischem Wissen dar, so dass das gesamte Werk auch als Nachschlagewerk dienen kann.

Zum Gedeihen dieser Reihe haben vor allem die Autoren beigetragen; ihnen allen sei hier gedankt. Dank gebührt auch dem Birkhäuser Verlag, insbesondere Frau L. Koechlin und den Herren H.-P. Thür, E. Mazenauer und G. Messmer.

Basel, Oktober 1995 DR. E. JUCKER

Progress in Drug Research, Vol. 45 (E. Jucker, Ed.)

Neuropeptides as native immune modulators

By Vijendra K. Singh
Department of Psychiatry, Psychoneuroimmunology Laboratory, University of Michigan Medical School, MSRB-I, Room A520B, Box 0656, Ann Arbor, Michigan 48109, USA

1 General introduction

Historically, all diseases in man have been considered to be interdependently related to such parameters as mental attitudes (neural factors), resistance to natural environment (immune factors), and population predisposition (genetic factors). Also, it has long been known that there are nervous system diseases that are mediated by the immune system but only recently it has become clear that the immune system itself may be regulated by the nervous system. So the cells of the immune system may function in a sensory capacity, presumably relaying foreign signals to the brain which would otherwise not be recognized by the more classical sensory system. Moreover, not only can the nervous system modulate immune responses (neuroimmunomodulation) but the immunocompetent cells may control the function of nerve cells (immunoneuromodulation), a reciprocal interrelationship between the two systems [1–3]. We previously [3] postulated that this relationship is of pathophysiologic significance as it fundamentally denotes the existence of immunologic abnormalities in neurologic or neuropsychiatric diseases. Now we also know that the evidence for neuroimmunomodulation is at virtually every level: structural, cellular, molecular, and physiological.

Psychoneuroimmunology (PNI), a rapidly emerging sub-specialty of neuropsychiatry and neuropsychology with immunologic involvement [4], has revealed extensive interconnections between the immune system and the nervous system. Much evidence now exists for viewing the interaction of psychological, neuroendocrine, and immune systems as a complex and integrated whole. Furthermore, several studies have demonstrated that there are associations between immunological parameters and psychological variables such as behavioral patterns and affective states. The general concept that the mind (and thus the behavior) can influence the course and perhaps the emergence of well-defined diseases.

Since the original report of stress-induced modulation of immune response [5], numerous studies have demonstrated that life-long stress suppresses the body's immunity [reviewed in ref. 6, 7]. The stressful events are commonly associated with a generalized suppression of immune functions. The psychological stressors such as bereavement following death of a spouse or relative, marital distress due to divorce or separation, and medical students with intense loneliness have been shown to suppress lymphocyte response to mitogens and natural killer (NK) cell activity. Similarly, the environmental stressors such as sleep deprivation, space-shuttle slashdown, enforced joblessness, and caregiving to Alzheimer's disease patients decrease T-cells, T-helper cells, lymphocyte response to mitogens, and NK-cell activity. On the other hand, situations such as physical exercise that reduce stress are known to restore immunity [8]. All of these findings suggest that modifying health habits, stress management, and developing better emotional support systems can be viewed as having equal importance to medicine in the prevention and treatment of today's health problems. More than that, the study of neuro-immune interactions is unfolding a new chapter in understanding a biological basis of mind-body relationships as in hope and faith [9]. This review article summarizes evidence that implicates neuropeptides as native mediators of immune response modulation.

2 Interplay between the nervous system and the immune system

Recent evidence suggests that the neuroendocrine and immune systems interact and respond to physiological and pharmacological stimuli in a coordinated manner. The relationships between nervous and immune systems are such that there exists a complete regulatory loop between the two systems [1, 10, 11]. The bidirectional communication between the ner-

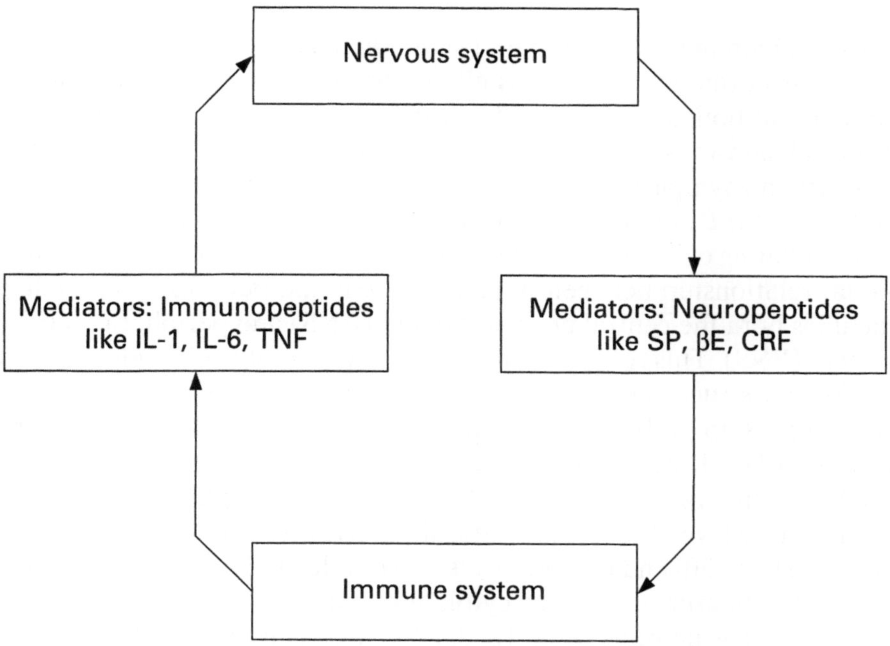

Fig. 1
Reciprocal relationship between the nervous system and the immune system

Table 1.
Antigenic expression common to both brain and immune cells

1.	Thy-1 antigen, a membrane glycoprotein of sequence homology with IgG.
2.	MRC OX-2 antigen, a glycoprotein of sequence homology with Ig light chains.
3.	Presence of Fc receptors, OKM1, and complement (C3, C4) proteins.
4.	Cytokines (IL-1, IL-6 and TNF) and their receptors [24].
5.	T-cell antigens such as CD4 and CD8.
6.	NKH-1 (Leu-7)-positive NK-cell antigen CD56.
7.	Ion-channels such as Na^+, K^+ and Ca^{++} ions.
8.	Receptors for neuropeptides (CRF, ACTH, substance P, etc.) and neurotransmitters (serotonin, dopamine, acetylcholine, etc.).
9.	Brain-derived proteins (MBP, S100, beta-APP, etc.) and peptide hormones (CRF, GH, ACTH, TRH, etc.).
10.	Enzymes of neurotransmitter metabolism such as acetylcholine esterase, choline acetyltransferase, etc.

(For individual references, see [3, 12 and 24])

vous and immune system (Figure 1) is mediated by soluble products (neuropeptide hormones, neurotransmitters, cytokines, and thymic hormones) common to both systems [12–15]. Autocrine or paracrine secretion and humoral pathways, and direct innervation of lymphoid tissue by primary sensory and sympathetic nerve fibers represent modes for the nervous system and the immune system to interact with each other [12, 13, 16]. Accumulating evidence suggests that there is a reciprocal structural-functional relationship between immune system and nervous system which includes both the central nervous system (CNS) and peripheral nervous system (PNS). This relationship is evident at virtually all levels of organization, i.e. structural, cellular, molecular and physiological. The structural relationship (Table 1) is exemplified by the fact that several antigenic proteins (Thy-1, Fc receptors, MBP, ACTH, endorphins, corticotropins, etc.) are commonly expressed in both brain and lymphoid cells [17–19]. At a cellular level, there is the natural occurrence of ion-channels for K^+, Na^+, and Ca^{++} [20] and receptor sites for soluble mediators (neuropeptide hormones, neurotransmitters, cytokines, and thymic hormones) in brain cells as well as immune cells [12, 20, 21]. Molecular studies showed that the genetic message encoding specific neuropeptides and interleukins is present in the cells of both nervous and immune system [12, 22]. And phys-

Table 2.
Functional interplay between the nervous system and the immune system

1.	IFN-γ and IL-3 [25] induce expression of Ia and MHC class II antigens by brain cells.
2.	IL-4 activates microglia but inhibits MHC class II antigen expression on these cells [26].
3.	Brain lesions modify immune responses directly or indirectly via neuroendocrine system.
4.	Immune responses invoke firing of CNS noradrenergic cells.
5.	Both monocytes and astrocytes present antigen to T-cells.
6.	Both neurons and lymphocytes synthesize neuropeptides (ACTH, βE, CRF, VIP, etc.).
7.	Several neuropeptides (VIP, SP, βE, CRF, ACTH, somatostatin, etc.) display immunomodulating properties.
8.	Interleukins such as IL-1 and IL-6 regulate hypothalamic synthesis and secretion of neuropeptide hormones.
9.	Many cytokines are synthesized in the brain and they modulate proliferation and differentiation of glial cells [24].
10.	Neuropeptide hormones such as TRH control thymus physiology including thymocyte development [27].
11.	Thymectomy impairs immune response and deteriorates learning and memory [28].

(For individual references, see [3, 12 and 24–28])

iologically speaking (Table 2), the cells of the two systems have a memory function and their soluble products act as growth factors with mitogenic activity [23, 24]. Thus there exists a very complex interplay between the nervous system and the immune system.

3 Immunomodulatory network

The immune system, like the nervous system, consists of specialized cell types that have unique functions and a specialized set of chemical messengers. There are two specific types of immune responses, namely the cell-mediated immune (CMI) response (cellular immunity) and the antibody-mediated immune (AMI) response or humoral immunity. A highly complicated network of immunoregulatory cells and cytokines, mainly

Table 3.
Cell-specificity of T- and B-cell mitogens

Mitogen	Responsive cell type
Phytohemagglutinin (PHA)	T-cells (human and mouse)
Concanavalin A (Con A)	T-cells (human and mouse, best for mouse)
Monoclonal Ab to CD3 (anti-CD3)	T-cells (human and mouse)
Pokeweed mitogen (PWM)	B-cells, T-cell-dependent (human but not for mouse)
S. aureus Cowain I strain (SAC)	B-cells, T-cell-independent (human)
Epstein-Barr Virus (EBV)	B-cells (human)
Lipopolysaccharide (LPS)	B-cells (mouse but not for human)

interleukins, provides an integrated line of defense mechanisms in higher organisms.The cellular immunity is primarily a function of T-lymphocytes, which are thymus-derived. A marker on all T-cells is the Thy-1 antigen which is also present in brain cells [17]. The function of T-cells is to induce a cellular immune response that occurs either by direct interaction with other cells or indirectly through the production and release of soluble mediators such as interleukins. T-lymphocytes are stimulated by T-cell mitogens such as PHA and Con A (Table 3). On interaction with T-cell mitogens, at least two events occur: (i) T-cell proliferation or blastogenesis, and (ii) production of cytokines. The two prominent T-cell-derived cytokines are IL-2 and IFN-γ. The IL-2 acts as an autocrine growth factor for T-lymphocytes (both helper and suppressor cells) whereas IFN-γ activates cytotoxic cells and macrophages and increases expression of MHC class II antigens by both lymphoid and brain cells. There are two major subsets of T-cells, namely helper (CD4+) and suppressor (CD8+) T-cells. After antigen (Ag) sensitization, the Ag-specific cytotoxic T-cells mediate cellular immunity.

The humoral immunity is a function of B-lymphocytes. The name for B-cells is derived from bursa in avian species and the bursa equivalent of bone marrow in mammals. Mature B-cells are marked by expression of cell surface membrane immunoglobulins (SmIg). The function of B-cells is to synthesize antibodies that are immunoglobulins (IgM, IgG, IgA, IgD and IgE). As schematically illustrated in Figure 2, the counterbalance of helper and suppressor T-cell function regulates B-cell response. In addition, T-cells produce and elaborate helper factors (IL-4, IL-5, etc.) which control the growth and differentiation of B-cells. The B-lymphocytes are

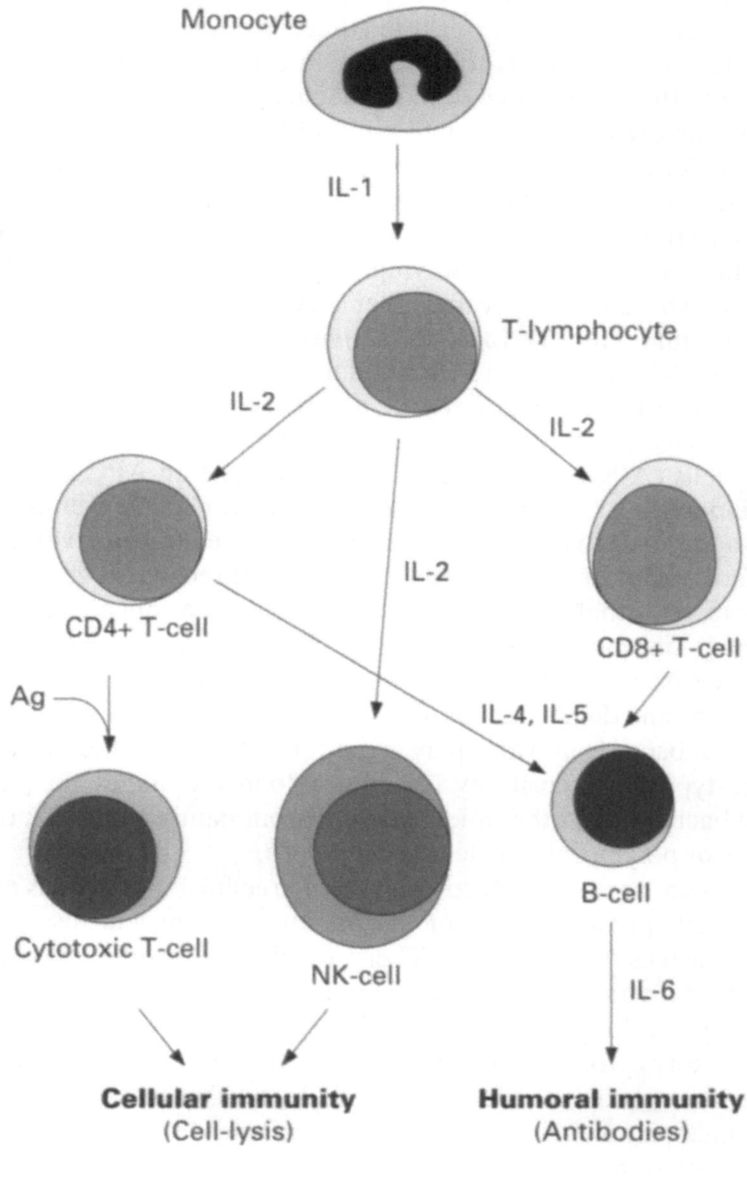

Fig. 2
Simplified sketch of immunoregulatory network

responsive to B-cell mitogens such as pokeweed mitogen (PWM) in human and lipopolysaccharide (LPS) in rodent (Table 3).The NK-cells are large granular lymphocytes (LGL) involved in cellular immunity. They cause spontaneous cell-mediated cytotoxicity in the absence of an antibody or prior antigen-sensitization. Because NK-cells provide natural resistance against tumors cells, virus- or microbe-infected cell and bone marrow transplants, they represent a primary mechanism of immune surveillance [29]. Certain cytokines such as IFN-α and IL-2 stimulate NK-cell activity. The killer (K) cells are also a subpopulation of lymphocytes without T- or B-cell surface marker but have Fc receptors. They provide immunity against tumor cells by antibody-dependent cell-cytotoxicity (ADCC). Incubation of peripheral blood lymphocytes with IL-2 results in the production of lymphokine-activated killer (LAK) cells which lyse tumor cells but not normal cells. The LAK cell activity is essentially a function of IL-2-activated NK cells that induce cellular immunity by ADCC [30].

Monocytes or macrophages are the accessory cells that present foreign antigens to lymphocytes. Hence they are referred to as the antigen-presenting cells (APC). The antigen interaction with an APC is a key step in the induction of an immune response. The APCs have a unique property of adherence to a polystyrene surface. They express a diverse nature of surface receptors (Fc receptors, complement receptors, growth factor receptors, etc.) that allows them to interact with a range of hormones, exogenous and endogenous proteins and lipids. There are cells other than monocytes or macrophages that can also function as APCs, for instance Langerhans and dendritic cells in the skin. Macrophages also cause phagocytosis of bacteria and also play an important role in inflammation and delayed-type hypersensitivity. In addition to macrophages, the phagocytosis of bacteria and other microbes is predominantly a function of granulocytes or polymorphonuclear (PMN) cells.

Cytokines are signaling molecules involved in cellular interactions between diverse cells predominantly of the immune system, but also of other systems such as skin and brain. There are about a dozen or so cytokines whose bioactivities have been well-characterized (Table 4).

Generally speaking, cytokines are divided into two categories: (i) proinflammatory cytokines that include IL-1, IL-6 and TNF; and (ii) immunoregulatory cytokines such as IL-2, IL-4, etc. The cytokine production is no longer restricted to the immune system since they are also produced by a variety of non-lymphoid cells including brain cells [24]. Cytokines are a group of low molecular weight proteins that are often glycosylated. Biologically speaking, they are extremely potent molecules generally acting at pico- to fentomolar concentrations. Most cytokines are multifunc-

Table 4.
Biological activities of diverse cytokines

Cytokine	Source	Biologic activity
IL-1	Monocytes, macrophages, dendritic cells, fibroblasts	Pro-inflammation; Augmentation of IL-2 and IFN-induced NK-cell activity; Induction of acute phase response (APR).
IL-2	T-cells	Stimulation of T-cell proliferation; Activation of NK, LAK and tumor infiltrating lymphocytes (TIL) cell-cytotoxicity.
IL-3	T cell lines, monocytes	Stimulation of differentiation of progenitor cells and pluripotent precursor cells.
IL-4	Th-2 subset of T-cells	B-cell activation and differentiation; Induction of IgG1 and IgE production; Suppression of Th-1 responses and antiinflammation; Inhibition of cell apoptosis.
IL-5	T-cells	B-cell activation and differentiation; Synergy with IL-4 for IgE production; Activation of differentiation of eosinophils.
IL-6	Monocytes, macrophages, endothelial cells	B-cell differentiation; Antibody switching; Enhancement of IL-3-dependent growth of multipotential hematopoietic progenitor cells; T cell differentiation; APR induction.
IL-7	Bone marrow stromal and thymic stromal cells	Growth and differentiation of precursor B-cells and early T-cell progenitors; Support growth of γ/δ T-cells.
IL-8	Activated T, monocytes, macrophages, fibroblasts, endo- and epithelial cells	Chemotactic factor for neutrophils; Stimulation of neutrophil activities; pro-inflammation.
IL-9	T-cell lines, PBL activated with mitogens	Induction of T-cell growth via IL-2- and IL-4-independent mechanisms.
IL-10	T-cells, monocytes	Growth and differentiation factor for activated B-cells.
IL-11	Bone marrow stromal cells	Enhancement of megakaryotopoietic and thrombopoietic activities; APR induction.
IL-12	Activated T-cells	Stimulation of NK- and LAK-cell activity; Enhancement of pro-inflammatory responses.
IL-13	Activated T-cells	Induction of B-cell differentiation; Anti-inflammatory.
TNF-α	Monocyte, macrophages	Pro-inflammation; Induction of APR; Activation of neutrophil-derived anti-viral activity.
IFN-γ	Activated T- and NK-cells	Th-1 cell response; MHC class I and II antigen expression; Macrophage activation; Stimulation of NK cell activity.
GM-CSF	Monocytes, macrophages, T-cells, endothelial cells	Potent stimulator of myelopoietic progenitor cells; Stimulation of neutrophil function.

tional and work together as a network called cytokine network. Cytokines interact with their target cells via highly specific receptors. Since cytokines are important in the regulation of the immune response, their over or under production may itself be associated with a disease pathology.

4 Neuromodulation of immune functions

It has long been known that myelin basic protein (MBP), a brain-specific protein, regulates T-lymphocyte function [31]. Furthermore, the MBP-sensitized T-lymphocytes passively transfer an autoimmune disease called experimental allergic encephalomyelitis (EAE), an animal model of human multiple sclerosis (MS) [31]. Recently, smaller fragments of MBP elicited immune responses [32], which suggests that MBP-derived neuropeptides also modulate immune responses. Neural modulation of immune response has also been demonstrated by many neuropeptides especially those of the hypothalamic-pituitary system. The immunomodulatory neuropeptides generally are low molecular weight peptides often derived from a larger precursor, for instance pro-opiomelanocortin (POMC) precursor for β-endorphin, α-MSH and ACTH.

Neuropeptides are ideal candidates for nervous system-mediated immune regulation since they are present in virtually all neurons. They are enriched in nerve endings at anatomic sites where they can influence immune function through neural innervation of lymphoid organs: thymus gland, spleen, liver, tonsils and lymph nodes. Indeed, many neuropeptides have been localized in nerve-terminals innervating both primary and secondary lymphoid organs [16]. The neuropeptide modulation of immune response depends on specific lymphoid organ, local concentration of neuropeptide, type and density of neuropeptide receptors, and co-signal factors. Some neuropeptides also influence microenvironment at a target tissue level, which is particularly important for the differentiation and development of the immune system [27]. The presence of neuropeptides and their receptors in bone marrow and thymus points to a trophic effect of neuropeptides on precursor immune cells. In addition, hypothalamic neuropeptides such as growth hormone and prolactin induce thymic hormone secretion by influencing the microenvironment of the thymus [33]. And, likewise, a TRH-mediated signal is essential for the extrathymic maturation of gut αβ T-lymphocytes [34]. Moreover, the genetic messages for the synthesis of diverse neuropeptides have been found in thymus, spleen and circulating immunocytes [12, 22]. The immunoregulatory properties of neuropeptides are generally assessed by a series of immune tests. Fundamentally, the approach is to determine if a neuropeptide influences cellular immunity or humoral immunity. This is important in identifying if the candidate neuropeptide has any role in the pathogenesis of a disease, for instance an immune-mediated inflammatory process. Immune effects of neuropeptides are evaluated both *in vivo* and *in vitro*. Initially, the enumeration of circulating immunocytes is performed to see whether neuropeptide alters the level of T-cells or B-cells or NK-cells or monocytes. Subsequently, functional analysis is performed to see whether neuropeptide influences the function of a specific cell type. Mature lymphocytes are resting cells but they undergo blastogenesis or cell proliferation following mitogenic stimulation. The index of lymphocyte proliferation is generally regarded as a measure of cellular immunity. Through this test, the nature of the affected immune response is indicated since different mitogens stimulate different lymphocytes (Table 3). The function of NK-cells is commonly evaluated by a cell-cytotoxicity assay. The B-cell function is assessed by antibody production. The cytokine production is an excellent way of assessing the nature of the immunocyte affected since there is some degree of specificity of cytokine elaborated by a cell, for instance IL-2 is a cytokine of T-cells whereas IL-1, IL-6 and TNF are produced by monocytes or macrophages. In addition, neuropeptide receptors are assayed by direct binding of radioactive ligands to immunocytes [35, 36]; this approach is particularly suited for neuropeptide receptors in live patients [11, 35], for instance Alzheimer's disease patients can be expected to donate a blood sample but not brain biopsies for research purposes. Through these immune tests, the immunomodulating properties of several neuropeptides have been identified (Table 5).

5 Immunomodulation by vasoactive intestinal peptide

Vasoactive intestinal peptide (VIP) is a twenty-eight amino acid-containing neuropeptide found in the CNS as well as PNS. Accumulating evidence suggests that VIP is an immunosuppressive neuropeptide. It inhibits T-cell proliferation and down regulates IL-2 production by interaction with TcR-CD3 complex, the T-cell antigen receptor [37]. The VIP concentrations resulting in significant inhibitions usually range between 10^{-9} to 10^{-7} M [38]. In regard to antibody synthesis, this neuropeptide inhibits IgA synthesis or increases IgM synthesis in lymphocytes from Payer's patches, but it has no influence on antibody production by lymphocytes from spleen and mesentric lymph nodes. VIP also inhibits T-cell mito-

Table 5.
Summary of immunoregulatory properties of neuropeptides

Neuropeptide	Immunologic activity
Corticotropin-Releasing Hormone (CRH)	Stimulates human NK-cell activity *in vitro* or suppresses it after i.c.v. injection in rodents; Induces immunocyte proliferation and especially stimulates Con A-induced lymphocyte proliferation; Increases IL-2R (Tac antigen) expression by T-cells; Suppresses antibody production by B-cells both *in vitro* and *in vivo*; Induces cytokines such as IL-1, IL-2, IL-6 and TNF.
Substance P (SP):	Augments human T-cell proliferation by PHA; Increases Con A-induced proliferation and IgA synthesis in lymphocytes of spleen, mesentric lymph nodes and Payer's patches; Increases histamine release from mast cells; Enhances macrophage phagocytosis and monocyte chemotaxis; Induces immune-mediated inflammation.
Vasoactive Intestinal Peptide (VIP):	Inhibits proliferation of lymphocytes from spleen, mesentric lymph nodes and Payer's patches; Inhibits IgA synthesis; Enhances IgM synthesis in lymphocytes from Payer's patches but not in lymphocytes from spleen or mesentric lymph nodes; Enhances NK-cell activity; Inhibits T-cell proliferation by PHA and Con A; Suppresses IL-2 production through TcR-CD3 complex.
Endorphins (END):	Decreases T-cell rosettes; Inhibits PHA response but increases Con A response to T-cell proliferation; Inhibits antigen-specific T-cell cytolysis; Inhibits phagocytosis and HLA-DR expression by monocytes; Increases anti-tetanus toxoid antibody production in human; Enhances NK cell activity; Augments chemotaxis of monocytes and PMN cells; Suppresses Con A-induced synthesis of IgM, IgG and IgA in lymphocytes of Payer's patches.
Alpha-Melanocyte-Stimulating Hormone (α-MSH):	Controls fever (antipyretic), acute phase response and inflammation; Modulates cytokine-induced responses; Suppresses IL-1-induced neutrophilia and synthesis of serum amyloid A.
Somatostatin (SOM):	Suppresses T-cell proliferation; Inhibits lymphocyte proliferation in mouse splenocytes; Suppresses colony-stimulating factor (CSF) activity; Inhibits Con A-induced proliferation of lymphocytes from mouse spleen, mesentric lymph nodes and Payer's patches; Suppresses synthesis of IgA, but not IgG and IgM, in the cells of spleen and Payer's patches.
Growth Hormone (GH):	Increases PHA-induced proliferation of T-lymphocytes; Modulates NK-cell activity; Enhances cytotoxic activity of T-cells; Increases differentiation of granulocytes from progenitor cells in bone marrow; Regulates macrophage function for TNF-α production.
Neuropeptide P (NYP):	Suppresses lymphocyte proliferation by PHA; Reduces NK activity.

genic responses (PHA and Con A) but not the B-cell response to LPS [39, 40]. Preincubation of immunocytes with VIP results in the enhancement of NK-cell activity, but without preincubation the NK-cell activity is inhibited by VIP [41]. This neuropeptide also modulates the trafficking of T-cells into GALT [42].

VIP shows high-affinity binding to human peripheral blood immunocytes with a kd of 0.47 nM [43]. The VIP-binding sites are about ten times more in Molt-4b leukemic T-lymphoblasts (15,000 sites/cell) than the number of sites in mature T-lymphocytes (1,500 sites/cell) [43–45]. The VIP receptors on human B-cells have not been studied but transformed B-cell lines (Nalm-6 pre-B-cell line, plasma cell line Dakiki and myeloma cell line U266) show high-affinity binding with kd values similar to those found in the Molt-4b T-cell line [see ref. 46]. Moreover, T-lymphoblasts and pre-B-lymphoblasts from patients with acute lymphoblastic leukemia (ALL) and common acute lymphoblastic leukemia (CALL) display high-affinity binding for VIP [47]. The immunomodulatory action of VIP involves activation of specific receptors that are functionally coupled to adenylate cyclase [43, 48]. This finding suggests that cyclic AMP serves as a second messenger in the transduction of VIP signal in human lymphocytes. This mode of action of VIP in lymphocytes resembles the action of this neuropeptide in brain [49]. Both immune cells as well as brain cells contain a protein band (47 kD) that may represent a receptor entity for this neuropeptide.

6 Immunomodulation by endorphins

A group of neuropeptides possessing opiate or morphine-like activity are commonly known as endorphins. They relieve pain and diarrhea or analgesia. They occur naturally in the CNS as well as in PNS. The brain opioid activity was originally identified in two pentapeptides, namely the Met-enkephalin (Tyr-Gly-Gly-Phe-Met) and Leu-enkephalin (Tyr-Gly-Gly-Phe-Leu) [50]. Moreover, the Met-enkephalin amino acid sequence is present as residues 61–65 in the structure of beta-lipoprotein hormone (β-LPH) of the anterior pituitary. This finding subsequently identified three neuropeptides known as α-endorphin, β-endorphin and γ-endorphin. All three had opiate-like activity. These neuropeptides are synthesized as part of the POMC precursor common to proteins encoded by three separate genes [51]; one of the proteins is the β-LPH which upon proteolytic cleavage yields all three molecular forms of endorphins.

The opioid receptors have been studied on a variety of immunocytes including human T-lymphocytes [36, 54, 65]. Multiple binding sites exist for opioid neuropeptides. The internalization of radioactive β-endorphin occurs in direct binding assays of immunocytes [66]. In addition, δ-opioid receptors are present in human and mouse leukocytes [36, 67]. By fluorescence-activated cell sorter (FACS) analysis, the β-endorphin binding is about 75% in T- (Lyt+) cells although some non-T- (Lyt–) cells also bind to this neuropeptide [68]. Also, it is noteworthy that many of the immunological actions of endorphins are sensitive to naloxone treatment [54, 69]. This suggests that the opioid receptors in immune cells, similar to brain cells, are pharmacologically sensitive. Recently, endorphin-induced immunomodulation was shown to involve a multitude of opioid receptors [70]. In this study, the i.c.v. injection in rat of opioid agonists and antagonists produced either immunopotentiation or immunosuppression. But the responses varied with the type of receptor involved, for instance δ-receptors in immunopotentiation and κ-receptors in immunosuppression. This is an intriguing observation pointing to a functional diversity of endorphin receptors.

7 Immunomodulation by substance P

Substance P (SP) is an eleven amino acid-containing peptide that functions as a neurotransmitter in the CNS as well as PNS. This neuropeptide is found mainly in the spinal cord, mesencephalon, hypothalamus, and preoptic area. It stimulates hypothalamic release of growth hormone and prolactin. In the PNS, this neuropeptide is released by sensory neurons innervating a wide variety of peripheral tissues such as gut-associated lymphoid tissues (GALT), skin, upper airways, joints, and smooth muscles.

Substance P is also involved in immunomodulation and inflammation. It stimulates mitogen-induced proliferation of human blood T-lymphocytes [71]. Irrespective of the absence or presence of T-cell-mitogens (PHA or Con A), the maximum effect occurs at around 10^{-8} M concentration of SP. Moreover, the SP-induced stimulatory effect is prevented by its antagonists ([D-Pro^2, D-Phe^7, D-Trp^9]-substance P), but not by α-endorphin [71]. The influence of SP on B-cells and monocytes remains to be clarified. In mice, SP increases Con A-induced proliferation of lymphocytes from spleen, mesentric lymph nodes, and Payer's patches [38]. These researchers also showed that SP increases Con A-induced synthesis of IgA, but not of IgG, by lymphocytes from spleen, mesentric lymph nodes, and Payer's patches. The IgM synthesis was only slightly increased in Payer's patches and spleen but unchanged in mesentric lymph nodes. SP also increases histamine release from mast cells, enhances phagocytosis, and activates macrophages. These activities are indicators of inflammatory response, which suggests that this neuropeptide has a role in inflammation [72]. Immune modulation by SP involves specific receptors present on different immunocytes. The high-affinity receptors for SP are present in human blood T-lymphocytes [73], IM-9 B-lymphoblasts [73], and mouse splenocytes [74]. Based on direct binding of ^{125}I-SP, mouse T-cells showed about twice the amount of specific binding in B-cells. The FACS analysis showed about an equal amount of bound SP in mouse helper and suppressor T-cells [74]. However, the specific binding in human T-cells was very small: about 20% in T helper-inducer cells and only 10% in T suppressor-cytotoxic cells [75]. The IM-9 cell line of human B-lymphoblasts had approximately 25,000 to 30,000 receptor sites for SP per cell, which is about three times greater than those found in human T-cells. In lymphocytes as well as other tissues, the action of SP is coupled to the phosphatidyl inositol (PI) pathway of signal transduction because it induces the hydrolysis of inositol phospholipid [76]. Analysis of ^{125}I-SP binding proteins in IM-9 B-lymphoblasts identified two proteins (58 kD and 33 kD) which are apparently derived from a larger (116 kD) receptor protein [76]. Based on its immunomodulating properties, SP may have a role in inflammatory diseases such as chronic arthritis, asthma, inflammatory bowel disease, and carcinoid tumors [72, 77]. In this respect, two findings are quite relevant: (i) SP stimulates mitogen-induced proliferation of synovial fluid T-lymphocytes from patients with rheumatoid arthritis [78]; and (ii) SP augments IL-1 synthesis by synovial fluid monocytes from chronic arthritis patients [78]. On the basis of these findings and other findings of our own, we propose a model for the inflammatory role of SP in the pathophysiology of chronic arthritis. In this model, we postulate that SP acts in synergy with CRH in synovium to induce chronic inflammation of the joints.

The CRH via IL-1 induction acts as an inducer of acute inflammation whereas SP via IL-1 augmentation acts as an amplifier to cause a chronic disease (see below).

CRH ----> IL-1----> Acute disease + SP ----> IL-1 amplification ----> Chronic disease

The model would predict a direct relationship between CRH, SP and IL-1 and, indeed, all three are significantly elevated in the synovial fluid of patients with chronic arthritis [78, 79]. And, CRH is known to induce IL-1 by monocytes [80] but SP is known to augment IL-1 production by monocytes especially in the synovium of chronic arthritis patients [78]. It is also interesting that the concentration of CRH required to induce IL-1 *in vitro*

[80] is about the same as found in synovial fluid of patients with chronic arthritis [79]. This model attempts to explain a putative role of immune modulation by neuropeptides such as SP and CRH, but it does not exclude other immune factors in the pathophysiology of chronic arthritis [81].

8 Immunomodulation by corticotropin-releasing hormone

Hypothalamic corticotropin-releasing hormone (CRH), a forty-one amino acid containing neuropeptide, is a key regulator of synthesis and secretion of pituitary hormones (ACTH, β-endorphin, GH, prolactin, MSH, etc.). CRH is the primary mediator of host's stress response and thus it is commonly referred to as "stress hormone" [82, 83]. In the CNS, it acts as a neurotransmitter [84] and, in the periphery, CRH functions as an immunomodulator [11, 12, 85]. Stress is well known to cause immunosuppression. And CRH, since it is a key mediator of stress, has been regarded as immunosuppressive. However, the CRH-induced immunomodulating activities are somewhat paradoxical, at least, in part due to a

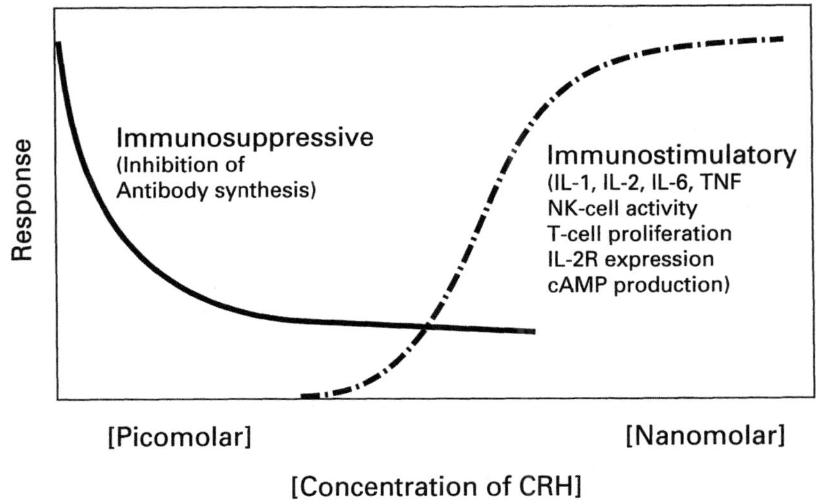

Fig. 3
Bimodal nature of immunomodulation by CRH

dosage problem. We recently demonstrated that CRH depending upon its concentration exerts a bimodal response *in vitro* [12, 85]. As schematically depicted in Figure 3, CRH in picomolar concentrations is immunosuppressive to humoral immunity (antibody synthesis), but in nanomolar concentrations it is immunostimulatory to cellular immunity (T-lymphocyte proliferation, NK-cell activity, cytokine induction and cyclic AMP production). This bimodal response to CRH-induced immunomodulation is consistent with low-dose (physiological) and high-dose (pharmacological) effects of this neuropeptide when it is administered directly into the brain [83].

We originally showed that CRH induces proliferation of human blood lymphocytes and monocytes [86]. Although this effect was a weaker effect, it is blocked by α-helical CRH which is a well-known antagonist of CRH [87]. In addition, CRH stimulates lymphocyte proliferation by T-cell mitogens (Con A and PHA), but not by B-cell responsive pokeweed mitogen (PWM) [86]. We also found that CRH did not influence anti-CD3-induced lymphocyte proliferation but it increased IL-2R (Tac antigen) expression [86] and induced IL-2 activity [81]. This was an important observation because it distinguished a mechanism of T-cell activation by CRH. Since anti-CD3 activates T-cells by interaction with T-cell antigen receptor (TcR-CD3 complex), the lack of an effect of CRH on anti-CD3 response indicated that CRH does not act via TcR-CD3 complex. On the other hand, CRH stimulated PHA- and Con A-induced T-cell proliferation which implied that this neuropeptide acts via IL-2R since these two mitogens act by IL-2 production and IL-2R expression. Indeed, CRF induces IL-2 [81] and increases IL-2R expression [86] by T-cells. We therefore conclude that CRH activates T-lymphocytes via IL-2R pathway, but not via T-cell antigen receptor (TcR-CD3) pathway.

CRH also modulates NK-cell activity in humans and animals. The i.c.v. injection of CRH or stress in animals inhibits splenic NK-cell activity [88]. This inhibitory effect is different from other studies which showed increase of NK-cell activity by CRH [89, 90]. The reason for this discrepancy is probably related to the nature of the study, i.e. inhibitory effect results from *in vivo* administration of CRH whereas stimulatory effect results from *in vitro* preincubation of effector cells with CRH. In order to elicit stimulation of NK-cell activity, the mouse splenocytes require 12 to 18 hours of preincubation with 10 nM CRH [89] whereas human blood immunocytes require 16 to 18 hours of preincubation with 0.1 nM CRH [90]. Because of a preincubation requirement, we suggested that CRH stimulates NK-cells indirectly via production of IL-1 and β-endorphin [90]. To support this contention, the rabbit-anti-IL-1 and rabbit-anti-β-endorphin block CRH-stimulated activity of human NK-cells [85, 90]. In addition, β-endorphin antagonist naloxone blocks mouse NK activity stimulated by CRH [89].

With regards to CRH and modulation of humoral immune response, we originally reported that it suppresses PWM-induced synthesis of IgG by human blood immunocytes [85]. Subsequently, we showed that the production of all three isotypes (IgM, IgG and IgA) was inhibited by CRH; maximum suppression occurred at 10^{-13} M [91]. Since our reports [85, 91], an animal study also showed that CRH after i.c.v. administration elicits suppression of antibody response [92]. The mechanism of suppression by CRH of antibody production is not well known but we postulated that it may involve enhanced function of suppressor/cytotoxic (CD8+) T-cells [12]. Indeed, we have found that CRH, under the same conditions as those for antibody production, increases suppressor-cytotoxic (CD8+) and suppressor-inducer (CD45R+ or 2H4+) T-cells, but helper and helper-inducer T-cells were not influenced (Figure 4). We previously showed that CRH stimulates IL-2 production [81], IL-2R expression [86], and Con A-induced lymphocyte proliferation [86], all of which especially Con A are known to induce suppressor-cytotoxic T-cell function. Thus, the mechanism of CRH-induced suppression of antibody production may involve induction of suppression-cytotoxic T-cells.

The high-affinity binding of ^{125}I-CRH with immunocytes [35, 93] suggests the presence of CRH receptors in lymphoid cells. The nature of CRH-binding sites in mouse splenic cells is similar to those found in pituitary cells [94]. In mouse, the binding of ^{125}I-CRH occurs mainly in splenic macrophages but not in T- or B-lymphocytes [93]. In humans, however, CRH receptors are present predominantly in monocytes and, to a lesser degree, in T-cells, B-cells and thymic cells [35]. With respect to CRH receptors, it should be noted that the α-helical CRH antagonist displays differential effects on different immunomodulating actions of CRH. They can be distinguished as follows: (i) all of the CRH-induced immunostimulating activities (immunocyte proliferation, NK enhancement, IL-6 induction and cyclic AMP production) are blocked by an antagonist at a 1:1 ratio of agonist:antagonist; and (ii) immunosuppressive activity (antibody synthesis) is not blocked by an antagonist at a ratio as high as 1:10,000 of agonist: antagonist. On the basis of this remarkable distinction, we speculate that CRH-induced modulation of immune response is mediated by multiple receptors in immune cells. To this end, the existence of multiple CRH receptors in brain was suggested by Fisher et al. [95], who also found marked differences in the ability of α-helical CRH to antagonize different actions of CRH in the nervous system. Furthermore, the presence of CRH recep-

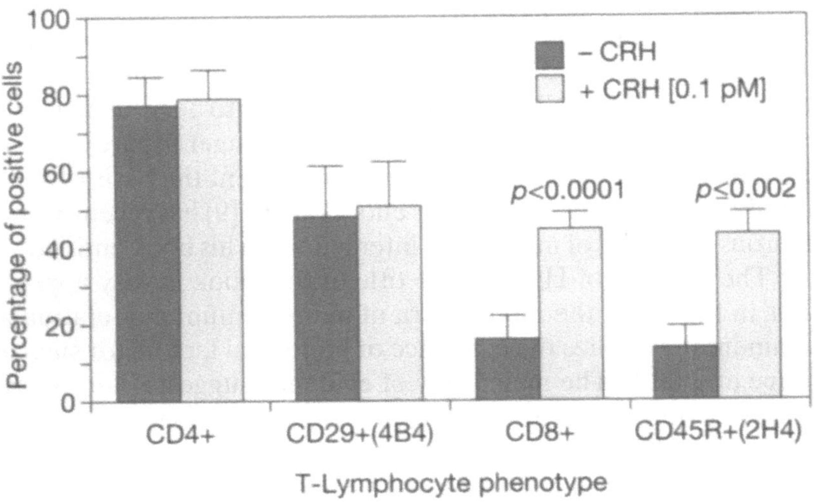

Fig. 4
T-cell subsets after CRH-mediated suppression of antibody synthesis
Peripheral blood immunocytes (1×10^6 MNC) were incubated with PWM in the absence (–CRH) or presence of CRH (10^{-13} M) as described previously [91]. After seven days, the cells were stained with monoclonal antibodies to T-cell antigens (CD4, CD29 or 4B4, CD8 and CD45R or 2H4 for helper, helper-inducer, suppressor-cytotoxic and suppressor-inducer cells, respectively). The FACS histogram showed two distinct populations: one with small cells and the other with large cells. The bitmap of larger cells showed a significant increase in the proportions of CD8+ and CD45R+ (or 2H4+) cells in cultures treated with CRH.

tors in immunocytes and antagonism by α-helical CRH suggests that the stimulation of immune response by CRH is a receptor-mediated process [96]. Indeed, CRH stimulates adenylate cyclase in mouse splenocytes [93] and induces cyclic AMP accumulation in human blood immunocytes [96]. Additionally, we noted a positive correlation (R = 0.972) between CRH-induced monocyte-derived IL-6 [97] and CRH-induced cyclic AMP accumulation in monocytes [96]. This observation leads us to conclude that CRH-signal transduction involves cyclic AMP as a second messenger, at least, in the stimulation of monocyte-derived cytokines such as IL-6 [96].

9 Conclusion

Recent advances in the field of neuroimmunology have demonstrated that the nervous system and immune system interface with each other in a reciprocal fashion. Their interactions display neuroimmunomodulation (NIM) from nervous system to immune system and, conversely, immunoneuromodulation (INM) from immune system to nervous system. Now, the stage is such that the NIM or INM is no longer regarded as a phenomenon. Instead, it may appropriately represent the basis of so-called "mind-body" relationships. To this end, Cousins [9] has recently outlined numerous examples of mind-body interactions in his book entitled "Head First: The Biology of Hope". The title of this book is very appropriate as it is in tune with the modern era of neuroimmunomodulation and it fundamentally implies the existence of biological factors for such things as hope and faith. The main body of evidence suggests that the regulatory interactions occur at virtually all levels, cellular to molecular. The mediators of NIM appeared to be neuropeptides whereas INM is mediated by immunopeptides such as cytokines and thymic hormones. The neuropeptides, which until recently were confined to the nervous system, are synthesized by the cells of the lymphoid organs. They exert biological activities via specific receptors present in immune cells. And, they act as autocrine or paracrine hormones in inflammatory reactions [98], suggesting their role in immune-mediated pathological conditions [79, 99]. Beyond their role in the nervous system, neuropeptides may function as native mediators of immune response. They may also regulate development and differentiation of immune responses because they are synthesized in primary lymphoid organs such as thymus, which also express neuropeptide receptors. Moreover, multiple forms of neuropeptide receptors exist in immunocytes which may explain functional diversity in terms of immune modulation. Some neuropeptides such as CRH [100] have soluble binding proteins that are different from receptors. And, there are neuropeptides that are pathologically relevant (e.g. β-amyloid $peptide_{1\text{-}40}$ in Alzheimer's disease), which modulate immunocyte proliferation [101]. Their role in neuropeptide modulation of immune response should be investigated. Moreover, there are some indications that neuropeptides interact with each other. These antagonistic and synergistic interactions may be important in elucidating the role of neuropeptides in immune modulation. In summary, it is expected that future research will uncover not only new pathways in which neuropeptides function as native mediators, but also explore mechanisms by which neuropeptides impact immune responses in the host.

References

1 J.E. Blalock: Immunology Today *15*, 504 (1994).
2 H.O. Besedovsky and A.F. del Ray: Front. Neuroendocrinology *13*, 61 (1992).
3 V.K. Singh and H.H. Fudenberg: J. Clin. Psychiatr. *47*, 592 (1986).
4 G.F. Solomon: Brain Behav. Immunity 7, 352 (1993).
5 A.A. Monjan and M.I. Collector: Science *196*, 307 (1977).
6 J.E. Hillhouse, J.K. Kiecolt-Glaser and R. Glaser: In: Stress and Immunity (eds. Plotnikoff, N., Murgo, A., Faith, R. and Wybran, J.), pp. 3 (1991), CRC Press, Inc., Boca Raton, Florida, USA.
7 D.O. Perkins, J. Lesserman, J.H. Gilmore, J.M. Petitto and D.L. Evans: In: Stress and Immunity (eds. Plotnikoff, N., Murgo, A., Faith, R. and Wybran, J.), pp. 167 (1991), CRC Press, Inc., Boca Raton, Florida, USA.
8 R.C. Hickman and J.B. Boone (Jr): In: Stress and Immunity (eds. Plotnikoff, N., Murgo, A., Faith, R. and Wybran, J.), pp. 211 (1991), CRC Press, Inc., Boca Raton, Florida, USA.
9 N. Cousins: In: Head First: The Biology Of Hope (ed. Cousins, N.), E. P. Dutton Publ., New York, N. Y., USA.
10 D.G. Payan and E.J. Goetzl: Ann. N.Y. Acad. Sci. *512*, 465 (1987).
11 V.K. Singh: Prog. Drug Res. *34*, 383 (1990).
12 V.K. Singh: Prog. Drug Res. *38*, 149 (1992).
13 J.E. Morley, N.E. Kay, G.F. Solomon and N.P. Plotnikoff: Life Sciences *41*, 527 (1987).
14 V. Geenen, F. Robert, J.J. Legros and P. Franchimont: In: Stress and Immunity (eds. Plotnikoff, N., Murgo, A., Faith, R. and Wybran, J.), pp. 481 (1991), CRC Press, Inc., Boca Raton, Florida, USA.
15 H.M. Johnson, M.O. Downs and C.H. Pontzer: In: Neuroimmunoendocrinology (ed. Blalock, J.E.), pp. 49 (1992), Karger Publ., Basel, Switzerland.
16 S.Y. Felton, D.L. Felton, D.L. Bellinger and J.A. Olschowka: In: Neuroimmunoendocrinology (ed. Blalock, J. E.), pp. 25 (1992), Karger Publ., Basel, Switzerland.
17 A.F. Williams and J. Gagnon: Science *216*, 696 (1982).
18 J. E. Blalock, D. Harbour-McMenamin and E.M. Smith: J. Immunol. *135*, 858s (1985).
19 E.M. Smith, A.C. Morrill, W.J. Meyer (III) and J.E. Blalock: Nature *321*, 881 (1986).
20 K.G. Chandy, T.E. DeCoursey, M.D. Cahalan and S. Gupta: J. Immunol. *135*, 787s (1985).
21 K.G. Coffey and J.W. Hadden: Fed. Proc. *44*, 112 (1985).
22 J.E. Blalock: In: Neuroimmunoendocrinology (ed. Blalock, J.E.), pp. 1 (1992), Karger Publ., Basel, Switzerland.
23 M.R. Hanley: Nature *315*, 14 (1985).
24 B. Schobitz, E.R. DeKloct and F. Holsboer: Prog. Neurobiology *44*, 398 (1994).
25 K. Imamura, A. Suzumura, M. Sawada, C. Mabuchi and T. Marunouchi: J. Neuroimmunol. *55*, 119 (1994).
26 A. Suzumura, M. Sawada, Y. Itoh and T. Marunouchi: J. Neuroimmunol. *53*, 209 (1994).
27 M. Dardenne and W. Savino: Immunology Today *15*, 518 (1994).
28 Y. Zhang, H. Saito and N. Nishiyama: Brain Res. *658*, 127 (1994).
29 R.B. Herberman and J.R. Ortaldo: Science *214*, 24 (1981).
30 J.H. Phillips and L.L. Lanier: J. Exp. Med. *164*, 814 (1986).
31 B.H. Waksman: Ann. N. Y. Acad. Sci. *540*, 13 (1988).
32 J. Inobe, T. Yamamura, T. Kunishita and T. Tabira: J. Neuroimmunol. *46*, 83 (1993).

33 J. Moreno, A. Vicente, I. Heijnen and A. G. Zapata: Immunology Today *15*, 524 (1994).
34 J. Wang and J.R. Klein: Science *265*, 1860 (1994).
35 V.K. Singh and H.H. Fudenberg: Immunology Lett. *18*, 5 (1988).
36 D.J.J. Carr: In: Neuroimmunoendocrinology (ed. Blalock, J. E.), pp. 84 (1992), Karger Publ., Basel, Switzerland.
37 Z. Xin, H. Tang and D. Ganea: J. Neuroimmunol. *54*, 59 (1994).
38 A.M. Stanisz, D. Befus and J. Bienenstock: J. Immunol. *136*, 152 (1986).
39 C.A. Ottaway and G.R. Greenberg: J. Immunol. *132*, 417 (1984).
40 C.A. Ottaway: Immunology *62*, 291 (1987).
41 M. Rola-Pleszczynski, D. Bolduc and S.St. Pierre: J. Immunol. *135*, 2569 (1985).
42 T.C. Moore: Immunology *52*, 511 (1984).
43 A. Danek, M.S. O'Dorisio, T.M. O'Dorisio and J.M. George: J. Immunol. *131*, 1173 (1983).
44 E.A. Beed, M.S. O'Dorisio, T.M. O'Dorisio and T.S. Gaginella: Regul. Pept. *6*,1 (1983).
45 P. Robberecht, M. Waelbroeck, P. De Neef, M. Tastenoy, P. Gourlet, J. Cogniaux and J. Christophe: FEBS Lett. *228*, 351 (1988).
46 G.D. Wenger, M.S. O'Dorisio and E.J. Goetzl: Ann. N. Y. Acad. Sci. *594*, 104 (1990).
47 B.T. Shanon, M.S. O'Dorisio, N.F. Grossman, A.F. Mulne and F.B. Ruymann: Ped. Res. *20*, 287A (1986).
48 M.S. O'Dorisio, N. Hermina, S.P. Balcerzak and T.M. O'Dorisio: J. Immunol. *127*, 2551 (1981).
49 M.S. O'Dorisio, J. Vasiloff, L.B. Campolito, M.S. Beattie and J.C. Bresnahan: Neuroscience Res. Commun. *2*,19 (1988).
50 J. Hughes, T.W. Smith, H.W. Kosterlitz, L.A. Fothergill, B.A. Morgan and H. Morris: Nature *258*, 579 (1975).
51 R.E. Mains, B.A. Eipper and N. Ling: Proc. Natl. Acad. Sci., USA *74*, 3014 (1977).
52 G.B. Stefano: Prog. Neurobiol. *33*, 159 (1989).
53 H. Teschemacher, G. Koch, H. Scheffler, A. Hildebrand and V. Brantl: Ann. N. Y. Acad. Sci. *594*, 66 (1990).
54 J. Wybran, T. Appelboom, J.P. Famaey and A. Govaerts: J. Immunol. *123*, 1068 (1979).
55 G.C. Miller, A.J. Murgo and N.P. Plotnikoff: Clin. Immunol. Immunopathol. *31*, 132 (1984).
56 C. De Carolis, G. De Sanctis, R. Perricone, C. Moretti, A. Fabbri, L. Gnessi, F. Fraioli and L. Fontana: Experientia *40*, 738 (1984).
57 H.W. McCain, I.B. Lamster, J.M. Bozzone and J.T. Grbic: Life Sci. *331*, 1619 (1982).
58 F. Puppo, G. Corsini, P. Mangini, L. Bottaro and T. Barreca: Immunopharmacology *10*, 119 (1985).
59 W. Gilmore and L.P. Weiner: Immunopharmacology *17*, 19 (1989).
60 W. Gilmore, M. Moloney and T. Berinstein: Brain Res. Bull. *24*, 687 (1990).
61 J. Prieto, M.L. Subira, A. Castilla, J.L. Arroyo and M. Serrano: Scan. J. Immunol. *29*, 391 (1989).
62 N.A. Munn and L.G. Lum: Clin. Immunol. Immunopathol. *52*, 376 (1989).
63 D.E. Van Epps and L. Saland: J. Immunol. *132*, 3046 (1984).
64 D.J.J. Carr, R.T. Radulescu, B.R. de Costa, K.C. Rice and J.E. Blalock: Life Sci. *47*, 1059 (1990).
65 P.M. Mathews, C.J. Froelich, W.L. Sibbitt (Jr.) and A.D. Bankhurst: J. Immunol. *130*, 1658 (1983).

66 R.E. Faith, H.J. Liang, A.J. Murgo and N.P. Plotnikoff: Clin. Immunol. Immunopathol. *31*, 412 (1984).
67 M. Kay, J. Allen and J.E. Morley: Life Sci. *35*, 53 (1984).
68 C.M. Ausciello and L.G. Roda: Cell Biol. Int. Rep. *8*, 353 (1984).
69 N.E. Falke and E.G. Fischer: Cell Biol. Int. Rep. *10*, 429 (1986).
69 D.J.J. Carr, C.H. Kin, B. De Costa, A.E. Jacobson, K.C. Rice and J.E. Blalock: Cell Immunol. *116*, 44 (1988).
70 J. Radulovic and B.D. Jankovic: Brain Res. *661*, 189 (1994).
71 D.G. Payan, D.R. Bewster and E.J. Goetzl: J. Immunol. *131*, 1613 (1983).
72 D.G. Payan: Ann. Rev. Med. *40*, 341 (1989).
73 D.G. Payan, J.P. McGillis and M.L. Organist: J. Biol. Chem. *261*, 14321 (1986).
74 A.M. Stanisz, R. Scicchitano, D.G. Payan and J. Bienenstock: Ann. N. Y. Acad. Sci. *496*, 217 (1987).
75 D.G. Payan, D.R. Brewster, A. Missirian-Bastin and E.J. Goetzl: J. Clin. Invest. *74*, 1532 (1984).
76 J.P. McGillis, M.L. Organist, K.H. Scriven and D.G. Payan: J. Neurosci. Res. *18*, 190 (1987).
77 E.S. Kimball: Ann. N. Y. Acad. Sci. *594*, 293 (1990).
78 M. Lotz, D.A. Carson and J.H. Vaughan: Science *235*, 893 (1987).
79 L.J. Crofford, H. Sano, K. Karalis, T.C. Friedman, H.R. Epps, E.F. Remmers, P. Mathem, G.P. Chrouses and R.L. Wilder: J. Immunol. *15*, 1587 (1993).
80 V.K. Singh and S.C. Leu: Neuroscience Lett. *120*, 151 (1990).
81 I. Wicks, G. McColl and L. Harrison: Immunology Today *15*, 553 (1994).
82 W.W. Vale, C. Rivier, M.R. Brown, J. Spies, J. Koob, L. Swanson, E. Blizikijan, F. Bloom and E. Rivier: Rec. Prog. Horm. Res. *39*, 245 (1983).
83 A.J. Dunn and C.W. Berridge: Brain Res. Rev. *15*, 71 (1990).
84 S.A. Joseph, W.H. Pilcher and K.M. Knigge: Fed. Proc. *44*, 100 (1985).
85 V.K. Singh: In: Immunobiology of Proteins and Peptides VI (ed. Atassi, M. Z.), pp. 289 (1991), Plenum Publ. Corp., N. Y., USA.
86 V.K. Singh: J. Neuroimmunol. *23*, 257 (1989).
87 J. Rivier, C. Rivier and W.W. Vale: Science *224*, 889 (1984).
88 M.R. Irwin, W. Vale and K.T. Britton: Brain Behav. Immun. *1*, 81 (1987).
89 D.J.J. Carr and J.E. Blalock: Ann. N. Y. Sci. *594*, 371 (1990).
90 S.C. Leu and V.K. Singh: J. Neuroimmunol. *33*, 253 (1991).
91 S.C. Leu and V.K. Singh: J. Neuroimmunol. *45*, 23 (1993).
92 M. Irwin: Endocrinology *133*, 1352 (1993).
93 E.L. Webster, D.E. Tracey, M.A. Jutila, S.A. Wolfe and E.B. De Souza: Endocrinology *127*, 440 (1990).
94 E.L. Webster and E.B. De Souza: Endocrinology *122*, 609 (1988).
95 L. Fisher, C. Rivier, J. Rivier and M. Brown: Endocrinology *129*, 1312 (1991).
96 V.K. Singh and S.C. Leu: Immunology Lett. *35*, 239 (1993).
97 S.C. Leu and V.K. Singh: Cell. Immunol. *143*, 220 (1992).
98 K. Karalis, H. Sano, J. Redwine, S. Litwak, R.L. Wilder and G.P. Chrousos: Science *254*, 421 (1991).
99 C. Jorgensen and J. Sany: Clin. Exptl. Rheumatol. *12*, 435 (1994).
100 D.P. Behan, E.A. Linton and P.J. Lowry: J. Endocrin. *122*, 23 (1989).
101 V.K. Singh: Molecular Neurobiol. *9*, 73 (1994).

Progress in Drug Research, Vol. 45 (E. Jucker, Ed.)

Calmodulin: Effects of cell stimuli and drugs on cellular activation

By Margaret E. Gnegy
Department of Pharmacology, 2220E MSRB III, University of Michigan Medical School, Ann Arbor, MI 48103-0632, USA

1. Introduction

Drugs, hormones and neurotransmitters affect cell Ca^{2+} in a variety of ways, by activating or blocking voltage- or ligand-dependent Ca^{2+} channels, membrane Ca^{2+} pumps, or Ca^{2+} release from intracellular stores. Upon elevation, Ca^{2+} usually acts either by directly stimulating enzymes such as protein kinase C (PKC) or calpain, a Ca^{2+} activated protease, or by binding to a Ca^{2+}-binding protein which will have restricted or multiple actions. Calmodulin (CaM) is a principal multifunctional mediator of Ca^{2+} signalling in cells. CaM acts as a Ca^{2+}-dependent regulator of cyclic nucleotide metabolism, protein phosphorylation-dephosphorylation cascades, Ca^{2+}- and other ion transport, cytoskeletal function, cell growth and proliferation [1-3]. Detailed knowledge of the *in vitro* activation of several target isoenzymes by CaM and its binding to cytoskeletal proteins is available, but knowledge concerning the *in vivo* or *in situ* activation of CaM-dependent processes in response to drugs, hormones and neurotransmitters is just emerging. Rapid activation of some CaM-dependent enzymes in response to elevated intracellular calcium ($[Ca^{2+}]i$) has been demonstrated *in situ* but it is unclear whether CaM-dependent enzymes are activated globally or selectively in the cell. Recent evidence suggests that Ca^{2+} and CaM-dependent physiological activities can be selectively altered depending upon cellular domains responding to stimuli. Limited information is available as to the *in situ* binding of CaM at resting Ca^{2+} levels in most cells and the importance of Ca^{2+}-independent CaM binding. Receptor-mediated activity can alter the sensitivity of CaM-dependent processes through phosphorylation of CaM-binding proteins. Persistent receptor activation or inhibition can elicit a redistribution of CaM within subcellular fractions that could enhance the sensitivity and activity of CaM-dependent processes. Alterations in cellular activity through hormonal or drug treatments can lead to changes in CaM content and, possibly, coordinate expression of CaM-binding proteins.

Drugs that alter receptor-mediated activity or cellular Ca^{2+} fluxes are likely to change CaM binding to cellular proteins resulting in altered sensitivity of Ca^{2+}-mediated processes. Knowledge of how stimuli affect CaM activation and content is key to an understanding of drugs' effects on CaM-sensitive systems and effectively targetting inhibition of CaM activities. The goal of this review is to discuss the regulation of CaM binding, localization and content in the cell by neurotransmitters, hormones and drugs that affect those stimuli. The binding of CaM at resting and elevated levels of Ca^{2+} will be discussed as well as the role of phosphorylation in affecting the response of CaM target proteins. This review focusses on mechanisms by which stimuli and drugs affect CaM and not on the use of CaM antagonist drugs. Several recent excellent and complete reviews on the subject of CaM antagonists are available [4–8]. Space demands preclude a discussion of every known CaM target protein and so a few select proteins will be emphasized in this review.

2 Calcium activation properties of CaM

CaM belongs to a family of Ca^{2+}-binding proteins exhibiting EF hands, defined by a select sequence of about 30 amino acids that folds into a helix-loop-helix pattern [9, 10]. Members of this family include troponin C, parvalbumins, myosin light chains, S-100 proteins, calbindins and the B-subunit of calcineurin, among others. Mammalian CaM, whose amino sequence has been highly conserved through evolution, has an approximate molecular weight of 16,500 kd and lacks cysteine and tryptophan residues. The crystal structure of CaM is that of a dumbbell containing N and C-terminal homologous globular domains, each containing two Ca^{2+}-binding sites, that are separated by a central extended 25 residue α-helix [11]. Inaccessable hydrophobic clefts in each domain are exposed after Ca^{2+} binding and are considered to be involved in binding to target proteins and pharmacological inhibitors and activation of various target enzymes [12–14]. The structure of CaM in solution, however, appears to be more globular and less extended than that of the crystal structure. Studies of CaM in solution utilizing nuclear magnetic resonance spectroscopy [15] and small angle X-ray scattering analysis [16] suggest that the central helix is very flexible and the two domains of the CaM molecule can actually bend around and enfold an α-helical target peptide [15, 17]. The central helix may function as a flexible tether [18]. The α-helical target peptide conformation appears to be stabilised by the two CaM domains that wrap around the peptide. For a discussion of CaM binding to target proteins, see [19, 20]. There is not a unique consensus sequence identifying a CaM-binding site in target proteins, but generally there is a characteristic basic amino acid amphiphilic helix structural motif in their CaM-binding domains [21]. The flexibility in the central helical region of CaM would allow it to bind to the variety of binding sequences.

Discrepant conclusions have been reached in direct binding and kinetic studies concerning binding constants for Ca^{2+} binding to CaM [22]. Direct binding and microcalorimetric studies suggest that there are four nearly independent binding sites for Ca^{2+} with very similar affinities. Kinetic data and some conformation studies favor a model suggesting two pairs of sites with pronounced positive cooperativity within each pair of sites but little cooperativity between the two globular domains [14, 23, 24]. The carboxy-terminal sites (sites III and IV) are higher affinity, with Kd's in the range of 10^{-6} M while the amino-terminal sites (sites I and II) are lower affinity with Kd's in the range of 10^{-5} to 10^{-6} M. The bulk of the conformational change occurs upon the binding of the first two Ca^{2+} molecules, which bind to sites III and IV in the C-terminal region of the molecule. Binding of three to four Ca^{2+} is required for CaM to activate most enzymes such as cyclic nucleotide phosphodiesterase, brain adenylyl cyclase, erythrocyte Ca^{2+}, Mg^{2+}-ATPase, skeletal muscle phosphorylase b kinase, CaM Kinase II and smooth and skeletal muscle myosin light chain kinase [22]. Binding of Ca^{2+} to CaM, however, is most relevantly examined in the presence of a target protein since the the presence of a binding protein can significantly change the Ca^{2+} and CaM binding characteristics. A cooperative enhancement in Ca^{2+} binding between the two domains has been observed in the presence of target peptides [25] involving an association of the opposing globular domains [15, 17]. In the presence of a target protein, binding of Ca^{2+} to the low affinity sites is increased by two orders of magnitude, while binding of Ca^{2+} to the high affinity sites is only moderately enhanced (2–10 fold) [24]. Thus Ca^{2+} increases the binding affinity of CaM for its target enzymes by several orders of magnitude while the presence of the target enzyme similarly enhances the affinity of CaM for Ca^{2+}. This highly cooperative interaction of Ca^{2+} with CaM has been demonstrated for several CaM-sensitive enzymes, and the degree of cooperativity is dependent upon the concentrations of Ca^{2+}, CaM, enzyme and substrates [22–24, 26]. For example, the mean dissociation constants for Ca^{2+} interaction with CaM in the absence and presence of myosin light chain kinase were 14 µM and 400 nM, respectively [26]. The strong degree of cooperativity means that CaM activation of enzymes exhibiting this property would occur over a very narrow and physiologically relevant range of Ca^{2+} concentrations, between 10^{-7} and 10^{-6} M. The degree of cooperative interaction could provide differential regulation of physiological functions of CaM as a function of subsaturating Ca^{2+}, Ca^{2+} fluxes, CaM concentrations and target protein availability.

3 Binding of CaM in a resting cell

An interesting and largely unanswered question is whether CaM is free or bound in the cell at resting Ca^{2+} levels. The issue gains importance when considering drug action since many drugs, even those not directly altering Ca^{2+}, could modify binding of CaM. In most cells a significant portion of CaM is soluble, some of which may be free, but much may be bound depending upon the properties of resident CaM binding proteins. The nature of the proteins to which CaM may bind at resting Ca^{2+} levels suggests that an alteration of CaM binding to these proteins would affect cytoskeletal structure, transport of cellular contents or even enzyme activity. Many cell types or tissues appear to contain significant concentrations of CaM-binding proteins which bind CaM in the absence of Ca^{2+} in suggesting that CaM could be highly bound at resting Ca^{2+} levels. This may be particularly true in brain. Although brain has a high CaM content (10–100 μM, [27]), the large number and high concentration of many Ca^{2+}-independent CaM binding proteins, such as neuromodulin, neurogranin and unconventional myosins, make it unlikely that CaM is predominantly free in neurons. This has been suggested experimentally [28]. In mammalian skeletal muscle 35–40% of the CaM is bound to phosphorylase kinase [29]. CaM is the δ subunit of phosphorylase kinase and is bound at that site independently of Ca^{2+}. In addition, cooperative effects and high Ca^{2+} sensitivity of some CaM target proteins, such as Type I CaM-stimulated adenylyl cyclase [30, 31], may enable some CaM to bind to select Ca^{2+}-requiring target proteins at resting Ca^{2+} levels. Cooperative effects may contribute to increased CaM binding to target proteins in cells such as neurons which, upon repetitive stimulation, retain residual Ca^{2+} and thus have higher baseline $[Ca^{2+}]i$ values.

An elegant series of studies exploring the question of CaM binding in quiescent and stimulated cells utilized an environmentally sensitive fluorescent analog of CaM, MeroCaM [32], together with steady state fluorescence anisotropy imaging microscopy. The distribution and activation of MeroCaM in serum-deprived fibroblasts in quiescent and serum-activated cells was examined. The results suggested that over 90% of CaM is unbound at low free Ca^{2+} in serum-deprived fibroblasts [33]. Upon stimulation of the serum-deprived fibroblasts with complete serum, 95% of the CaM became bound in direct correlation with the time course of the elevation and decline of the free Ca^{2+} concentration. Interpretation of these results is dependent on the assumption that the CaM fluorophore would freely exchange with any endogenous bound CaM. On the other hand, Van Eldik et al. [34] immunoprecipitated CaM/CaM-binding protein complexes from ^{35}S labeled chick embryo fibroblasts with an antibody capable of immunoprecipitating CaM bound to target proteins. The combined levels of the CaM-associated proteins were estimated to be higher than the levels of CaM alone, suggesting that there is not a large excess of CaM in these cells compared to CaM binding proteins. The Ca^{2+}

and CaM binding characteristics are likely to be cell specific and would vary depending upon the type of CaM-binding proteins in each cell. There is an ever-increasing list of proteins to which CaM preferentially binds in the absence of Ca^{2+} or to which binding is independent of Ca^{2+}. Proteins to which CaM binds in the absence of Ca^{2+} are neuromodulin (GAP-43, B-50, F1 and pp46) [35–37], neurogranin (BICKS, RC3) [35, 38, 39], gap junction protein [40], and several of the unconventional myosins [41]. At least four enzymes contain CaM as a subunit bound in a Ca^{2+}-independent manner: macrophage inducible nitric oxide synthase [42], *Bordetella Pertussis* adenylyl cyclase [43], phosphorylase kinase [44], and a bovine lung cyclic nucleotide phosphodiesterase [45]. Neuromodulin, neurogranin, and the unconventional myosins contain IQ-domains which are extremely basic ~ 23 amino acid units whose conserved core usually fits the consensus IQXXXRGXXXR. Variable numbers of repeats of IQ motifs are contained in the neck region of all myosins [41] but this domain is also present in neuromodulin and neurogranin [38, 46]. The IQ motif is felt to provide a binding site for Ca^{2+}-binding proteins containing EF-hands but is not specific for Ca^{2+}-independent binding [41].

Neuromodulin and neurogranin are neural specific proteins both of which are present in concentrations in brain that may equal or surpass those of CaM [37]. Neuromodulin is involved in the regulation of neurite outgrowth, adult neuronal plasticity, neurotransmitter release and polyphosphoinositide metabolism and Go function [35, 36, 47, 48]. Neurogranin may enhance Ca^{2+} mobilization in spines [49]. Neuromodulin is primarily localized to neuronal axons and terminals while neurogranin is concentrated in perikarya and dendrites [36, 38, 50]. Neuromodulin binds actin [51] and phospholipid [52], and can exist in actin-rich membrane skeletons [53]. In PC12 cells, however, neuromodulin was mainly localized to lysosomal structures, including Golgi apparatus, and was absent from the plasma membrane until NGF-induced differentiation of the cells [54]. The high concentration of neuromodulin in brain (1 μM) and CaM-binding properties have led to the hypothesis that neuromodulin sequesters CaM along the cytoplasmic surface of neuronal membrane domains [37]. Neurogranin may serve the same function postsynaptically. Phosphorylation within the IQ domains at ser^{41} for neuromodulin and at ser^{36} for neurogranin by PKC or phosphorylase kinase completely abrogates CaM binding [38, 55, 56]. Increased $[Ca^{2+}]i$ also decreases CaM binding to these proteins although at physiological levels of K^+, binding of CaM to neuromodulin appears independent of Ca^{2+} [37]. *In vitro*, neuromodulin was able to block activation of nitric oxide synthase by CaM at physiologic concentrations of both neuromodulin and Ca^{2+}, most likely by binding

to CaM [57]. The inhibition by neuromodulin was reversed by phosphorylation with PKC. Similar *in vitro* inhibition of a CaM target enzyme activity by neurogranin has been demonstrated [58]. Thus neuromodulin and neurogranin may regulate the binding of CaM to target proteins by sequestering CaM under conditions of low [Ca^{2+}]i until a PKC-activating stimulus or rise in intracellular Ca^{2+} forces a dissociation of CaM. This has never been demonstrated *in vivo*, although CaM can crosslink to neuromodulin in brain membranes [59]. This crosslinking, however, was performed in a buffer containing high concentrations of EGTA, rather than a buffer containing physiological concentrations of ions.
Sources of Ca^{2+}-independent CaM binding which could prove to be crucial for controlling the subcellular distribution of CaM and mediating some of its physiological responses are unconventional myosins. Much can be learned concerning the cellular activities and regulation of CaM from an investigation of unconventional myosins. These myosins exhibit structural diversity from the classical group I and II myosins. A prominent, abundant unconventional myosin is myosin-V, originally identified as a 190 kd CaM-binding protein present in actomyosin preparations in mammalian brain [60–62]. The protein contains six IQ motifs in the neck region to which four CaM light chains are bound in the absence of Ca^{2+} [61]. Myosin-V has actin-activated magnesium-ATPase activity which is further activated in the presence of exogenous CaM and Ca^{2+}. It is unclear whether additional CaM would be required to activate the ATPase *in vivo* or whether some CaM chains are lost during purification [62]. Since it is so abundant, accounting for 0.3% of brain protein [62], and binds four CaM light chains per myosin, myosin-V would serve as a significant source of CaM binding at both basal and stimulated levels of intracellular Ca^{2+}. In brain, CaM binding to myosin-V could be a significant source of CaM identified in the cytosol since myosin-V colocalizes with perinuclear organelles [61]. Myosin-V is a member of a structural class of unconventional myosins that includes gene products encoded by the dilute gene of mouse and the MYO2 gene of *Saccharomyces cerevisiae* [41]. Yeast cells carrying a mutation of a CaM gene blocking binding of CaM to MYO2 cannot translocate secretory vesicles along actin cables to fusion sites in the bud of the yeast [63].
Rat myr 4, an unconventional myosin of ~100 kDa, is also highly expressed in brain tissue [64]. Rat myr 4 binds CaM light chains to two separate IQ motifs which, interestingly, differ slightly in amino acid sequence and Ca^{2+} sensitivities. The IQ motif in the amino terminal bound CaM well only in the absence of free Ca^{2+} whereas the the carboxy-terminal motif bound only in the presence of Ca^{2+}. In the carboxy terminal myr 4 IQ motif, the

motif IQXXXRGXXXR is altered such that glutamine and glycine residues are exchanged for an isoleucine and an arginine, respectively. Whether this accounts for the difference in Ca^{2+} requirement for binding is unclear.

Almost nothing is known about the regulation of CaM binding to myr 4 or myosin-V. On the other hand, hormonal regulation of CaM binding to the unconventional myosin, brush border myosin I (BBMI) (110kDa), has been demonstrated. One of the first mammalian unconventional myosins found to bind CaM [65], BBMI is a major CaM binding protein in the intestinal microvilli; binding of CaM is independent of Ca^{2+}. BBMI exists as a helical array of cross-bridges linking the plasma membrane and actin filament bundle in microvilli and activates magnesium-ATPase activity. BBMI binds three to four CaM light chains and has at least three IQ motifs in the neck region. Calcitriol increased CaM binding to BBMI-enriched chicken brush border membrane vesicles in a manner paralelling increased Ca^{2+} uptake [66]. Recently, calcitriol treatment was shown to increase CaM binding to ATP-releasable myosin I in both whole brush borders and brush border membrane vesicles [67] most likely by an increase in the amount of BBMI or its ATP releasability rather than via phosphorylation. BBMI is a PKC substrate when bound to membranes or vesicles through phosphatidylserine [68]. The site of phosphorylation is not the CaM binding site but phosphorylation could regulate binding of BBMI to CaM or phosphatidylserine. In a manner similar to neuromodulin and neurogranin, CaM is released from BBMI upon a rise in $[Ca^{2+}]i$ [68, 69]. The physiological significance of this dissociation is unclear, however, since, in the microvillus, the CaM concentration is 1–10 mM, which may preclude such a dissociation [41]. An alternative model proposes that increases in Ca^{2+} would induce an allosteric regulation of myosin activity through interactions between heavy and light chains (CaM) that remain bound to each other [41].

Myosins can be crucial for determination of CaM's subcellular localization. CaM content and localization in *Drosophila* photoreceptor cells was absolutely dependent upon the unconventional myosins *Nina*C splice forms p174 in the rhabdomere and p132 in the cytosol [70]. Since there is a defect in vision when CaM was not concentrated in rhabdomeres, CaM may have a role in fly phototransduction.

Therefore the concept of CaM binding to proteins at resting Ca^{2+} levels and the alteration of CaM binding upon cellular activation becomes quite important to understand the physiological regulation of CaM. Ca^{2+}-independent CaM-binding proteins could be important as CaM cellular "storehouses" awaiting cell stimulus, but also could serve as regulators of subcellular localization of CaM and participate in cellular activities such as protein or vesicle trafficking. Actin binding and ATPases could be important activities regulated by this binding. The importance of Ca^{2+}-independent binding of CaM is underscored by the finding that inactivation of all the Ca^{2+}-binding sites in yeast CaM did not abolish the ability of the protein to support growth [71] although CaM itself was essential for yeast viability [72]. This suggests that, despite the attention given to Ca^{2+}-dependent enzymatic activities of CaM, CaM may perform essential functions in cell growth without acting as a Ca^{2+} receptor.

4 Stimuli-mediated activation of CaM-sensitive enzymes

Ca^{2+}-dependent activation of CaM target proteins is clearly a response to a variety of hormones, neurotransmitters and drugs that would increase intracellular Ca^{2+}. Key regulators would be stimuli that act through receptors that mobilize intracellular Ca^{2+}, activators of ligand-gated ion channels that increase Ca^{2+} permeability, such as the glutamate receptor agonists, N-methyl D-aspartate (NMDA), α-amino-3-hydroxy-5-methyl-isoxazole-4-proprionate (AMPA) and kainate and dihydropyridine Ca^{2+} channel activators. CaM activates isozymes of enzymes such as adenylyl cyclase [73, 74], cyclic nucleotide phosphodiesterase (PDE) [75, 76], myosin light chain kinase MLCK [77], Ca^{2+}, Mg^{2+} ATPase [78], calcineurin [79], nitric oxide synthase [80], guanylate cyclase from Paramecium [81], NAD kinase [82], phosphofructokinase [83], RNA replitase [84], inositol trisphosphate kinase [85] and at least four Ca^{2+}/CaM-dependent protein kinases [86]. CaM also binds, Ca^{2+}-dependently, to a number of other, predominantly membrane or cytoskeletal proteins, including microtubule-associated protein-2 (MAP-2) [87], fodrin (spectrin) [88], Na^+/H^+ exchanger isoform 1 [89], kinesin light chains [90], myristoylated alanine-rich C kinase substrate (MARCKS) [91], caldesmon [92], adducin [93], synapsin I [94], protein 4.1 [95], synaptotagmin [96], NAP-22 [97], tau [87], tubulin [98] and the heat shock proteins, hsp90 [99] and hsp100 [100], and clathrin light chains [101–103] (see review [1]). The dissociation constants for binding of Ca^{2+}\CaM to the various target proteins vary from 10^{-11} – 10^{-5} M. For example, the affinity of CaM for cyclic nucleotide PDE is 0.1 nM [1] while that of neuromodulin is 200 nM [104] and that for brain adducin is 1.3 μM [105]. The highest known affinity of CaM for a target protein (60 pM) is that of CaM for the autonomous, phosphorylated multifunctional CaM-dependent protein kinase II (CaM-Kinase II) [104].

Although it is often postulated that stimuli-mediated increases in cellular Ca^{2+} will induce binding of CaM to various CaM target proteins, *in vivo* activation of CaM-dependent proteins has been demonstrated for relatively few. Clear data are obtained with Ca^{2+}-dependent protein kinases since specific substrates or specific sites on substrates for phosphorylation/dephosphorylation can often be identified. Some enzymes, such as MLCK or the constitutive CaM-dependent NOS have no activity in the absence of CaM and Ca^{2+} and are readily activated upon increases in $[Ca^{2+}]i$. The role of CaM in various physiological activities has been predominantly examined by incubation of cells or tissues with CaM inhibitors. While most inhibitors are not specific for CaM and may even affect Ca^{2+} transport in cells [4, 5], some more specific inhibitors do exist. The immunosuppressant drugs FK506 and cyclosporin A are fairly specific for calcineurin [106]. Mediation of the α-adrenergic stimulation of Na^+, K^+-ATPase activity by calcineurin in renal tubule cells was demonstrated with the use of FK506 and a calcineurin inhibitory peptide [107]. CaM inhibitors have also been useful in demonstrating activation of CaM-dependent PDE in response to muscarinic agonists in dog thyroid slices [108] and 1321 cells [109] and in response to δ-opioid receptor stimulation in neuroblastoma x glioma NG108-15 cells [110]. More selective inhibitors of CaM-dependent protein kinases and CaM PDEs that bind specifically to the enzyme have been synthesized [6–8].

In this section, receptor-mediated activation of type I adenylyl cyclase, CaM Kinase II and nitric oxide synthase (NOS) activities will be discussed. All three enzyme activities are affected by neurotransmitter receptor activation and Ca^{2+} channel activity and, through their localization and activation characteristics, may play important roles in synaptic plasticity.

4.1. CaM-activated adenylyl cyclase

Ca^{2+}/CaM and cAMP can interact through direct effects of CaM on enzymes of cyclic nucleotide metabolism. CaM was discovered as a Ca^{2+}-binding activator of cyclic nucleotide-dependent PDE and adenylyl cyclase [1]. Of the cloned adenylyl cyclases, Types I, III and the newly-identified Type VIII are CaM-activated enzymes [111–114] and Type I, which was originally purified as a CaM-sensitive adenylyl cyclase (115 kDa) is neural specific [115]. Although CaM-activated adenylyl cyclase responds to a Ca^{2+} stimulus, the concentration of Ca^{2+} required to half maximally activate the enzyme in brain is so low, approximately 100 nM [30, 31, 116], that CaM may be partially bound to the enzyme at resting Ca^{2+} levels. The increased Ca^{2+} sensitivity is most apparent at low but physiological levels of Mg^{2+} (1–3 mM) [31, 117]. The $[Ca^{2+}]$i levels are slightly greater, however, when measured with fura-2 [30]. This suggests the enzyme would be highly and rapidly responsive to increased $[Ca^{2+}]$i levels either through mobilization of intracellular Ca^{2+} or influx of extracellular Ca^{2+}.

Earlier studies in brain membranes showed that Gs-coupled neurotransmitter receptors activated CaM-dependent adenylyl cyclase activity and there were synergistic interactions between neurotransmitters, Gs and CaM [30, 117–120]. Recent *in situ* studies using 293 cells stably transfected with type I [120] or Type VIII [114] adenylyl cyclase demonstrated that Ca^{2+} and CaM activation is requisite for enzyme activation through Gs-coupled receptors and that Gs or forskolin was requisite for type III activation by Ca^{2+}\CaM [113]. The synergistic stimulation resulting from the combination of stimuli is likely due to a Ca^{2+}/CaM-induced conformational change in the enzyme and not a phosphorylation [30, 120]. A role for CaM-dependent adenylyl cyclases in neuroplasticity is demonstrated by their localization in the hippocampus in brain [114, 121] and roles in models of learning and memory, such as the *Drosophila* learning mutant, *rutabaga,* classical conditioning in *Aplysia* and long-term potentiation (see [122] for review). Recently, the role for type I adenylyl cyclase in long-term potentiation and learning has been demonstrated more clearly in mice in which the type I gene was inactivated by targeted mutagenesis. These mice had decreased synaptic responses in long-term potentiation and altered performance in a test of spatial memory [123]. The synergistic interaction between Ca^{2+} signals and Gs-coupled neurotransmitters seems to be important in the temporal aspects of classical conditioning in *Aplysia* [124] and may serve as Ca^{2+} and neurotransmitter coincidence detectors in neuronal systems [125].

4.2 CaM-Kinase II

The clearest demonstration of stimuli-dependent activation of a neuronal CaM-stimulated kinase is shown for the multifunctional CaM-dependent protein kinase, CaM-Kinase II [126, 127]. CaM-Kinase II exists as a homomultimer or heteromultimer of 6–12 kinase subunits each; the neuronal specific isoforms are: α (54 kDa), β (60 kDa) and β' (59 kDa). Other isoforms include γ (Mr 59,038) and δ (Mr 60,080). Its substrates include enzymes such as tyrosine hydroxylase, tryptophan hydroxylase, pyruvate kinase, myosin light chains, casein and cytoskeletal proteins such as synapsin 1, MAP-2, tau, tubulin and transcription factors such as CREB (cAMP response element binding protein) and C/EBPβ, a member of the bZip family of transcription factors [86, 127]. Stimulus-induced activation of CaM-Kinase II can be detected either by determining the phosphorylation of a specific site on a substrate (e.g. the tail region of synapsin I [128]) or by measuring the Ca^{2+}/CaM-dependent and CaM-independent enzyme activity after *in vivo* activation using a specific peptide substrate [129]. Direct activation of CaM-Kinase II has been demonstrated *in situ* in response to the Ca^{2+}-mobilizing hormones bradykinin and muscarine [129, 130], by stimulation of ligand-gated Ca^{2+} channels for ATP and acetylcholine, by caffeine [130] and activation of voltage-gated Ca^{2+} channels [131, 132].

Even though CaM-Kinase II may be activated by multiple signals in a cell, diverse physiological responses could result from those signals. For example, Ca^{2+} entry through either the ionotropic glutamatergic NMDA receptors or L-type Ca^{2+} channels in hippocampus leads to CaM Kinase II activation and expression of the *c-fos* gene [131, 132]. Although CaM Kinase II activation can result in fos expression in the hippocampus its activation was critical only for propagating the signal from the L-type Ca^{2+} channel to the nucleus but not that from the NMDA receptor. Similar results were reported in hippocampal dentate gyrus cells where Ca^{2+} entry through kainate receptors led to a CaM-dependent production of *c-fos*, while NMDA-mediated Ca^{2+} entry activated *c-fos* through a CaM-independent mechanism [133]. This suggests that Ca^{2+} activation of distinct signaling pathways depends upon spatially discreet sites of entry into neurons [132].

CaM-Kinase II possesses a unique mechanism to maintain activation of the enzyme following a decline in a Ca^{2+} pulse. Although enzyme activity principally correlates with the spike of Ca^{2+} released from intracellular stores, the enzyme can remain active for several minutes in the absence of elevated Ca^{2+} [129]. CaM kinase consists of three domains, a catalytic domain, a regulatory domain and an association domain responsible for the heteromultimeric structure. The regulatory domain consists of an autoinhibitory site (amino acids 281 to 303) and a CaM binding site (296–309). Initial binding of Ca^{2+}/CaM displaces the autoinhibitory segment and fully activates the enzyme. The enzyme then locks itself into an activated state by autophosphorylation of a threonine (Thr^{286}) in the autoinhibitory segment, which markedly reduces the dissociation rate of CaM independent of the Ca^{2+} concentration. Autophosphorylation increases the affinity of CaM-Kinase II for CaM from 45 nM in the unphosphorylated enzyme to 60 pM in the phosphorylated enzyme [104]. CaM must also be bound to the subunit for continued intermolecular autophosphorylation and CaM trapping, a cooperative process that is inefficient at low CaM [134]. CaM acts both to activate the kinase subunit and to present the substrate unit for autophophorylation. The trapping and autonomy effect of CaM-Kinase II could make it more sensitive to Ca^{2+} oscillations that can occur in cells [135] as well as highly sensitive to rapid alterations in Ca^{2+} that occur in neurons. This ability of the enzyme to remain active at sub-threshold levels of Ca^{2+} makes it an attractive candidate to play a role in sensitization or memory processes, such as long-term potentiation [127, 136].

4.3 Nitric oxide synthase

Nitric oxide (NO), shown to be the endothelium-derived relaxing factor, an important mediator in macrophages and endothelial cells, has recently been recognized as a prominent neuronal messenger [137]. Nitric oxide synthase (NOS) transforms arginine into NO and citrulline. NO increases cGMP formation by binding to the iron in the heme of guanylyl cyclase, causing a conformational change that activates the protein [138]. Constitutive CaM-dependent NO activity, highly localized in brain, is readily measured in response to neurotransmitter stimulation since the enzyme has virtually no activity in the absence of Ca^{2+} and CaM. The enzyme can be activated in response to ligand- or voltage-gated Ca^{2+} channels or to increases in $[Ca^{2+}]i$. In brain, NOS is highly responsive to glutamate, via the NMDA or kainate receptors and increases NO and cGMP levels 10-fold [138–140], see references in [137]. Activation of the Ca^{2+}-dependent enzyme in cultured cells by neurotensin and antiotensin II has been demonstrated [141, 142]. Antipsychotic drugs have been shown to inhibit NOS activity in cerebellum and N1E-115 neuroblastoma cells, but the inhibition is due to their binding of CaM [143]. NO has been proposed as a mediator in two models of synaptic plasticity, long-term potentiation and long-term depression, both of which are blocked by NOS inhibitors. NO is extremely attractive as a candidate for a retrograde mediator of hippocampal long-term potentiation since it could readily diffuse from postsynaptic to presynaptic sites. NO is also postulated to play a role in neurotoxicity; NOS inhibitors completely prevent NMDA-induced neurotoxicity [137, 138].

5 Stimuli-induced regulation of CaM binding through phosphorylation of CaM target proteins

Receptor stimuli or drugs that alter second messenger activity could profoundly alter CaM responses through activation of phosphorylation pathways. Phosphorylation may serve to increase the availability of CaM in the cell and to decrease activation of some CaM target enzymes. Most CaM-binding proteins are substrates for one or more protein kinases, including PKC, protein kinase A (PKA) and CaM Kinase II. While phosphorylations by PKA and CaM-Kinase II have been demonstrated to affect the affinity of CaM for target proteins, in many cases PKC-mediated phosphorylations completely abolish binding by CaM. PKC-mediated phosphorylations of neuromodulin [37], neurogranin [38], MARCKS [91], p68 RNA helicase [84], neural tissue-enriched acidic protein, NAP-22 [144], caldesmon [145], adducin [146, 147] and Ca^{2+}, Mg^{2+} ATPase [148–150] appear to abrogate CaM binding.

5.1 Phosphorylation-mediated changes in CaM localization and binding to target proteins

Stimulus-induced redistribution of CaM from the membrane fraction to cytosol in response to phosphorylation has been demonstrated. The redistribution begins within minutes after stimulus and sometimes lasts hours. Neurotransmitter-stimulated translocation of CaM was originally demonstrated in rat striatal membranes in response to cyclic AMP and dopamine [151, 152]. The redistribution resulted in a reduction in dopamine-stimulated adenylyl cyclase activity and an activation of a cytosolic EGTA-sensitive PDE [151–153]. Although a role for PKA in the dopamine-mediated translocation was suggested, no clear substrate for PKA mediating the decreased binding of CaM was found.
PKC activation, however, actively decreases binding of CaM to several CaM-binding proteins which could result in an altered CaM distribution within the cell. Activation of M3 muscarinic receptors by carbachol in human neuroblastoma SK-N-SH cells led to a four- to five-fold increase in CaM in the cytosol, with an accompanying decrease in the membrane-bound CaM [154]. The action of carbachol was blocked by a PKC antagonist and was mimicked by TPA and ionomycin, showing a role for PKC in the redistribution. In PC12 cells, the Ca^{2+}-mobilizing hormone, bradykinin elicited a rapid increase in soluble CaM, resulting in a heightened activation of CaM Kinase II [155]. Differential binding of CaM to target

proteins following phosphorylation could occur depending upon local concentrations of $[Ca^{2+}]i$, since different CaM target proteins have different Ca^{2+} requirements, and the number of CaM-binding proteins phosphorylated. Using the active photoreactive CaM derivative, calmodulin-diazopyruvamide (CaM-DAP), [156] demonstrated a carbachol-stimulated increase in photoaffinity labeling of three distinct CaM binding proteins in SK-N-SH cells. The time course of labeling was distinct for the proteins as was the retention of label. This suggests a coordinated regulation of activation of CaM target proteins in response to a hormone or neurotransmitter stimulus. Due to the Ca^{2+}/CaM synergism, an increase in localized CaM could significantly increase Ca^{2+} sensitivity of target enzymes.

PKC-mediated phosphorylation of several CaM-binding proteins, most notably neuromodulin, neurogranin, MARCKS and NAP-22, would result in a dissociation of CaM and may serve a regulatory function in a cell by leading to an increased availability of CaM for other processes. These cytoskeletal proteins share physicochemical characteristics of relative heat stability, solubility in 2.5% perchloric acid solution, low hydrophobicity and anomalous behavior in SDS-PAGE [35, 38, 144, 157, 158]. MARCKS is a filamentous actin crosslinking protein of wide cellular distribution whose activity is regulated by PKC-mediated phosphorylation and CaM binding [91, 157]. Less is known about NAP-22 except that it is a neural specific protein concentrated in growth cones [36, 144]. Unlike that for neuromodulin or neurogranin, Ca^{2+} is required for binding of CaM to MARCKS [91] and NAP-22 [97, 144]. The Ca^{2+}-sensitivity of binding is reflected in the affinities of the proteins for CaM; the affinity of CaM for MARCKS and NAP-22 is 4.6 nM [159] and 1.2 nM [97], respectively, while that for neuromodulin is 200 nM in the presence of low KCl [37]. MARCKS is a highly prominent PKC substrate in cells since it has two to four PKC substrate sites in the molecule. Phosphorylation of neuromodulin, neurogranin and MARCKS obviates CaM binding because the PKC phosphorylation site is near to or overlaps with the CaM-binding site within the protein [38, 157, 160]. The PKC substrate site in NAP-22 is ser^6 but at this time it is unknown whether this is near the CaM-binding site [97]. Both MARCKS and neuromodulin are in SK-N-SH cells and may contribute to the PKC-induced redistribution of CaM in those cells [161].

Although it has been postulated that the relatively high concentrations of MARCKS and NAP-22 make them candidates for binding significant amounts of CaM in an unstimulated cell, the Ca^{2+} requirement for binding of CaM to these proteins should make this role less probable unless significant Ca^{2+}\CaM synergism existed. MARCKS or NAP-22 would have to bind CaM at resting levels of Ca^{2+} to serve as a CaM reservoir. Overexpression of MARCKS in rat1 cells, however, increased the sensitivity of the inhibition of DNA synthesis to CaM-binding CaM inhibitors [162] without altering the levels of cellular CaM. The data were interpreted that the increased MARCKS resulted in increased sequestered CaM, making it unavailable to other cellular processes and increasing the sensitivity of CaM inhibitors. Although transfected MARCKS could be phosphorylated, which should dissociate CaM, the effects of the phosphorylation on CaM inhibitor activity was not assessed. The resting Ca^{2+} level in the transfected cell, which would affect CaM binding, is similarly unknown. These results do suggest, however, that the level of CaM-binding proteins in the cell can alter the responsiveness of the cell to CaM-dependent processes and would alter the responsiveness to CaM inhibiting drugs.

Following dissociation, CaM might rebind to proteins relatively close the phosphorylated protein, either localized in the membrane or in more soluble locations. *In vitro* phosphorylation of the MARCKS/CaM complex by PKC resulted in a dissociation of bound CaM with a subsequent binding to MLCK, and activation of phosphodiesterase and calcineurin with a t1/2 of 1.2 to 1.7 min [163]. Some physiological consequences of phosphorylation-mediated release of CaM have been demonstrated, such as CaM Kinase II activation [155]. PKC-mediated phosphorylation of MARCKS in IC2 mast cells enhanced cAMP formation mediated through the prostacyclin receptor, but not basal or fluoride-stimulated activity [164]. Important factors in the receptor activation were phosphorylation-induced dissociation of MARCKS from the actin cytoskeleton and release of CaM. CaM appeared to mediate the enhancement of receptor activity by affecting the interaction of prostacyclin receptor and Gs.

PKC-mediated phosphorylation of caldesmon, a protein involved in skeletal muscle contraction, reduced its binding to CaM as well as F-actin and myosin [145]. In the erythrocyte, binding of CaM affects the ability of adducin, a cytoskeletal protein, to regulate spectrin-actin interactions [105]. Phosphorylation of β-adducin by PKA has been reported to inhibit binding of CaM [147] while Ca^{2+} and CaM can protect adducin against PKC-mediated phosphorylation [146]. Binding of CaM to the nuclear protein, p68 RNA helicase, is abolished by phosphorylation by PKC [84]. p68 RNA helicase exhibits RNA-dependent ATPase activity, binds CaM in a Ca^{2+}-dependent manner and is a member of the IQ domain-containing family. Thus there can be a significant amount of cross talk and interaction in the effect of PKC and Ca^{2+} regarding CaM binding to these cytoskeletal and nuclear

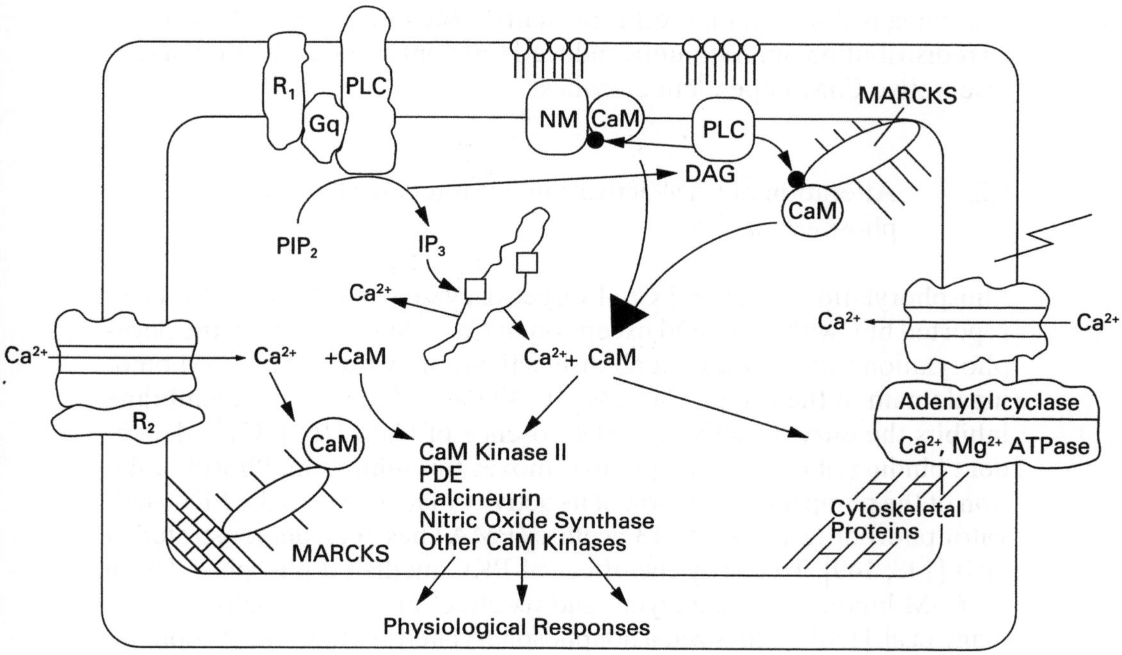

Fig. 1
Representation of a cell demonstrating various ways in which intracellular $[Ca^{2+}]i$ can be elevated leading to binding of CaM to target proteins. Elevation of $[Ca^{2+}]i$ through voltage- or ligand (R2)-gated ion channels or through Ca^{2+}-mobilizing receptors (R1) will lead to immediate activation of CaM-dependent target enzymes and binding of CaM to cytoskeletal proteins such as MARCKS. CaM activation of Ca^{2+}, Mg^{2+}, ATPase would participate in removal of Ca^{2+} from the cell. Stimulation of a phospholipase C (PLC)-coupled receptor would lead to release of $[Ca^{2+}]i$ through production of inositol trisphosphate (IP_3) and activation of PKC through production of diacylglycerol (DAG). PKC-mediated phosphorylation of CaM-binding proteins such as MARCKS and neuromodulin (NM) would dissociate CaM. The newly-released CaM can greatly enhance the activity of cytosolic or membrane target proteins even under conditions of declining Ca^{2+} due to synergistic activation with Ca^{2+}, CaM and target enzymes. Physiological responses to activation of CaM target enzymes could depend upon the mechanism or cellular domain by which Ca^{2+} enters the cell.

proteins and their properties on actin binding, cytoskeletal and nuclear function. These phosphorylations, however, have largely been demonstrated *in vitro*, and the *in vivo* CaM binding and phosphorylation of these proteins by a physiological stimulus activating PKC has not been determined.

A schema is shown in Figure 1 representing the binding of CaM in a cell, its redistribution upon stimulus-induced Ca^{2+} entry and activation of representative CaM-dependent enzymes.

5.2 Alteration of CaM activation of target enzymes through phosphorylation

Phosphorylation of several CaM target enzymes by PKC has also been reported but, with the noted exception of Ca^{2+}, Mg^{2+}, ATPase, the phosphorylation usually does not abolish activation by CaM. The CaM binding domain of the P-type Ca^{2+}, Mg^{2+}, ATPase of the plasma membrane inhibits the enzyme activity in the absence of CaM [165]. Ca^{2+}-dependent binding of CaM to the pump removes this inhibition. Phosphorylation of the pump and reduction of its activity in response to the PKC-activator phorbol 12-myristate 13-acetate (PMA) has been demonstrated *in vivo* [148, 149]. To clarify the effect of PKC-mediated phosphorylation on CaM binding to the enzyme and its effect on ATPase activity, Hofmann et al. [150] synthesized a nonphosphorylated peptide and phosphothreonine-containing peptide representing the CaM binding site of the enzyme. The phosphothreonine-containing synthetic CaM binding domain was much less efficient as an inhibitor of ATPase activity than the unphosphorylated peptide and could not bind CaM. PKC-mediated phosphorylation of nitric oxide synthase (NOS) has been demonstrated [141, 166] but its relationship to CaM binding is unknown. Both increases [141] and decreases [166] in activity as a consequence of PKC stimulation have been reported. Ca^{2+}/CaM protect against phosphorylation of calcineurin by PKC, but PKC-mediated phosphorylation of calcineurin does not affect the binding or activation by CaM [167].
CaM-binding proteins are also substrates for PKA, PKG and CaM-Kinase II although phosphorylation by these enzymes does not usually completely abolish CaM binding. These phosphorylations, however, may mediate subtle regulation of the CaM-dependent enzymes by Ca^{2+} or cAMP levels in the cell. PKA-mediated phosphorylation of the Type I 61-kDa subunit of PDE at ser^{120}, which may be within a postulated second CaM-binding domain of PDE, reduced its affinity for PDE by 20-fold [168, 169]. In neurons in particular, a Ca^{2+} pulse increasing cyclic AMP through activation of adenylyl cyclase could sustain its signal by desensitizing PDE. Phosphorylation of the 63-kDa PDE by CaM Kinase II produced a more modest two-fold decrease in affinity for Ca^{2+} in the activation by CaM [170, 171]. Physiological regulation of PDE in response to a Ca^{2+} pulse in the

cell would depend upon the local CaM concentration as well as the time- and Ca^{2+}-dependence of activation and affinity of the enzymes involved. In response to a Ca^{2+} pulse, the 63-kDa PDE might be phosphorylated in the cell before CaM could bind to it and activate it. However, the synergism between PDE, Ca^{2+} and CaM suggest that at low Ca^{2+} concentrations, the PDE may be selectively activated since CaM Kinase II requires higher Ca^{2+} levels for activation. PDE will bind CaM *in situ* in unstimulated cells. In human neuroblastoma SK-N-SH cells, scrape-loaded photoreactive CaM-DAP cross-linked to PDE in the absence of a Ca^{2+} stimulus [156]. Basal levels of Ca^{2+}, measured using fura-2, were 25 nM in unscraped cells and 70 nM in cells scraped-loaded with CaM-DAP. This suggests that PDE can be activated at Ca^{2+} levels well below those required to activate the enzyme *in vitro* [23, 24]. The abundance of CaM and Ca^{2+} sensitivity of the enzyme makes the physiological consequences of modest changes in CaM binding to PDE unclear. However, CaM may be spatially limited with PDE depending upon the activation status of the cell and increased competition for CaM with another closely localized high-affinity protein might exist.

Although phosphorylation of CaM-binding proteins and target enzymes has been extensively demonstrated in response to a number of protein kinases *in vitro*, receptor-mediated phosphorylation of a specific site in response to a specific enzyme has rarely been demonstrated *in vivo*. *In vivo* phosphorylation of smooth muscle myosin light chain kinase (MLCK) and its physiological consequences in response to hormone stimulation has been demonstrated. MLCK is a high specificity protein kinase which phosphorylates only myosin II. Its activity is totally dependent upon CaM which it binds with high affinity (1 nM) [172, 173]. The enzyme is inactive or nearly inactive at resting Ca^{2+} in the smooth muscle cell but is activated by the rise in $[Ca^{2+}]i$ mediated by certain neurotransmitters, hormones or growth factors. MLCK is phosphorylated by PKA, CaM-Kinase II and PKC at a specific site (site A, Ser^{815} in the CaM-binding domain) which reduces the sensitivity of the enzyme for CaM 10–20-fold [173–175]. Activation of tracheal smooth muscle by carbachol and KCl but not isoproterenol, which induces relaxation, decreased the affinity for CaM and increased phosphorylation of MLCK [176]. Carbachol and KCl stimulated phosphorylation of Ser^{815} solely through activation of CaM Kinase II, as opposed to PKC or PKA [175]. Phosphorylation of myosin light chain and MLCK may be differentially separated by Ca^{2+} levels and time. Higher Ca^{2+} is required for MLCK phosphorylation, (CaM-Kinase II activation) than is required for myosin light chain phosphorylation (MLCK activity). CaM Kinase II is half maximally activated at 0.1 μM to 1 μM Ca^{2+} while MLCK can be

Table 1.
Phosphorylated sites in select CaM-binding target proteins

CaM-binding protein	CaM-binding site	Phosphorylated site	Phosphorylating enzyme	Reference
Ca, Mg ATPase (autoinhib. domain)	QILWFRGLNRIQTQI RVVNAFRSS	QIWFRGLNRIQTQIR VVNAFRSS-NH2	PKC	[165, 150]
Calcineurin	ARKEVIRNKIRAIGK MARVFSVLR	MARVFSVLRGGSGS MARVFSVLR	CaM Kinase II	[167]
h-caldesmon	WEKGNVF (659-665)	PKC site: S^{726}	PKC	In: [172]
sm musc MLCK (autoinhib. domain)	MARRKWQKTGHAV RAIGRLSS	ARRKWQKTGHAVR AIGRLSS (S^{815})	CaM Kinase II	In: [172] [246]
MARCKS	KRFSFKKSFKLSFGS FKK	KRFSFKKSFKLSFGS FKK	PKC	In: [247]
Neuromodulin	IQASFRGHMARKKI KS	IQASFRGHITRKKLK GEKK	PKC	[160]
Neurogranin	IQASFRGHMARKKIKS KS	IQASFRGHMARKKI KS	PKC	[38]
β-Adducin	KQQKEKTRWLNTPN TYLRVNVADEVQRN MGSPRPKTT (aa425-462)	KQQKEKTRWLNTPN TYLRVNVADEVQRN MGSPRPKTT	PKA (T461)and CaM Kinase II (S455)	[147]
Type I 61 kDa cAMP PDE	QTEKMWQRLKGILR CLVKQL (aa 22-41)	PRFRSIVHVV(ser^{120}) reduces binding affinity for CaM	PKA	[169, 248]
CaM-Kinase II (autoinhib domain)	RRKLKGAILTTMLA (aa 296-309)	RRKLKGAILTTMLA (Thr^{305} and Thr^{306})	CaM Kinase II	In:[172]

half maximally activated at 170 nM to 250 nM Ca^{2+} depending upon the phosphorylated state of the protein [173]. The process of light chain phosphorylation is so sensitive to Ca^{2+} that it is maximal by 230 ms in response to tracheal smooth muscle depolarization while the cytosolic Ca^{2+} concentrations were not maximal until 9 sec. As the Ca^{2+} concentration rose, MLCK became phosphorylated. This phosphorylation may be responsible for the partial, rather than complete, phosphorylation of myosin light chains in response to depolarization.

The phosphorylated sites affecting CaM binding for several CaM-binding proteins are shown in Table I. Non-phosphorylated peptides have been used as inhibitors on CaM-dependent enzyme activities. They would be especially useful when activities can be measured in permeabilized cells [107] or when the peptides can be microinjected. While the peptides appear to be fairly specific for CaM-mediated activities, they are not specific for the enzyme whose CaM-binding site they represent since they act by binding CaM [150, 177, 178]. For instance, synthetic peptides based on the CaM-binding domain of skeletal muscle myosin light chain kinase inhibit the 61 kDa cyclic nucleotide PDE, brain adenylyl cyclase, *Bordetella pertussis* adenylyl cyclase, red cell membrane Ca^{2+}, Mg^{2+} ATPase, calcineurin and skeletal muscle phosphorylase b kinase [177]. This demonstrates that, although the amino acid sequences of the binding domains may be quite different in the various proteins, the target enzymes compete for a common binding determinant or domain on CaM. It also suggests that the hydrophobic character and amphipathicity of the CaM binding domain plays a large role in the binding of CaM. A more selective CaM peptide inhibitor is one based on the autoinhibitory domain of CaM kinase II [179, 180]. Peptides encompassing both the CaM-binding domain and the autoinhibitory domain potently block CaM action and at higher concentrations block kinase activity.

6 CaM localization and content in response to persistent stimuli or drug treatment

Persistent hormone or drug treatment can increase CaM content and alter its localization in a cell. Alterations in CaM localization not specifically related to rapid phosphorylation have been demonstrated in cell culture or peripheral tissues in response to angiotensin II [181], gonadotropin releasing hormone [182], and calcitriol [183, 184]. Elevations in CaM in the nucleus have been noted in response to estrogen [185] or during proliferation of rat liver cells [186] and human T lymphocytes [187]. In rat liver cells activated by partial hepatectomy, the increase in total cellular CaM was largely located in the nuclear matrix which contains the replitase complexes [188]. This suggests a role for nuclear CaM in the triggering or progression of DNA replication [189]. Increases in nuclear CaM are also expressed in response to ACTH in the adrenal cortex [190], estrogen in chicken liver cells [191] and the convulsant agents lindane or Ca^{2+}-channel agonists in brain [192]. CaM-binding proteins identified in the nucleus are MLCK, α-spectrin, CaM-Kinase II, calcineurin, basic helix-loop-helix proteins such as E2A, the hnRNA-associated proteins, hnRNP A2 and hnRNP C, p68 replitase and other proteins of unknown function [84, 189]. CaM takes part in DNA synthesis, the onset and progression of mitosis, gene expression and DNA repair [189]. Recently, a facilitated ATP-independent transport of CaM into the nucleus in tissue culture cells has been identified [193].

6.1 Psychoactive drugs and sensitization

Neuroactive drugs have demonstrated effects on CaM localization and content. Translocation of CaM from membranes to cytosol has been demonstrated in rats in response to acute treatment with amphetamine [153, 194, 195], dopamine [152], morphine [196], and leu-enkephalin in NG 108-15 cells [197]. Cocaine [198] and ethanol [199] elicit a redistribution of CaM from cytosol to membranes. In addition to altering the localization of CaM, the content of CaM in rat brain was increased in response to repeated treatment with haloperidol [153, 200–202], amphetamine [195, 200, 203], cocaine [198] and morphine [204]. The role of the increase in CaM is unknown but it should be noted that all of the drugs listed above elicit plasticity or sensitization states especially when administered intermittently. On the other hand, continuous administration of the dopamine D2 agonist, quinpirole, which down-regulates stereotyped behavior, decreases Ca^{2+}/CaM-dependent phosphorylation of striatal membranes [205]. CaM could play a role in several neurochemical changes reported to result from repeated treatment with the sensitizing psychoactive drugs, such as an increase in stimulus-induced neurotransmitter release [206] or morphological changes in synaptic structures [207–209]. Roles for CaM in neurotransmitter release have been demonstrated through its activation of CaM-Kinase II and calcineurin or other proteins involved in vesicular trafficking. CaM-Kinase II phosphorylates the actin-binding protein synapsin I, proposed to relax cytoskeletal constraints and allow more vesicles to migrate toward the active zone in the terminal [128]. Calcineurin dephosphorylates dynamin, a microtubule-binding protein with GTPase activity, in an action that may stimulate synaptic vesicle recycling [210]. CaM could also affect vesicular trafficking by activating kinesin ATPase activity [90] which can increase fast axonal transport in nerves and by binding to clathrin-coated vesicles, which are agents for receptor-mediated transport of macromolecules [103]. By increasing the transport, availability or recycling of synaptic vesicles, CaM could be making a contribution to enhanced neurotransmitter release. A role for CaM in vesicle trafficking is supported by a study of a phenotype of a specific mutation of the yeast CaM gene, CMD1. This phenotype specifically caused defects in actin organization which disrupted transport of secretory vesicles to the bud to produce localized growth [63]. The mutant CaM may be unable to bind and regulate the unconventional myosin MYO2, also involved in this process.

Another role for CaM in the sensitization process is to alter transcription, which is shown to be important in plasticity states [211]. CaM can directly alter transcription through the activation of CaM-dependent protein kinases or increased production of cyclic AMP leading to phosphorylation of the transcription factors CREB [212–214] and C/EBPBβ [215, 216]. Amphetamine, cocaine, dopamine, morphine and antipsychotic drugs rapidly increase transcription of immediate early genes [217–220].

An increase in CaM and cytoskeletal binding proteins could be involved with drug-induced morphological alterations [207–209] through regulation of the shape of nerve cells and synapses and the movement of cytosolic components within the cell [221, 222]. Recently, an increase in MLCK immunoreactivity was identified to accompany the increase in CaM in response to repeated haloperidol treatment [202]. Drug-induced changes in MLCK could enhance myosin-actin interactions in the dendritic spine [221], inducing movement of cytoplasm within the spine. Increases in both MLCK and CaM have also been detected in response to estrogen treatment in rabbit myometrium [185] and chick liver [223], and in proliferating rat liver nuclei [186]. Homeostatic increases in CaM binding proteins are not a generalized consequence to rises in $[Ca^{2+}]i$ and CaM, however. Treatment of PC12 cells with nerve growth factor (NGF), which increases $[Ca^{2+}]i$ and CaM content [224], results in a down-regulation of CaM-Kinase III that could result in a decrease in phosphorylation of eEF-2 [225]. This could permit cells to stop dividing and differentiate from the G1 stage [226]. Reserpine, a psychoactive drug which alters neuronal activity and depletes monoamines in the brain, increased expression of the 4.0 kb form of the CaM I gene in rat brain stem two days after single subcutaneous injection [227]. Reserpine also increases mRNA species of proteins involved in catecholamine biosynthesis [228, 229], a process known to involve Ca^{2+} and CaM [230]. Five mRNAs for CaM have been found in rat, mouse and human tissues that are derived from three different genes [231, 232] and all code for a CaM identical in amino acid sequence. Selective regulation of CaM mRNAs has been reported [224, 227, 233, 234].

6.2 Ethanol

Ethanol, at concentrations of 50 to 200 mM, inhibited binding of $[^{125}I]$CaM to rat synaptic plasma membranes maximally by 50% [199]. The inhibition was correlated with a decreased membrane affinity for $[^{125}I]$CaM and a decreased dissociation of $[^{125}I]$CaM-membrane complexes. The inhibition was readily reversible upon washing the membranes, indicating that the direct interaction of ethanol with the membranes was required for inhibition. Animals receiving ethanol for 3 weeks were resistant to the inhibitory effects of acute ethanol on synaptic plasma membrane $[^{125}I]$CaM binding. Since the synaptic plasma membranes were washed extensively, the resistance to ethanol inhibition was not due to endogenously bound CaM. There was a higher membrane affinity for $[^{125}I]$CaM after chronic ethanol suggesting CaM could be more tightly bound in membranes from ethanol-treated rats. The endogenous concentration of CaM in synaptic plasma membranes from ethanol-treated rats was not measured, however. Binding of $[^{125}I]$CaM was altered by lipid transition of the membrane and a higher transition temperature of the membranes was found in chronic ethanol-treated rats. The effect of ethanol on CaM binding to synaptic plasma membranes was manifested by the effect of ethanol on Ca^{2+}, Mg^{2+} ATPase activity [235]. In untreated rats, ethanol inhibited Ca^{2+}, Mg^{2+} ATPase activity, resulting from a decreased affinity of the enzyme for CaM. As with $[^{125}I]$CaM binding, the inhibition was readily reversible upon washing the membranes. In chronic ethanol-treated rats, ethanol no longer could inhibit Ca^{2+}, Mg^{2+} ATPase activity and the enzyme exhibited a higher affinity for CaM, as compared to membranes from untreated rats. The enzyme activity was affected by lipid transition of the membrane in a manner similar to that for $[^{125}I]$CaM binding. Since the Ca^{2+}, Mg^{2+} ATPase is important for lowering Ca^{2+} in the cell, ethanol could have a pronounced effect on cell excitability and synaptic activity by affecting this enzyme. The altered effect in chronically-treated rats suggests that the effects of ethanol on CaM binding and Ca^{2+}, Mg^{2+} ATPase activity could play a role in alcohol tolerance and dependence.

6.3 Glucocorticoids

Glucocorticoids have a pronounced effect on CaM localization, target enzyme activation and mRNA content in various tissues. Corticosterone, incubated with purified rat cortical synaptic plasma membranes for 30 to 60 min, increased Ca^{2+}-dependent membrane binding of ^{125}I-CaM and membrane CaM content [236, 237]. The EC50 for corticosterone was 140 nM which is nearly identical to the Kd of specific binding of corticosterone to synaptic plasma membranes [237]. In *in vivo* studies, however, measurable increases in cortical synaptic plasma membrane CaM, bound Ca^{2+}-dependently, were detected within 10 min after an injection of 2 mg/kg corticosterone. This suggests that glucorticoids can, rather rapidly, modulate CaM binding in the cell. It is possible that corticosterone acts by stabilizing membrane conformation. Measurement of membrane-bound CaM after adrenalectomy would also help determine whether endogenous corticosteroid levels tonically regulate CaM binding. CaM appears, however, to be directly involved in the activation of the glucocorticoid receptor. CaM can interact in a Ca^{2+}-dependent manner with the untransformed glucocorticoid receptor complex which contains hsp90, hsp70 and hsp56 [238]. CaM inhibits binding of hsp90/glucocorticoid receptor complexes to actin [99, 239] perhaps by altering the ATPase activity of hsp90 [240] to which CaM can bind [99]. By inhibiting binding to the actin cytoskeleton, CaM may functionally help to maintain the untransformed glucocorticoid receptor in a state responsive to hormone activation [238].

Removal of endogenous corticosteroids through adrenalectomy alters activation of CaM-dependent adenylyl cyclase and CaM mRNAs in select areas of brain. Adrenalectomy reduced the CaM-dependent adenylyl cyclase activity in rat hippocampus, an area enriched in Type I and Type VIII adenylyl cyclases [122]. There was no change in cerebral cortex and the basal and forskolin-stimulated adenylyl cyclase activities were much less affected than the CaM-dependent activity [241]. Adenylyl cyclase in the hippocampus could be important for learning and memory [122, 123]. Adrenalectomy decreased the level of the CaM III gene mRNA in rat hippocampus and cerebral cortex [242]. Levels of CaM were not measured, so it is not known how the alteration of the CaMIII mRNA altered CaM levels. The effect of adrenalectomy on hippocampal CaM-dependent adenylyl cyclase activity and mRNA levels was prevented by prior corticosterone administration. This study demonstrates that cell stimuli and drugs can differentially regulate CaM genes, even though all of the CaM genes make the same product. The effect of glucorticoids in the hippocampus is another example of a coordinate regulation between CaM levels and target protein responsiveness. In pituitary corticotrope cells, 10 nM dexamethasone increased CaM mRNA within 45 min of incubation and increases in both CaM mRNA and CaM were detected in the cells after 90 min of incubation [243]. Early induction of CaM mRNA in response to glucocorticoids has also been reported in lymphocytes [244, 245]. These studies have suggested that CaM could play a role in glucocorticoid action in various cells, such as apoptosis [245], inhibition of ACTH release in pituitary [243] and glucorticoid action in brain.

7 Summary

The activity, localization and cellular content of CaM can be regulated by drugs, hormones and neurotransmitters. Regulation of physiological responses of CaM can depend upon local Ca^{2+}-entry domains in the cells and phosphorylation of CaM target proteins, which would either decrease responsiveness of CaM target enzymes or increase CaM availability for binding to other target proteins. Despite the abundance of CaM in many cells, persistent cellular activation by a variety of substances can lead to an increase in CaM, reflected both in the nucleus and other cellular compartments. Increases in CaM-binding proteins can accompany stimuli-induced increases in CaM. A role for CaM in vesicular or protein transport, cell morphology, secretion and other cytoskeletal processes is emerging through its binding to cytoskeletal proteins and myosins in addition to the more often investigated activation of target enzymes. More complete knowledge of the physiological regulation of CaM can lead to a greater understanding of its role in physiological processes and ways to alter its actions through pharmacology.

References

1 A.S. Manalan, C.B. Klee: Adv. Cyclic Nucleotide Protein Phosphorylation Res. *18*, 227 (1984).
2 J.C. Stoclet, D. Gerard, M.C. Kilhoffer, C. Lugnier, R. Miller, P. Schaeffer: Prog. Neurobiol. *29*, 321 (1987).
3 A.R. Means: FEBS Lett. *347*, 1 (1994).
4 M.L. Veigl, R.E. Klevit, W.D. Sedwick: Pharmacol. Ther. *44*, 181 (1989).
5 J. Ovadi: Prog. Drug. Res. *33*, 353 (1989).
6 H. Hidaka, M. Hagiwara: Adv. Second Messenger Phosphoprotein Res. *25*, 241 (1992).
7 H. Hidaka, M. Hagiwara, H. Tokumitsu: Adv. Exp. Med. Biol. *269*, 159 (1990).

8 H. Hidaka, T. Ishikawa: Cell Calcium *13*, 465 (1992).
9 R.H. Kretsinger: Adv. Cyclic Nucl. Res. *11*, 2 (1979).
10 D.M. Watterson, F. Sharieff, T.C. Vanaman: J. Biol. Chem. *255*, 962 (1980).
11 Y.S. Babu, J.S. Sack, T.J. Greenhough, C.E. Bugg, A.R. Means, W.J. Cook: Nature *315*, 37 (1985).
12 M.P. Walsh: Rev. Clin. Basic Pharmacol. *5*, 35 (1985).
13 C.B. Klee, T.C. Vanaman: Adv. Protein Chem. *35*, 213 (1982).
14 T. Tanaka, H. Hidaka: J. Biol. Chem. *255*, 11078 (1980).
15 M. Ikura, G.M. Clore, A.M. Gronenborn, G. Zhu, C.B. Klee, A. Bax: Science *256*, 632 (1992).
16 D.B. Heidorn, J. Trewhella: Biochemistry *27*, 909 (1988).
17 W.E. Meador, A.R. Means, F.A. Quiocho: Science *262*, 1718 (1993).
18 A. Persechini, R.H. Kretsinger: J. Biol. Chem. *263*, 12175 (1988).
19 K. Török, M. Whitaker: BioEssays *16*, 221 (1994).
20 H. Weinstein, E.L. Mehler: Annu. Rev. Physiol. *56*, 213 (1994).
21 K.T. O'Neil, W.F. DeGrado: Trends Biochem. Sci. *15*, 59 (1990).
22 J.A. Cox: Biochem. J. *249*, 621 (1988).
23 C.Y. Huang, V. Chau, P.B. Chock, J.H. Wang, R.K. Sharma: Proc. Natl. Acad. Sci. USA *78*, 871 (1981).
24 C.B. Klee: Calmodulin. Molecular Aspects of Cellular Regulation, v .5, Ed. by P. Cohen, C.B. Klee. Elsevier, Amsterdam 1988, p. 35.
25 M. Yazawa, M. Ikura, K. Hikichi, L. Ying, K. Yagi: J. Biol. Chem. *262*, 10951 (1987).
26 B.B. Olwin, A.M. Edelman, E.G. Krebs, D.R. Storm: J. Biol. Chem. *259*, 10949 (1984).
27 S. Kakiuchi, S. Yasuda, R. Yamazaki, Y. Teshima, K. Kanda, R. Kakiuchi, K. Sobue: J. Biochem. 92, 1041 (1982).
28 R.J. Grand, S.V. Perry: Biochem. J. *183*, 285 (1979).
29 P. Cohen, C.B. Klee: Calmodulin. Molecular Aspects of Cellular Regulation, v. 5, Ed. by P. Cohen, C.B. Klee. Elsevier, Amsterdam 1988, p. 357.
30 J.K. Harrison, G.H.K. Hewlett, M.E. Gnegy: J. Biol. Chem. *264*, 15880 (1989).
31 Y. Yovell, E.R. Kandel, Y. Dudai, T.W. Abrams: J. Neurochem. *59*, 1736 (1992).
32 K.M. Hahn, A.S. Waggoner, D.L. Taylor: J. Biol. Chem. *265*, 20335 (1990).
33 A.H. Gough, D.L. Taylor: J. Cell Biol. *121*, 1095 (1993).
34 L.J. Van Eldik, W.E. Zimmer, S.W. Barger, D.M. Watterson: Adv. Exp. Med. Biol. *269*, 111 (1990).
35 P.J. Coggins, H. Zwiers: J. Neurochem. *56*, 1095 (1991).
36 J.H.P. Skene: Ann. Rev. Neurosci. *12*, 127 (1989).
37 K.A. Alexander, B.M. Cimler, K.E. Meier, D.R. Storm: J. Biol. Chem. *262*, 6108 (1987).
38 J. Baudier, J.C. Deloulme, A. Van Dorsselaer, D. Black, H.W. Matthes: J. Biol. Chem. *266*, 229 (1991).
39 K.P. Huang, F.L. Huang, H.C. Chen: Arch. Biochem. Biophys. *305*, 570 (1993).
40 M.J. Welsh, J.C. Aster, M. Ireland, J. Alcala, H. Maisel: Science *216*, 642 (1982).
41 R.E. Cheney, M.S. Mooseker: Curr. Opin. Cell Biol. *4*, 27 (1992).
42 H.J. Cho, Q. Xie, J. Calaycay, R.A. Mumford, K.M. Swiderek, T.D. Lee, C. Nathan: J. Exp. Med. *176*, 599 (1992).
43 D. Ladant, S. Michelson, R. Sarfati, A.-M. Gilles, R. Predeleanu, O. Bârzu: J. Biol. Chem. *264*, 4015 (1989).

44 S. Shenolikar, P.T. Cohen, P. Cohen, A.C. Nairn, S.V. Perry: Eur. J. Biochem. *100*, 329 (1979).
45 R.K. Sharma, J.H. Wang: J. Biol. Chem. *261*, 14160 (1986).
46 K.A. Alexander, B. Wakim, G.S. Doyle, K.A. Walsh, D.R. Storm: J. Biol. Chem. *263*, 7544 (1988).
47 W.H. Gispen, H.B. Nielander, P.N.E. De Graan, A.B. Oestreicher, L.H. Schrama, P. Schotman: Mol. Neurobiol. *5*, 61 (1991).
48 P.J. Robinson: Mol. Neurobiol. *5*, 87 (1991).
49 R.W. Cohen, J.E. Margulies, P.M. Coulter, J.B. Watson: Brain Res. *627*, 147 (1993).
50 J.B. Watson, J.G. Sutcliffe, R.S. Fisher: Proc. Natl. Acad. Sci. USA *89*, 8581 (1992).
51 J.J.H. Hens, F. Benfenati, H.B. Nielander, F. Valtorta, W.H. Gispen, P.N.E. De Graan: J. Neurochem. *61*, 1530 (1993).
52 D. Houbre, G. Duportail, J.-C. Deloulme, J. Baudier: J. Biol. Chem. *266*, 7121 (1991).
53 K.F. Meiri, P.R. Gordon-Weeks: J. Neurosci. *10*, 256 (1990).
54 C.O. Van Hooff, P.N. De Graan, A.B. Oestreicher, W.H. Gispen: J. Neurosci. *9*, 3753 (1989).
55 D.D. Gerendasy, S.R. Herron, J.B. Watson, J.G. Sutcliffe: J. Biol. Chem. *269*, 22420 (1994).
56 H.K. Paudel, H. Zwiers, J.H. Wang: J. Biol. Chem. *268*, 6207 (1993).
57 J.R. Slemmon, M.R. Martzen: Biochemistry *33*, 5653 (1994).
58 M.R. Martzen, J.R. Slemmon: J. Neurochem. *64*, 92 (1995).
59 P.N.E. De Graan, A.B. Oestreicher, M. De Wit, M. Kroef, L.H. Schrama, W.H. Gispen: J. Neurochem. *55*, 2139 (1990).
60 R.E. Larson, F.S. Espindola, E.M. Espreafico: J. Neurochem. *54*, 1288 (1990).
61 E.M. Espreafico, R.E. Cheney, M. Matteoli, A.A.C. Nascimento, P.V. De Camilli, R.E. Larson, M.S. Mooseker: J. Cell Biol. *119*, 1541 (1992).
62 R.E. Cheney, M.K. O'Shea, J.E. Heuser, M.V. Coelho, J.S. Wolenski, E.M. Espreafico, P. Forscher, R.E. Larson, M.S. Mooseker: Cell *75*, 13 (1993).
63 Y. Ohya, D. Botstein: Science *263*, 963 (1994).
64 M. Bahler, R. Kroschewski, H.E. Stoffler, T. Behrmann: J. Cell Biol. *126*, 375 (1994).
65 J.R. Glenney,Jr., K. Weber: J. Biol. Chem. *255*, 10551 (1980).
66 D.D. Bikle, S. Munson: J. Clin. Invest. *76*, 2312 (1985).
67 R. Kaune, S. Munson, D.D. Bikle: Biochim. Biophys. Acta Bio-Membr. *1190*, 329 (1994).
68 H. Swanljung-Collins, J.H. Collins: J. Biol. Chem. *267*, 3445 (1992).
69 K. Collins, J.R. Sellers, P. Matsudaira: J. Cell Biol. *110*, 1137 (1990).
70 J.A. Porter, M. Yu, S.K. Doberstein, T.D. Pollard, C. Montell: Science *262*, 1038 (1993).
71 J.R. Geiser, D. Van Tuinen, S.E. Brockerhoff, M.M. Neff, T.N. Davis: Cell *65*, 949 (1991).
72 T.N. Davis, M.S. Urdea, F.R. Masiarz, J. Thorner: Cell *47*, 423 (1986).
73 W.Y. Cheung, L.S. Bradham, T.J. Lynch, Y.M. Lin, E.A. Tallant: Biochem. Biophys. Res. Commun. *66*, 1055 (1975).
74 C.O. Brostrom, Y.C. Huang, B.M. Breckenridge, D.J. Wolff: Proc. Natl. Acad. Sci. U. S. A. *72*, 64 (1975).
75 S. Kakiuchi, R. Yamazaki, Y. Teshima, K. Uenishi, E. Miyamoto: Biochem. J. *146*, 109 (1975).
76 W.Y. Cheung: J. Biol. Chem. *246*, 2859 (1971).
77 R. Dabrowska, D. Aromatorio, J.M. Sherry, D.J. Hartshorne: Biochem. Biophys.

Res. Commun. *78*, 1263 (1977).
78 V. Niggli, P. Ronner, E. Carafoli, J.T. Penniston: Arch. Biochem. Biophys. *198*, 124 (1979).
79 S.-D. Yang, W.Y. Cheung: Biochem. Biophys. Res. Commun. *106*, 1419 (1982).
80 D.S. Bredt, S.H. Snyder: Proc. Natl. Acad. Sci. U. S. A. *87*, 682 (1990).
81 S. Klumpp, G. Kleefeld, J.E. Schultz: J. Biol. Chem. *258*, 12455 (1983).
82 J.M. Anderson, M.J. Cormier: Biochem. Biophys. Res. Commun. *84*, 595 (1978).
83 B. Buschmeier, H.E. Meyer, G.W. Mayr: J. Biol. Chem. *262*, 9454 (1987).
84 M.K. Buelt, B.J. Glidden, D.R. Storm: J. Biol. Chem. *269*, 29367 (1994).
85 K. Yamaguchi, M. Hirata, H. Kuriyama: Biochem. J. *244*, 787 (1987).
86 P.I. Hanson, H. Schulman: Annu. Rev. Biochem. *61*, 559 (1992).
87 Y.C. Lee, J. Wolff: J. Biol. Chem. *259*, 1226 (1984).
88 K. Sobue, K. Kanda, J. Adachi, S. Kakiuchi: Proc. Natl. Acad. Sci. USA *80*, 6868 (1983).
89 B. Bertrand, S. Wakabayashi, T. Ikeda, J. Pouysségur, M. Shigekawa: J. Biol. Chem. *269*, 13703 (1994).
90 H.J.G. Matthies, R.J. Miller, H.C. Palfrey: J. Biol. Chem. *268*, 11176 (1993).
91 J.M. Graff, T.N. Young, J.D. Johnson, P.J. Blackshear: J. Biol. Chem. *264*, 21818 (1989).
92 R. Kakiuchi, M. Inui, K. Morimoto, K. Kanda, K. Sobue, S. Kakiuchi: FEBS Lett. *154*, 351 (1983).
93 S.M. Mische, M.S. Mooseker, J.S. Morrow: J. Cell Biol. *105*, 2837 (1987).
94 N.V.L. Hayes, A.F. Bennett, A.J. Baines: Biochem. J. *275*, 93 (1991).
95 G.M. Kelly, B.D. Zelus, R.T. Moon: J. Biol. Chem. *266*, 12469 (1991).
96 J.M. Trifaro, S. Fournier, M.L. Novas: Neuroscience *29*, 1 (1989).
97 S. Maekawa, H. Murofushi, S. Nakamura: J. Biol. Chem. *269*, 19462 (1994).
98 H. Kumagai, E. Nishida, H. Sakai: J. Biochem. (Tokyo) *91*, 1329 (1982).
99 E. Nishida, S. Koyasu, H. Sakai, I. Yahara: J. Biol. Chem. *261*, 16033 (1986).
100 S. Koyasu, E. Nishida, Y. Miyata, H. Sakai, I. Yahara: J. Biol. Chem. *264*, 15083 (1989).
101 C.D. Linden, J.R. Dedman, J.G. Chafouleas, A.R. Means, T.F. Roth: Proc. Natl. Acad. Sci. U. S. A. *78*, 308 (1981).
102 L.A. Silveira, D.H. Wong, F.R. Masiarz, R. Schekman: J. Cell Biol. *111*, 1437 (1990).
103 U.M. Pley, B.L. Hill, C. Alibert, F. Brodsky, P. Parham: J. Biol. Chem. *270*, 2395 (1995).
104 T. Meyer, P.I. Hanson, L. Stryer, H. Schulman: Science *256*, 1199 (1992).
105 V. Bennett, K. Gardner, J.P. Steiner: J. Biol. Chem. *263*, 5860 (1988).
106 D.A. Fruman, C.B. Klee, B.E. Bierer, S.J. Burakoff: Proc. Natl. Acad. Sci. USA *89*, 3686 (1992).
107 A. Aperia, F. Ibarra, L.-B. Svensson, C. Klee, P. Greengard: Proc. Natl. Acad. Sci. USA *89*, 7394 (1992).
108 F. Miot, C. Erneux, J.N. Wells, J.E. Dumont: Mol. Pharmacol. *25*, 261 (1984).
109 L.I. Tanner, T.K. Harden, J.N. Wells, M.W. Martin: Mol. Pharmacol. *29*, 455 (1986).
110 P.Y. Law, H.H. Loh: Mol. Pharmacol. *43*, 684 (1993).
111 W.-J. Tang, J. Krupinski, A.G. Gilman: J. Biol. Chem. *266*, 8595 (1991).
112 H.A. Bakalyar, R.R. Reed: Science *250*, 1403 (1990).
113 E.-J. Choi, Z. Xia, D.R. Storm: Biochemistry *31*, 6492 (1992).
114 J.J. Cali, J.C. Zwaagstra, N. Mons, D.M.F. Cooper, J. Krupinski: J. Biol. Chem. *269*, 12190 (1994).
115 Z. Xia, E.-J. Choi, F. Wang, C. Blazynski, D.R. Storm: J. Neurochem. *60*, 305 (1993).

116 M. Gnegy, G. Treisman: Mol. Pharmacol. *19*, 256 (1981).
117 J.K. Harrison, C.K. Mickevicius, M.E. Gnegy: J. Neurochem. *51*, 345 (1988).
118 A. Malnoe, J.A. Cox: J. Neurochem. *45*, 1163 (1985).
119 M.E. Gnegy: Annu. Rev. Pharmacol. Toxicol. *32*, 45 (1993).
120 G.A. Wayman, S. Impey, Z. Wu, W. Kindsvogel, L. Prichard, D.R. Storm: J. Biol. Chem. *269*, 25400 (1994).
121 Z.G. Xia, C.D. Refsdal, K.M. Merchant, D.M. Dorsa, D.R. Storm: Neuron *6*, 431 (1991).
122 E.-J. Choi, Z. Xia, E.C. Villacres, D.R. Storm: Curr. Opin. Cell Biol. *5*, 269 (1993).
123 Z.L. Wu, S.A. Thomas, E.C. Villacres, Z. Xia, M.L. Simmons, C. Chavkin, R.D. Palmiter, D.R. Storm: Proc. Natl. Acad. Sci. USA. *92*, 220 (1995).
124 Y. Yovell, T.W. Abrams: Proc. Natl. Acad. Sci. USA *89*, 6526 (1992).
125 S. Impey, G. Wayman, Z. Wu, D.R. Storm: Mol. Cell. Biol. *14*, 8272 (1994).
126 J.A.P. Rostas, P.R. Dunkley: J. Neurochem. *59*, 1191 (1992).
127 H. Schulman: Curr. Opin. Cell Biol. *5*, 247 (1993).
128 P. De Camilli, P. Greengard: Biochem. Pharmacol. *35*, 4349 (1986).
129 M. MacNicol, A.B. Jefferson, H. Schulman: J. Biol. Chem. *265*, 18055 (1990).
130 M. MacNicol, H. Schulman: FEBS Lett. *304*, 237 (1992).
131 K. Fukunaga, T.R. Soderling, E. Miyamoto: J. Biol. Chem. *267*, 22527 (1992).
132 H. Bading, D.D. Ginty, M.E. Greenberg: Science *260*, 181 (1993).
133 L.S. Lerea, J.O. McNamara: Neuron *10*, 31 (1993).
134 P.I. Hanson, T. Meyer, L. Stryer, H. Schulman: Neuron *12*, 943 (1994).
135 M.J. Berridge: Adv. Second Messenger Phosphoprotein Res. *24*, 108 (1990).
136 A.J. Silva, Y. Wang, R. Paylor, J.M. Wehner, C.F. Stevens, S. Tonegawa: Cold Spring Harbor Symp. Quant. Biol. *57*, 527 (1992).
137 D.S. Bredt, S.H. Snyder: Annu. Rev. Biochem. *63*, 175 (1994).
138 S.H. Snyder: Science *257*, 494 (1992).
139 P. Marin, J.F. Quignard, M. Lafon-Cazal, J. Bockaert: Neuropharmacology *32*, 29 (1993).
140 L. Kiedrowski, E. Costa, J.T. Wroblewski: J. Neurochem. *58*, 335 (1992).
141 U. Forstermann, L.D. Gorsky, J.S. Pollock, K. Ishii, H.H. Schmidt, M. Heller, F. Murad: Mol. Pharmacol. *38*, 7 (1990).
142 S. Chaki, T. Inagami: Mol. Pharmacol. *43*, 603 (1993).
143 J. Hu, J.-H. Lee, E.E. el-Fakahany: Psychopharmacology (Berl) *114*, 161 (1994).
144 S. Maekawa, M. Maekawa, S. Hattori, S. Nakamura: J. Biol. Chem. *268*, 13703 (1993).
145 H. Umekawa, H. Hidaka: Biochem. Biophys. Res. Commun. *132*, 56 (1985).
146 A. Waseem, H.C. Palfrey: Eur. J. Biochem. *178*, 563 (1988).
147 D.A. Scaramuzzino, J.S. Morrow: Proc. Natl. Acad. Sci. USA *90*, 3398 (1993).
148 K.K. Wang, L.C. Wright, C.L. Machan, B.G. Allen, A.D. Conigrave, B.D. Roufogalis: J. Biol. Chem. *266*, 9078 (1991).
149 L.C. Wright, S. Chen, B.D. Roufogalis: Arch. Biochem. Biophys. *306*, 277 (1993).
150 F. Hofmann, J. Anagli, E. Carafoli, T. Vorherr: J. Biol. Chem. *269*, 24298 (1994).
151 M.E. Gnegy, P. Uzunov, E. Costa: Proc. Natl. Acad. Sci. USA *73*, 3887 (1976).
152 M. Memo, W. Lovenberg, I. Hanbauer: Proc. Natl. Acad. Sci. USA *79*, 4456 (1982).
153 I. Hanbauer, S. Pradham, H.-Y.T. Yang: Ann. NY Acad. Sci. *356*, 292 (1980).
154 L.A. Mangels, M.E. Gnegy: Mol. Pharmacol. *37*, 820 (1990).
155 M. MacNicol, H. Schulman: J. Biol. Chem. *267*, 12197 (1992).
156 L.A. Mangels, M.E. Gnegy: J. Biol. Chem. *267*, 5847 (1992).
157 A. Aderem: Trends Biochem. Sci. *17*, 438 (1992).

158 P.J. Blackshear: J. Biol. Chem. *268*, 1501 (1993).
159 G.M. Verghese, J.D. Johnson, C. Vasulka, D.M. Haupt, D.J. Stumpo, P.J. Blackshear: J. Biol. Chem. *269*, 9361 (1994).
160 E.R. Chapman, D. Au, K.A. Alexander, T.A. Nicolson, D.R. Storm: J. Biol. Chem. *266*, 207 (1991).
161 A.M. Goldsmith, M.E. Gnegy: Soc. Neurosci. Abstracts *20*, 1173 (1994).
162 T. Herget, S. Broad, E. Rozengurt: Eur. J. Biochem. *225*, 549 (1994).
163 B.K. McIlroy, J.D. Walters, P.J. Blackshear, J.D. Johnson: J. Biol. Chem. *266*, 4959 (1991).
164 T. Sawai, M. Negishi, N. Nishigaki, T. Ohno, A. Ichikawa: J. Biol. Chem. *268*, 1995 (1993).
165 P. James, T. Vorherr, J. Krebs, A. Morelli, G. Castello, D.J. McCormick, J.T. Penniston, A. De Flora, E. Carafoli: J. Biol. Chem. *264*, 8289 (1989).
166 D.S. Bredt, C.D. Ferris, S.H. Snyder: J. Biol. Chem. *267*, 10976 (1992).
167 Y. Hashimoto, T.R. Soderling: J. Biol. Chem. *264*, 16524 (1989).
168 R.K. Sharma, J.H. Wang: Proc. Natl. Acad. Sci. USA *82*, 2603 (1985).
169 V.A. Florio, W.K. Sonnenburg, R. Johnson, K.S. Kwak, G.S. Jensen, K.A. Walsh, J.A. Beavo: Biochemistry *33*, 8948 (1994).
170 Y. Hashimoto, R.K. Sharma, T.R. Soderling: J. Biol. Chem. *264*, 10884 (1989).
171 R.K. Sharma, J.H. Wang: J. Biol. Chem. *261*, 1322 (1986).
172 M.P. Walsh: Mol. Cell. Biochem. *135*, 21 (1994).
173 J.T. Stull, M.G. Tansey, D.-C. Tang, R.A. Word, K.E. Kamm: Mol. Cell. Biochem. *127–128*, 229 (1993).
174 M.A. Conti, R.S. Adelstein: J. Biol. Chem. *256*, 3178 (1981).
175 J.T. Stull, L.C. Hsu, M.G. Tansey, K.E. Kamm: J. Biol. Chem. *265*, 16683 (1990).
176 M.G. Tansey, R.A. Word, H. Hidaka, H.A. Singer, C.M. Schworer, K.E. Kamm, J.T. Stull: J. Biol. Chem. *267*, 12511 (1992).
177 D.K. Blumenthal, H. Charbonneau, A.M. Edelman, T.R. Hinds, G.B. Rosenberg, D.R. Storm, F.F. Vincenzi, J.A. Beavo, E.G. Krebs: Biochem. Biophys. Res. Commun. *156*, 860 (1988).
178 T. Vorherr, L. Knöpfel, F. Hofmann, S. Mollner, T. Pfeuffer, E. Carafoli: Biochemistry *32*, 6081 (1993).
179 P.T. Kelly, R.P. Weinberger, M.N. Waxham: Proc. Natl. Acad. Sci. USA *85*, 4991 (1988).
180 R.W. Tsien, H. Schulman, R. Malinow: Adv. Second Messenger Phosphoprotein Res. *24*, 101 (1990).
181 K. Kushiku, Y. Araki, T. Furukawa, T. Iwasa, N. Inoue, E. Miyamoto: J. Pharmacol. Exp. Ther. *245*, 311 (1988).
182 P.M. Conn, J.G. Chafouleas, D. Rogers, A.R. Means: Nature *292*, 264 (1981).
183 D.D. Bikle, S. Munson, J. Chafouleas: FEBS. Lett. *174*, 30 (1984).
184 A.R. deBoland, V. Massheimer, L.M. Fernandez: Calcif. Tissue Int. *43*, 370 (1988).
185 K. Matsui, K. Higashi, K. Fukunaga, K. Miyazaki, M. Maeyama, E. Miyamoto: J. Endocrinol. *97*, 11 (1983).
186 M.J. Pujol, M. Soriano, R. Aligue, E. Carafoli, O. Bachs: J. Biol. Chem. *264*, 18863 (1989).
187 J. Colomer, A. López-Girona, N. Agell, O. Bachs: Biochem. Biophys. Res. Commun. *200*, 306 (1994).
188 J. Serratosa, M.J. Pujol, O. Bachs, E. Carafoli: Biochem. Biophys. Res. Commun. *150*, 1162 (1988).

189 O. Bachs, N. Agell, E. Carafoli: Cell Calcium *16*, 289 (1994).
190 J.F. Harper, R.W. Wallace, W.Y. Cheung, A.L. Steiner: Adv. Cyclic Nucleotide. Res. *14*, 581 (1981).
191 R.C. Simmen, B.S. Dunbar, V. Guerriero, J.G. Chafouleas, J.H. Clark, A.R. Means: J. Cell Biol. *99*, 588 (1984).
192 M. Vendrell, M.J. Pujol, J.M. Tusell, J. Serratosa: Brain Res. Mol. Brain Res. *14*, 285 (1992).
193 M. Pruschy, Y. Ju, L. Spitz, E. Carafoli, D.S. Goldfarb: J. Cell Biol. *127*, 1527 (1994).
194 N. Popov, H. Matthies: Eur. J. Pharmacol. *172*, 205 (1989).
195 M.E. Gnegy, G.H.K. Hewlett, S.L. Yee, M.J. Welsh: Brain Res. *562*, 6 (1991).
196 I. Hanbauer, J. Gimble, K. Sankaran, R. Sherard: Neuropharmacology *18*, 859 (1979).
197 D. Baram, R. Simantov: J. Neurochem. *40*, 55 (1983).
198 M. Memo, S. Pradhan, I. Hanbauer: Neuropharmacology *20*, 1145 (1981).
199 P.Y. Sze, Z. Iqbal: J. Pharmacol. Exp. Ther. *268*, 1183 (1994).
200 N. Popov, S. Schulzeck, D. Nuss, A.-U. Vopel, C. Jendrny, H. Struy, H. Matthies: Biomed. Biochim. Acta *47*, 435 (1988).
201 M. Gnegy, P. Uzunov, E. Costa: J. Pharmacol. Exp. Ther. *202*, 558 (1977).
202 M.E. Gnegy, A. Agrawal, K. Hewlett, E. Yeung, S. Yee: Mol. Br. Res. *27*, 195 (1994).
203 J.M. Roberts-Lewis, M.J. Welsh, M.E. Gnegy: Brain Res. *384*, 383 (1986).
204 R. Nehmad, H. Nadler, R. Simantov: Mol. Pharmacol. *22*, 389 (1982).
205 S.-P. Zhang, L.-W. Zhou, N. Natsukari, B. Weiss: Neurochem. Int. *23*, 361 (1993).
206 T.E. Robinson: Taniguchi Symposia on Brain Sciences, vol 14, Biological Basis of Schizophrenic Disorders, Ed. by T. Nakazawa. Japan Scientific Societies Press, Tokyo 1991, p. 185.
207 N.A. Uranova, A.J. Klintzova, V.V. Istomin, U. Haselhorst, H. Schenk: J. Hirnforsch. *30*, 45 (1989).
208 A.J. Klintzova, U. Haselhorst, N.A. Uranova, H. Schenk, V.V. Istomin: J. Hirnforsch. *30*, 51 (1989).
209 F.M. Benes, P.A. Paskevich, J. Davidson, V.B. Domesick: Brain Res. *329*, 265 (1985).
210 J.-P. Liu, A.T.R. Sim, P.J. Robinson: Science *265*, 970 (1994).
211 P. Goelet, V.F. Castellucci, S. Schacher, E.R. Kandel: Nature *322*, 419 (1986).
212 T.B. Shea, N.I. Perrone-Bizzozero, M.L. Beermann, L.I. Benowitz: J. Neurosci. *11*, 1685 (1991).
213 R.F. Power, J.P. Lydon, O.M. Conneely, B.W. O'Malley: Science *252*, 1546 (1991).
214 H. Enslen, P. Sun, D. Brickey, S.H. Soderling, E. Klamo, T.R. Soderling: J. Biol. Chem. *269*, 15520 (1994).
215 M. Wegner, Z. Cao, M.G. Rosenfeld: Science *256*, 370 (1992).
216 D.D. Ginty, H. Bading, M.E. Greenberg: Curr. Opin. Neurobiol. *2*, 312 (1992).
217 G.S. Robertson, S.R. Vincent, H.C. Fibiger: Brain Res. *523*, 288 (1990).
218 A.M. Graybiel, R. Moratalla, H.A. Robertson: Proc. Natl. Acad. Sci. USA *87*, 6912 (1990).
219 E.J. Nestler, B.T. Hope, K.L. Widnell: Neuron *11*, 995 (1993).
220 J.C. Miller: J. Neurochem. *54*, 1453 (1990).
221 E. Fifkova, M. Morales: Ann. NY Acad. Sci. *568*, 131 (1989).
222 G. Lynch, M. Baudry: Br. Res. Bull. *18*, 809 (1987).
223 P. Cohen: Eur. J. Biochem. *111*, 563 (1980).
224 G. Bai, B. Weiss: J. Cell. Physiol. *149*, 414 (1991).
225 A.C. Nairn, R.A. Nichols, M.J. Brady, H.C. Palfrey: J. Biol. Chem. *262*, 14265 (1987).
226 A.G. Ryazanov, A.S. Spirin: New Biol. *2*, 843 (1990).

227 B. Ni, I.R. Brown: Neurochem. Res. *18*, 185 (1993).
228 N.F. Biguet, M. Buda, A. Lamouroux, D. Samolyk, J. Mallet: EMBO J. *5*, 287 (1986).
229 I.B. Black, D.M. Chikaraishi, E.J. Lewis: Brain Res. *339*, 151 (1985).
230 H. Fujisawa, T. Yamauchi, H. Nakata, S. Okuno: Fed. Proc. *43*, 3011 (1984).
231 H. Nojima: J. Mol. Biol. *208*, 269 (1989).
232 R. Fischer, M. Koller, M. Flura, S. Mathews, M.-A. Strehler-Page, J. Krebs, J.T. Penniston, E. Carafoli, E.E. Strehler: J. Biol. Chem. *263*, 17055 (1988).
233 A.R. Means: Recent Prog. Horm. Res. *44*, 223 (1988).
234 G. Bai, R.A. Nichols, B. Weiss: Biochim. Biophys. Acta Gene Struct. Expression *1130*, 189 (1992).
235 Z. Iqbal, P.Y. Sze: Neurochem. Res. *19*, 475 (1994).
236 P.Y. Sze, Z. Iqbal: J. Steroid Biochem. Mol. Biol. *48*, 179 (1994).
237 P.Y. Sze, Z. Iqbal: Neurochem. Res. *19*, 1455 (1994).
238 Y.-M. Ning, E.R. Sánchez: Biochem. Biophys. Res. Commun. *208*, 48 (1995).
239 Y. Miyata, I. Yahara: J. Biol. Chem. *266*, 8779 (1991).
240 K. Nadeau, A. Das, C.T. Walsh: J. Biol. Chem. *268*, 1479 (1993).
241 M.N. Gannon, T. Akompong, M.L. Billingsley, B.S. McEwen: Endocrinology *134*, 853 (1994).
242 M.N. Gannon, B.S. McEwen: Mol. Brain Res. *22*, 186 (1994).
243 M.J. Shipston, F.A. Antoni: Biochem. Biophys. Res. Commun. *189*, 1382 (1992).
244 G. Baughman, M.T. Harrigan, N.F. Campbell, S.J. Nurrish, S. Bourgeois: Mol. Endocrinol. *5*, 637 (1991).
245 D.R. Dowd, P.N. MacDonald, B.S. Komm, M.R. Haussler, R. Miesfeld: J. Biol. Chem. *266*, 18423 (1991).
246 R.B. Pearson, R.E. Wettenhall, A.R. Means, D.J. Hartshorne, B.E. Kemp: Science *241*, 970 (1988).
247 A. Aderem: Cell *71*, 713 (1992).
248 H. Charbonneau, S. Kumar, J.P. Novack, D.K. Blumenthal, P.R. Griffin, J. Shabanowitz, D.F. Hunt, J.A. Beavo, K.A. Walsh: Biochemistry *30*, 7931 (1991).

Progress in Drug Research, Vol. 45 (E. Jucker, Ed.)

Recent advances in benzodiazepine receptor (BZR) binding studies

By S.P. Gupta

Department of Chemistry, Birla Institute of Technology and Science, Pilani 333031, India

1 Introduction

The discovery of benzodiazepines (BZs) **1** and their receptors have opened a new era in the discovery and characterization of drugs acting on the central nervous system (CNS). The pioneering and explorative synthetic work

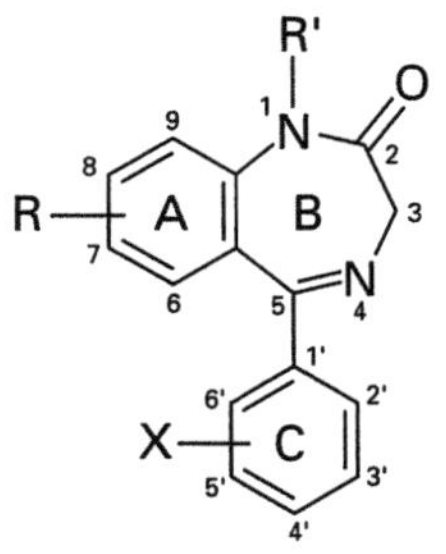

1

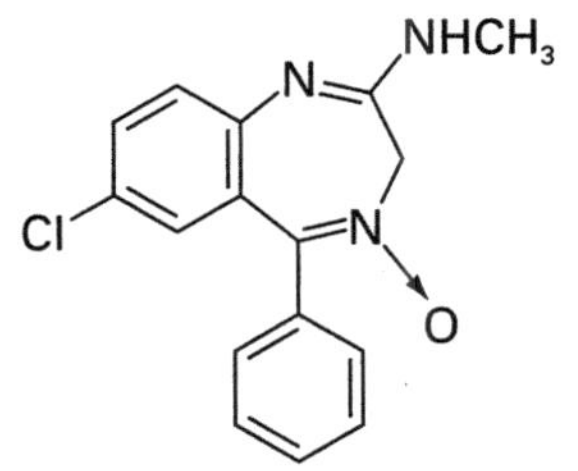

2

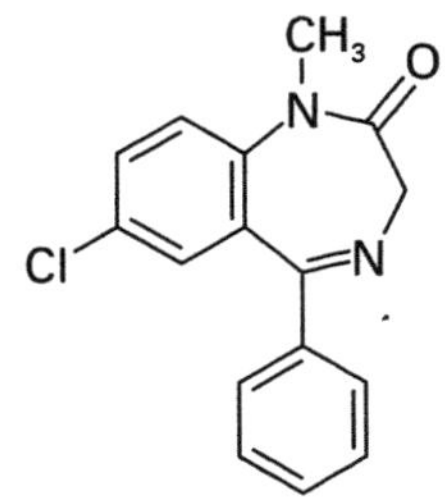

3

of Sternbach in the early days of the BZ era led to the development of compound **2** with its unusual pharmacological profile. The story of its development as narrated by Sternbach himself is very interesting [1a–c]. While its structure was studied by Sternbach and Reeder [1d], its sophisticated pharmacological tests were done by Randall and his staff [2]. It was given the generic name chlordiazepoxide and was launched under the trade name Librium®. The synthesis of this compound was rapidly followed by its derivative diazepam **3**, which was given the trade name Valium®. These two drugs, which appeared on the market in rapid succession, soon became the most frequently prescribed CNS drugs. The success of these two drugs led Sternbach and his group to synthesize a number of related products (for examples see papers in ref. [3]) and, by the end of 1983, about 35 benzodiazepine drugs were available for therapy. The BZ drugs have a wide range of therapeutic applications [4]. They can be used in the pharmacotherapy of anxiety and related emotional disorders, in the treatment of sleep disorders, status epileptics, and other convulsive states. They also act as centrally acting muscle relaxants and can be drugs of choice for medication and for inducing agents in anesthesiology. However, the mechanisms of action of these unusually well-tolerated and broadly effective drugs remained obscure for years, as the discovery and characterization of benzodiazepine receptors (BZRs) from the brain tissue came much later [5] than the synthesis of chlordiazepoxide or diazepam. The recognition of the BZRs was rapidly followed by the development of the *in vitro* binding assay [6] which was capable of expeditiously screening a large number of compounds regardless of the structural type.

The BZR, in fact, is not an independent receptor, but is coupled to the γ-aminobutryric acid (GABA) receptor and is a part of the $GABA_A$-controlled chloride ion channel. Thus, the BZs and related compounds are not directly responsible for their observed biological activity but act as modulators of GABA binding to its receptor, which then directly alters the gating of the GABA-dependent transmembrane chloride ion channel [7, 8]. GABA acts on at least two different receptor types [9–13]; the action of BZs seems to be restricted to synaptic effects of GABA that are mediated by the so-called $GABA_A$ receptors.

The benzodiazepine receptors may be, like other pharmacological receptors, proteins, glycoproteins, or nucleic acids. However, little is known about the chemical structure of BZ binding sites. It has been proposed that tyrosinyl residue in or very close to the binding site plays a crucial role in the recognition and binding of ligands [14]. It has also been concluded, however, that histidine might be involved as an essential contact residue [15]. Additionally, BZRs have also been found to possess glycoprotein qualities [16], where carbohydrate moieties are supposed to affect the biological response of BZ ligands, but it has not been decided yet whether the carbohydrate moieties are involved in the binding of BZs or whether they influence the conformation of the binding site.

The BZR, however, no longer signifies a receptor that selectively interacts with ligands belonging only to the BZ class of compounds. Certain purines, cyclopyrrolones, triazolopyridazines, phenylquinolinones, β-carbolines, and some other structurally different non-BZ molecules have been identified as endogeneous ligands for BZR [17], and there are BZs that interact highly specifically with a completely different receptor, such as tifluadom with the opiate κ receptor [18–20].

2 Types of BZR ligands

Basically three different types of ligands have been identified for BZR; they have been termed by Haefely [21] as full agonists, full antagonists, and full inverse agonists. The first and third types act as allosteric modulators of the $GABA_A$ receptor complex, producing mirror biological effects, and the second type acts as a true antagonist at the receptor for the former, but shows no effect on the binding of GABA (Fig. 1) [22]. Therefore, the ligands that exert a positive cooperative effect on GABA binding to its receptor complex, resulting in a full biological response over the complete agonist profile (positive intrinsic efficacy) are known as full agonists, and the ligands that exert a negative cooperative effect on GABA binding to its receptor and, when compared to agonists, show a mirror image biological response over the full inverse profile of activity (negative intrinsic efficacy) are known as full inverse agonists. Finally, full antagonists are the ligands with high affinity for BZR, having no modulatory effect on GABA binding to its receptor complex, and showing no relevant biological effects of their own, but blocking the effects of both agonist and inverse agonist ligands (no intrinsic efficacy).

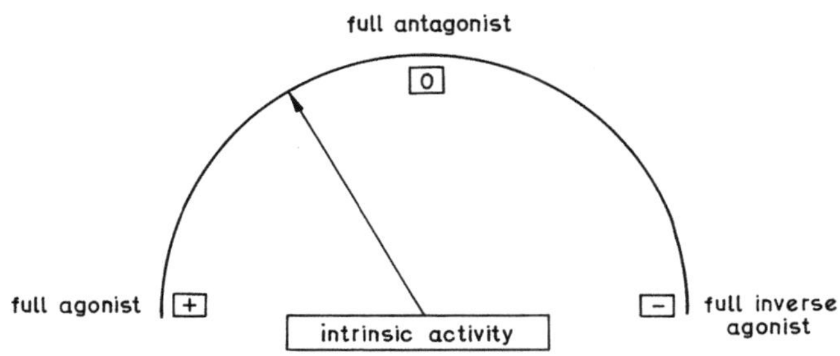

Fig. 1
A schematic representation of the three different types of ligands [22].

While some compounds are known to be full agonists, full antagonists, or full inverse agonists, the majority of compounds that have been synthesized and found to bind to the BZR, regardless of structure, show properties combining agonistic with antagonistic or inverse agonistic with antagonistic features. Such compounds are known as partial agonists or partial inverse agonists [17].

Thus all the terms coined to typify the ligands are provisionally best considered as purely based on phenomenology and thus there seems no general rule that would help us to decide which of the BZR ligands is an agonist, antagonist, and inverse agonist. One has, therefore, to wait for the eventual identification of a possible endogenous ligand of the BZR in order to know if it acts as an agonist, antagonist, or inverse agonist.

3 Interrelationship of ligands and homogeneity of BZR

The three types of ligands exhibit an interrelationship, which can be explained on the basis of changes in the conformation of the receptor from its unoccupied resting state [23, 24]. After primary recognition of the essential binding pharmacophores, the receptor will undergo a shift to either an agonist or an inverse agonist conformation, based on the geometry and hydrophobic nature of the ligand. This conformational change, probably energy driven, then allosterically modulates the binding of GABA to $GABA_A$ receptor. It is proposed that no conformational shift takes place when a full antagonist binds to the resting state of the BZR, and it would therefore be expected that such a ligand-receptor complex would show no efficacy at the GABA receptor [22]. This model for explaining the interrelationship of ligands is known as the three-state receptor model. An alternative two-state receptor model has also been proposed, in which the unoccupied receptor is in equilibrium with agonist and inverse agonist conformations [25].

It has been observed that there exists a homogeneity in BZR binding sites for all the three types of ligands. This homogeneity is defined purely in the chemical sense, i.e., it is the amino acid sequence for the receptor protein that should be identical for all three sites. The homogeneity of BZR binding sites has been demonstrated for compounds having only minor structural modifications, which showed similar binding interactions but which displaced activities across the full spectrum from agonist to antagonist to inverse agonist. While Figure 2 presents an example for the imidazobenzodiazepin-6-one series [26], analogous observations have been made for β-carbolines [27–29], pyrazoloquinolines [30–33], and triazolopyridazines [34, 35]. Several structure-activity relationship studies have also supported the homogeneity of BZR [36].

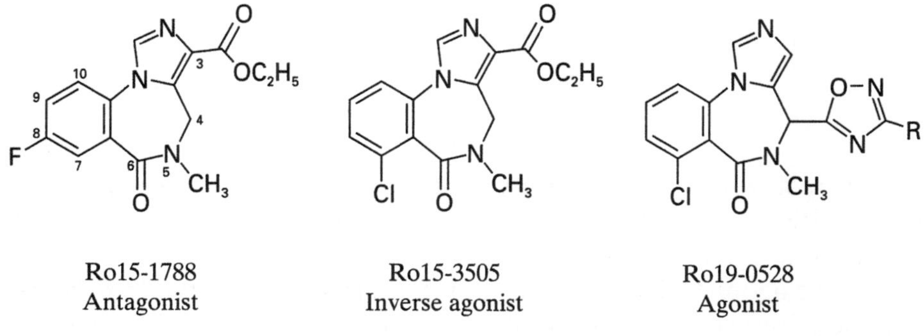

Fig. 2
Change in the nature of the ligand belonging to the imidazobenzodiazepin-6-one series by a minor modification in the structure.

4 Compounds studied for BZR binding

The benzodiazepine receptors, as such, exhibit a very high specificity for pharmacologically and clinically active BZs, and the minimum structural requirements for bindings in BZs are only the aromatic ring A and the carbonyl group in position 2 (Fig. 3) [22]. The substituents at ring A, the 4,5-(methyleneimino) group, the substituted or unsubstituted N(1), and the 5-phenyl ring have been shown to produce little effect on *in vitro* binding [22]. The aromatic ring is believed to undergo π/π stacking, probably with amino acid residues, within the receptor, and the carbonyl oxygen acts as a proton acceptor and is arbitrarily labelled as π_1 [24, 37, 38].

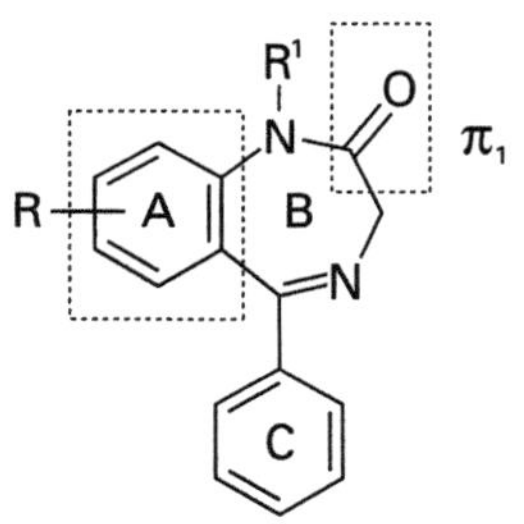

Fig. 3
The minimum structural requirements (encircled by dotted lines) in BZs for binding with BZR.

There are now, however, a variety of nonbenzodiazepine molecules that bind to BZRs in the same molar range (generally nanomolar) as BZs and exhibit *in vivo* biological response either as agonists, antagonists, or inverse agonists [39–42]. It becomes, therefore, essential to find the common features of ligands that allow for recognition by the receptor regardless of the type of *in vivo* activity and gross structural features. For this purpose, the following families of nonbenzodiazepines (non-BZs), in addition to those of BZs, were studied for their *in vitro* binding with BZRs:

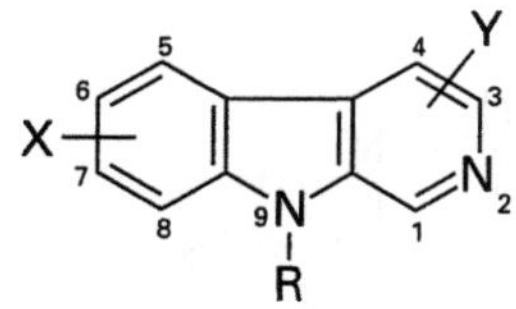

β-Carbolines
4

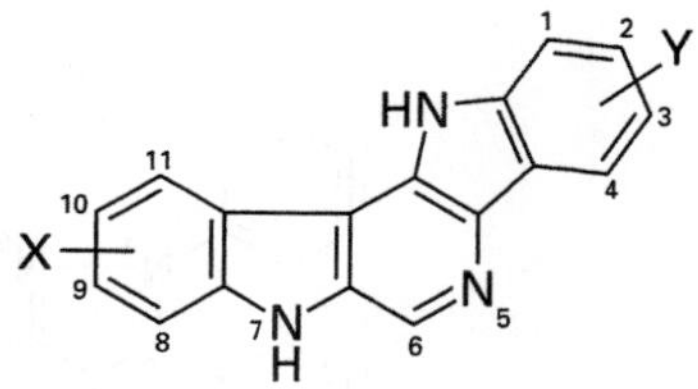

Pyridodiindoles
5

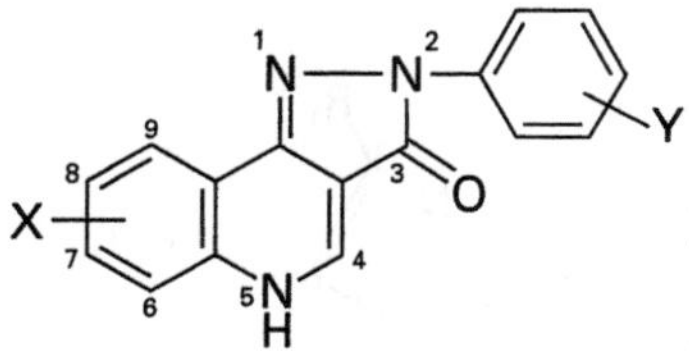

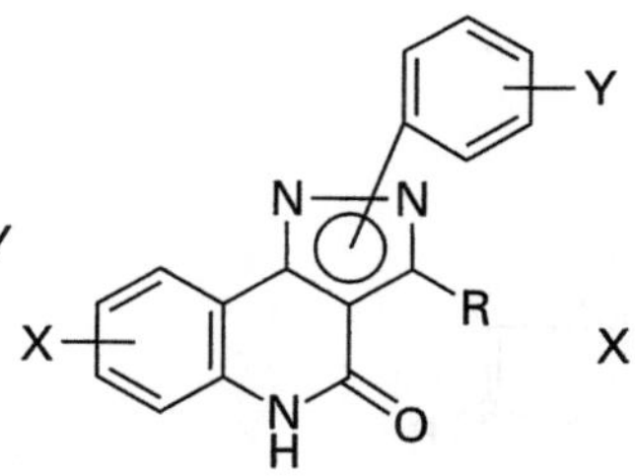

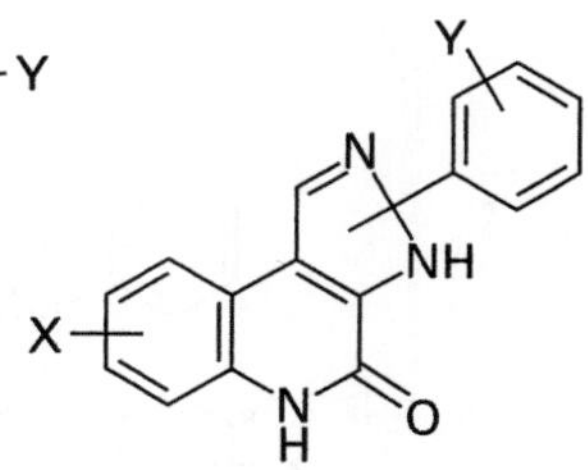

Pyrazoloquinolines

6 **7** **8**

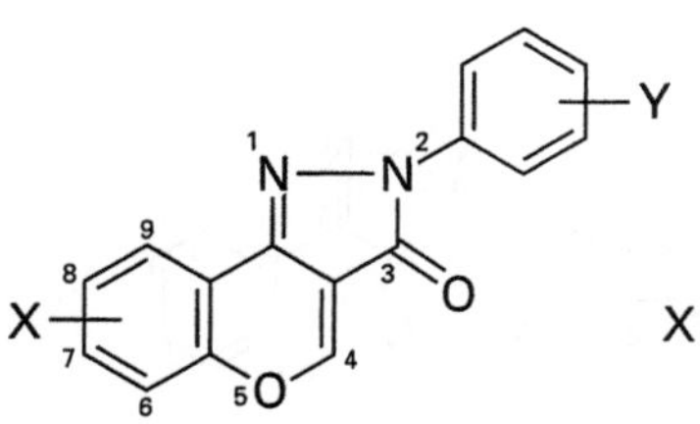

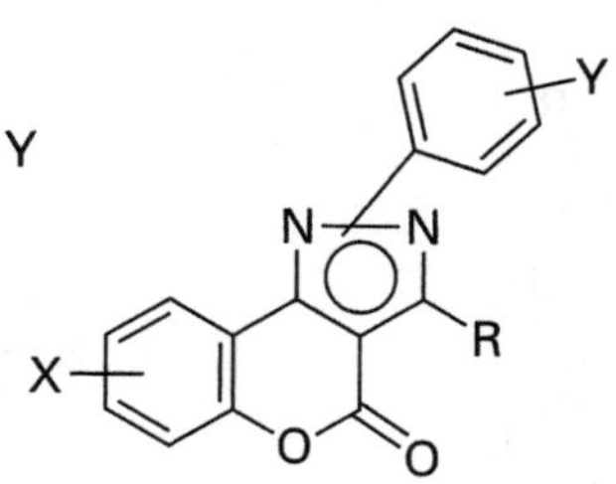

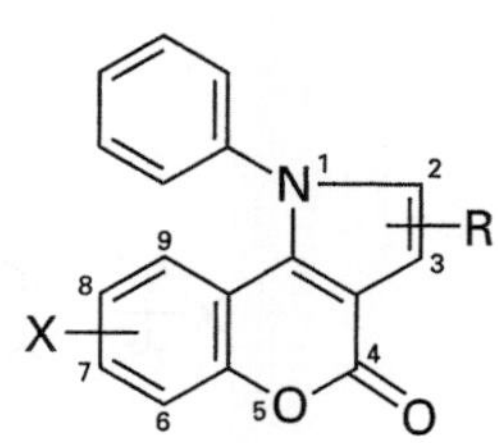

[1]Benzopyranopyrazolines
9 **10**

[1]Benzopyranopyrroles
11

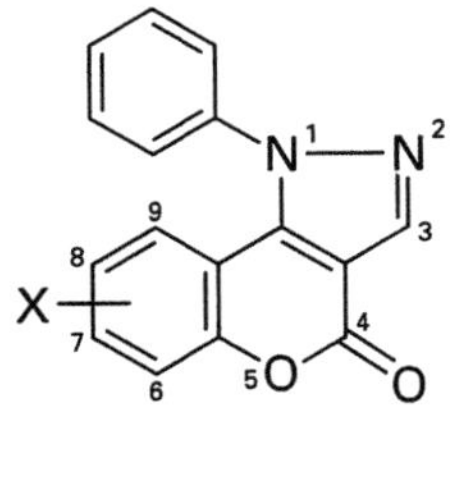

[1]Benzopyranotriazoles
12

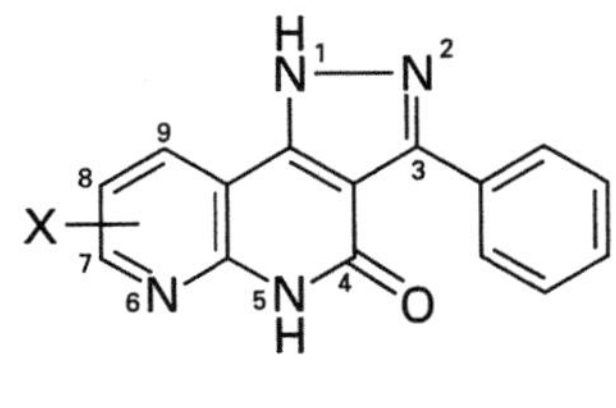

Pyrazolonaphthyridines
13

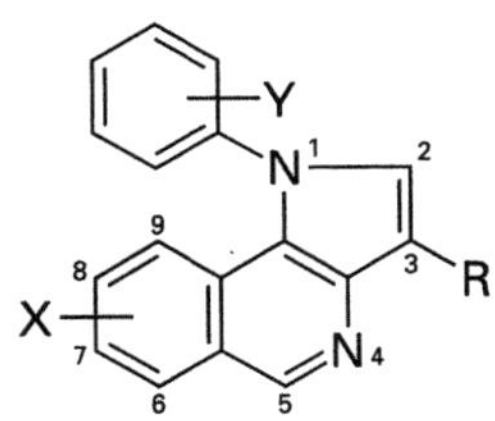

Pyrazoloisoquinolines
14

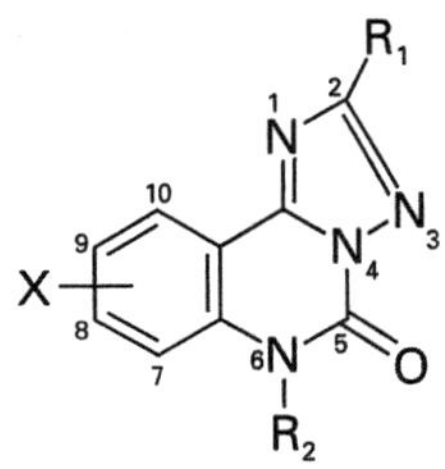

[1,2,4]Triazoloquinazolines
15

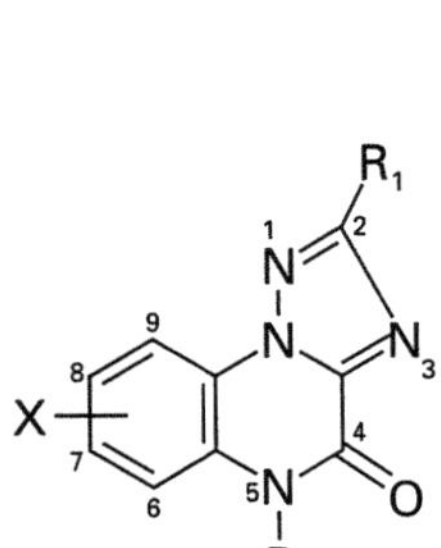

[1,2,4]Triazoloquinoxalines
16

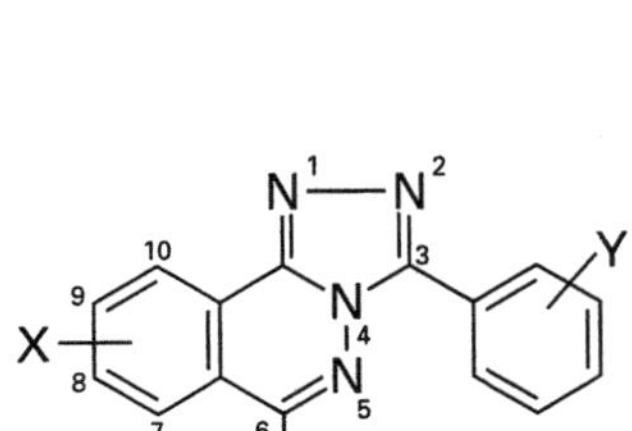

[1,2,4]Triazolophthalazines
17

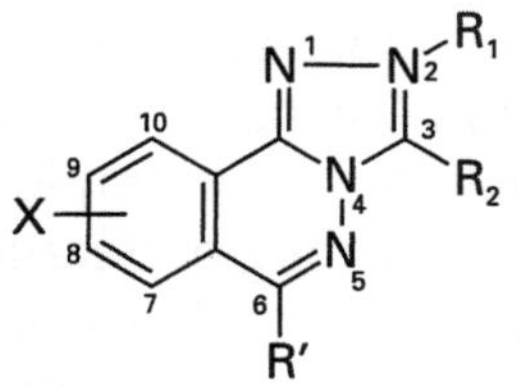

Imidazophthalazines
18

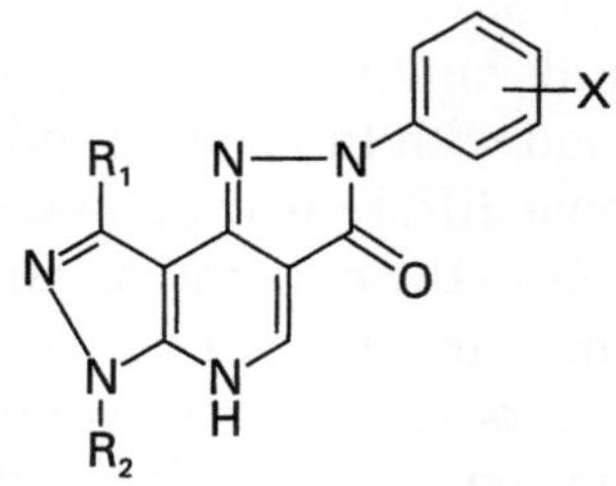

Dipyrazolopyridines
19

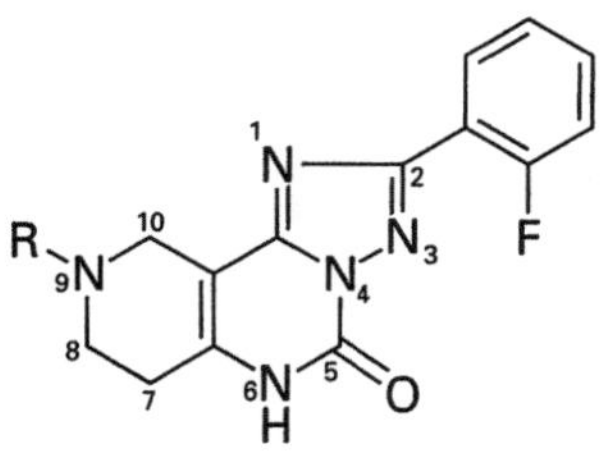

[1,2,4]Triazolopyrimidines
20

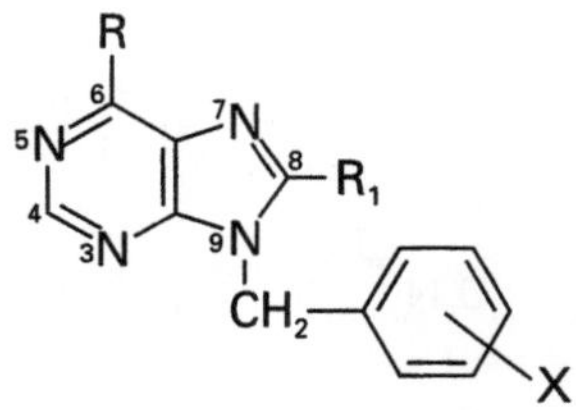

9-Benzyl-9H-purines
21

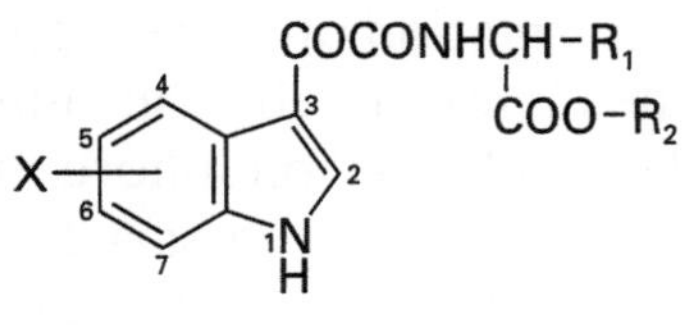

Indolylglyoxylylamino acid derivatives
22

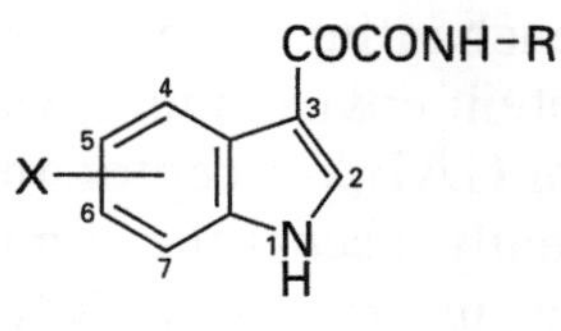

Indolylglyoxylylamine derivatives
23

5 Structure-activity relationship (SAR) studies

There have been many structure-activity relationship (SAR) studies on ligands binding to BZRs [17, 22]. The early studies were, however, concerned with the compounds of BZ series, but more recently all of the known different structural classes of compounds capable of binding to BZRs in the nanomolar range have been included. The simple *in vitro* binding test is relatively well suited for the screening of a large series of compounds and proves useful in detecting compounds acting directly on the receptor, distinguishing them from compounds requiring *in vivo* metabolic transformation in order to become active (prodrugs). Because of this metabolic transformation of many compounds before they become active, the *in vivo* data are not found to be useful for SAR studies. The *in vitro* data usually refer to the molar concentration of drugs leading to a 50% inhibition of [^{3}H]diazepam **3** or [^{3}H]flunitrazepam **24** binding to BZR and are generally expressed by IC_{50} or I_{50}.

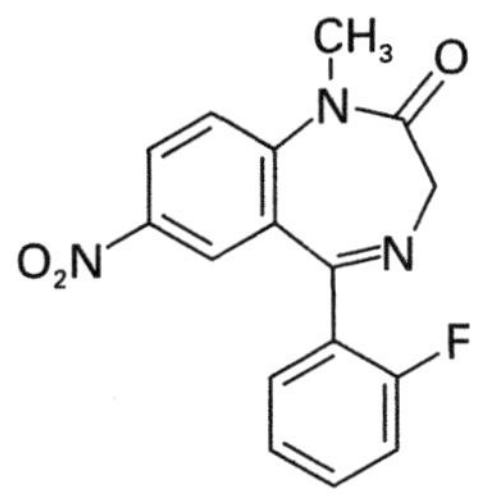

24

For a meaningful SAR study, it is necessary to distinguish between the agonistic, antagonistic, and inverse agonistic activities of the ligands. Usual conditions of the binding test, however, do not allow one to make such a differentiation among the ligands. Tentatively, it could be assumed that different ligands exert their effects by interacting at the same site, each influencing differently the conformation of the receptor glycoprotein environment, which modulates allosterically the supramolecular GABA-receptor, the BZR, and the chloride ionophore. Before we finally discuss the common structural features necessary for BZR binding in structurally different ligands and analyse various interaction models proposed, we present here the recent SAR studies available on them. Some SAR studies are purely qualitative and some quantitative. This latter one is designated as QSAR and presents a quantitative correlation between the activity and various physico-chemical, electronic, and steric properties of the compounds.

5.1 Benzodiazepines

Some fundamental SAR studies [15, 16, 43–47] on BZs (1) have suggested that the presence of a seven-membered imino ring (B) is essential and that substitution is advantageous only at positions 1, 3, 7 and 2'. In particular, the electronegative substituents at 7- and 2'-positions were observed to markedly increase the activity. A Free-Wilson QSAR analysis by Borea et al. [48] of *in vivo* data (antipentetrazol activity in mice) of 55 BZs led to the following rank orders for the individual group contributions to activity at the 7- and 2'-positions.

7-Position:
$NO_2 > CF_3 > Br > CN > Cl > N(CH_3)_2 > SOCH_3 > SBu > SCH_3 > CH_3 > H > SO_2CH_3 > Ph > F$

2'-Position:
$Cl > F > Br > NO_2 > CF_3 > H > OCH_3 > CH_3$

This study underscores the importance of highly electron-withdrawing groups at these two positions for pharmacological potency and generally the negative effect of substitution at other positions. Squires et al. [3] had observed that any kind of substitution at 4'-position would provoke a dramatic decrease both in biological activity and in receptor binding affinity. A similar observation was made regarding the 4'-substituent (para substituent of 5-phenyl ring) in pyrazolodiazepines **25** by Baraldi et al. [49].

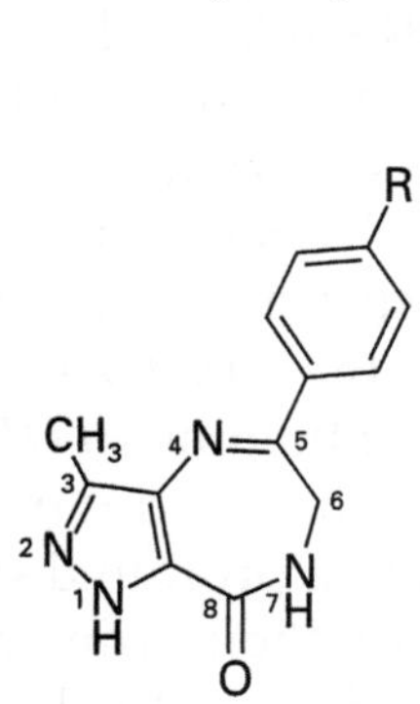

25

The importance of the substituents at the 7- and 2'-positions was, however, reaffirmed by a recent QSAR study [50], where the binding data for a series of 50 BZs was correlated with hydrophobic and electronic constants, π and σ, respectively, of these substituents, as shown by eq. (1).

$$\log(1/IC_{50}) = 0.449\ (\pm 0.143)\pi_7 + 1.114\ (\pm 0.361)\sigma_7 + 2.174\ (\pm 0.537)\sigma'_2 - 0.870\ (\pm 0.387)I_6 + 6.988$$
$$n = 50,\ r = 0.91,\ s = 0.31,\ F(4,45) = 52.38 \qquad (1)$$

In this equation, n refers to the number of data points, r is the correlation coefficient, s is the standard deviation, F is the F-ratio between the variances of calculated and observed activities, and the data within parentheses are 95% confidence intervals. Judging from the values of these statistical parameters, the correlation expressed by eq. (1) is found to be highly significant, exhibiting significant roles of the electronic nature (electron-withdrawing) of the 2'-substituent and both the electronic as well as the hydrophobic nature of the 7-substituent. The parameter I_6, which is a dummy parameter used to account for the role of chlorine at the 6-position with a value of unity, expresses the negative role of the chlorine at this position.

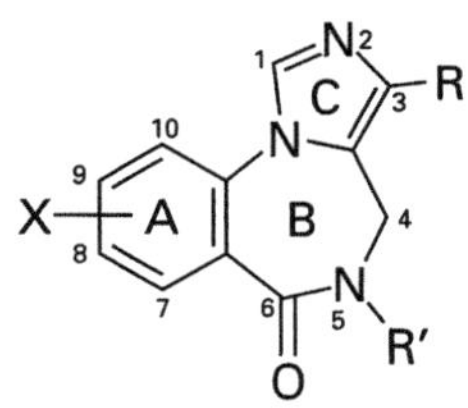

26

In the BZ-series, there have been several SAR studies [51–56] on imidazobenzodiazepines **26**. These compounds were studied for their binding to diazepam-sensitive (DS) as well as diazepam-insensitive (DI) subtypes of BZR. The DI subtype of BZR is characterized by the low affinity for the prototypical 1,4-BZs, such as diazepam or flunitrazepam, which exhibit high affinity for the DS BZR subtype [57–60]. The structural requirements for ligand binding to DI appear far more restrictive than to DS. An SAR study on a series of imidazobenzodiazepines **26** by Gu et al. [54] revealed a profound steric effect of the 3-position ester side chain moiety on their affinity for DI, while there was a less robust effect on DS binding. A further reduction in the binding affinity for both DI and DS subtype BZRs was observed [53] by replacement of the ester group of the 3-position by a carbamate, acetylamino, formylamino, isothiocyanato, 2-oxazolinyl, 2-benzoxazolyl, or p-tolylsulfonyl group. It was also observed that a substitution at N (5) was sterically constrained since groups bulkier than a methyl group caused significant reduction in affinities for both BZR isoforms [56]. However, incorporation of a benzyl group at this position yielded ligands with moderate to high affinities for DS, suggesting the presence of a hydrophobic pocket at the receptor site capable of accepting this group.

Regarding the substituent effect at other positions, it was reported [53] that chlorine at the 7-position could enhance the ligand affinity for DS but decreased at the 8-position. On the other hand, the same substituent at either the 7- or 8-position increased the DI affinity.

Annelation of a four- or five-membered ring (ring D) onto ring B of **26**, e.g. **27**, was shown to decrease the DI binding affinity but to produce no effect on DS binding affinity [55]. However, the replacement of the benzene A ring by thiophene **28** was found to increase the ligand affinity for both DS and DI with enhanced selectivity for the latter [55].

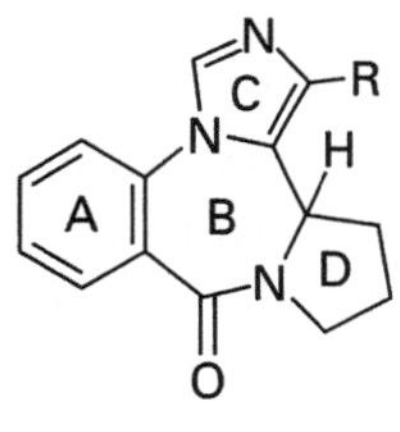

27

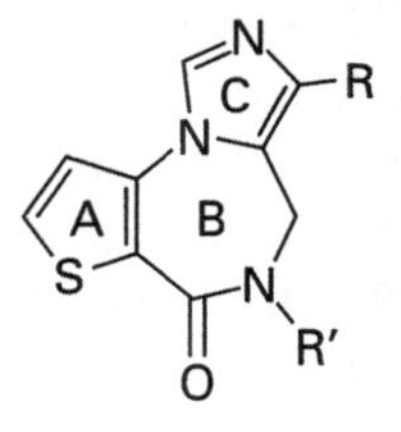

28

Fryer et al. [56] have studied the enantiomeric effect (C_4-chirality) of the analogues of **27** and found that S-enantiomers displayed affinities for both DI and DS BZRs at least two orders of magnitude higher than the corresponding R-enantiomers.

The effect of substitution of an oxadiazole ring (**29a** or **b**), instead of an ester group, at the 3-position in **26** or in **30** was also studied [51] and observed that, though oxadiazole rings were isosteric to the ester groups, they led to the better receptor efficacy than the latter.The effect of substitution at the oxadiazole ring and other positions in the derivatives were also discussed [51] and quantified in a recent study by Sharma et al. [61], deriving eqs. (2) and (3), where the former is meant for the derivatives of **26** and the latter for the derivatives of **30**.

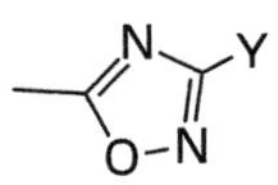

29a

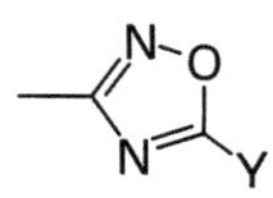

29b

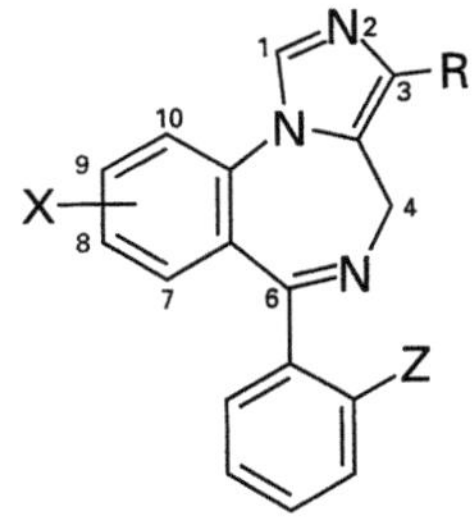

30

$$\log(1/IC_{50}) = 4.73\ (\pm 0.35)V_{w,7} - 0.83\ (\pm 0.12)V_{w,Y} + 7.24$$
$$n = 32,\ r = 0.94,\ s = 0.15,\ F(2,29) = 113.32 \quad (2)$$

$$\log(1/IC_{50}) = 2.09\ (\pm 0.28,\ \sigma_7 - 1.97\ (\pm 0.48)V_{w,8} - 0.74\ (\pm 0.17)V_{w,Y} + 0.35\ (\pm 0.09)I_Z + 7.82$$
$$n = 43,\ r = 0.90,\ s = 0.24,\ F(4,38) = 40.45 \quad (3)$$

In these equations, the V_w refers to the van der Waals volume of the substituent. Thus both equations express a steric effect of the substituent at the 3-oxadiazole ring. Since a positive coefficient of V_w denotes the dispersion interaction, the 7-substituent at ring A in oxadiazole derivatives of **26** is shown by eq. (2) to produce a dispersion effect, while in the derivatives of **30**, eq. (3) exhibits an electron-withdrawing effect of this substituent along with a steric effect of the 8-substituent. The indicator parameter I_Z in eq. (3) accounts for the influence of chlorine present at the ortho position of 6-phenyl ring in **30**. In both equations, the IC_{50} is against the [^{3}H]-Ro15-1788 (**26**; X = 8-F, R = CO_2Et, R' = CH_3), a BZR antagonist.
Some benzothiazepine derivatives **31**, **32** were also studied for their binding to BZRs [62–65], which exhibited micro- or nanomolar affinity against [^{3}H]PK 11195 **33**. An SAR analysis [65] for the series belonging to **32** revealed that the 6,7-double bond, the carbamoyloxy, alcanoyloxy, and mesyloxy side chains at the 7-position, and the prospective chloro substitution at the 4-position were the most important structural features improving the affinity.

5.2 β-Carbolines

Among the various non-BZ series of BZR ligands, the β-carbolines **4** are the most important [66–70]. Quite remarkable BZR affinities were report-

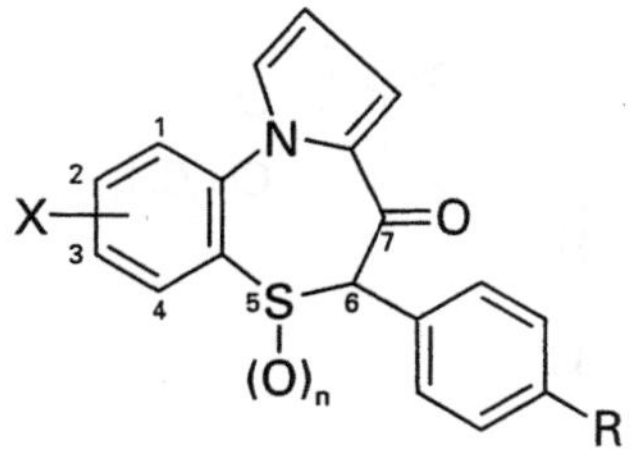

31

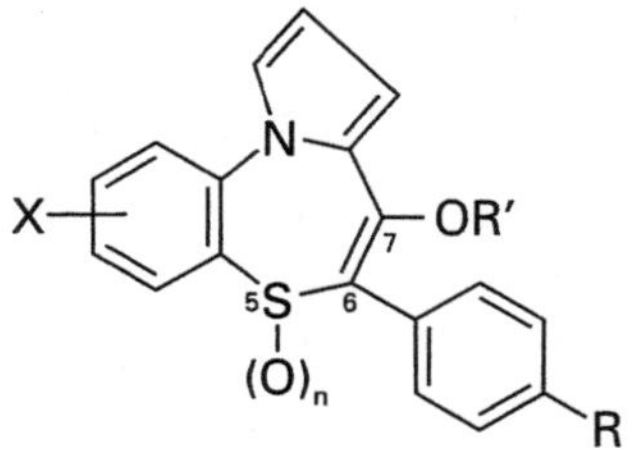

32

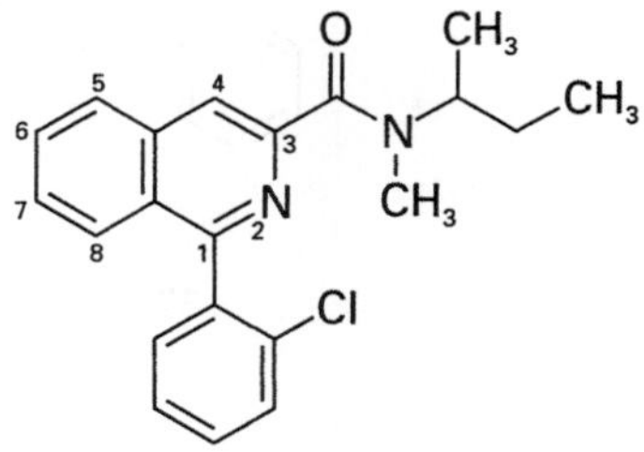

33

ed for some β-carboline-3-carboxylates **34** (low nanomolar range) that were about three orders of magnitude higher than that of the parent compound, β-carboline-3-carboxylic acid [70] (35), making these β-carboline derivatives important tools with which to study BZR functions [71–74]. The β-carboline structure, of course, has become an important basis for the design of new BZ-related drugs.

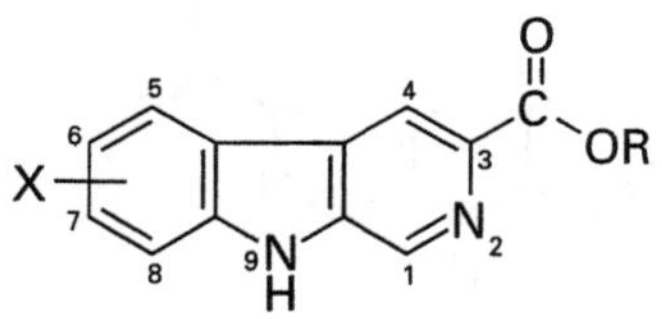

34

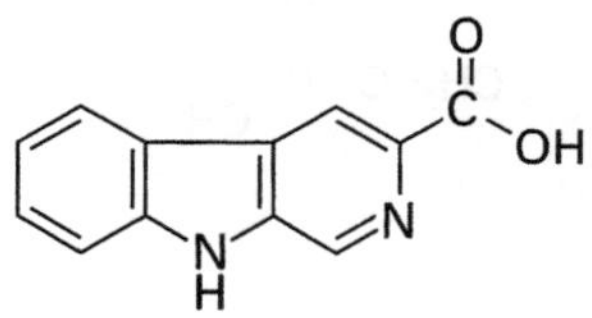

35

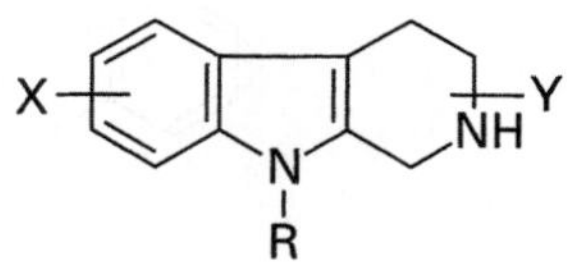

36

It was found [75] that full aromatic β-carbolines **4** were more potent than their corresponding tetrahydro-β-carboline derivatives **36**. When substituents possessing a carbonyl group, such as CO_2Me, $COCH_3$, or CHO, were introduced at the 3-position of β-carboline, the *in vitro* activity was augmented, but alcohol substituents (CH_2OH, $CHOHCH_3$) led to a decrease in potency [75]. Somewhat similar observations were made for isoquinolines **37** [75]. It was concluded in a later study by Lippke et al. [76] that the potency of β-carboline-3-carboxylates was profoundly dependent on molecular size of the ester group and that if the 3-substituent was an ester alcohol component, e.g., $CO_2CH_2CH_2OCH_3$, the hydrophobic and electronic parameters too were important. Guzman et al. [77], however, observed that maximum binding affinity of β-carbolines is achieved when the carbonyl group at the 3-position is attached directly to the aromatic

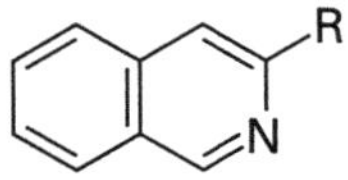

37

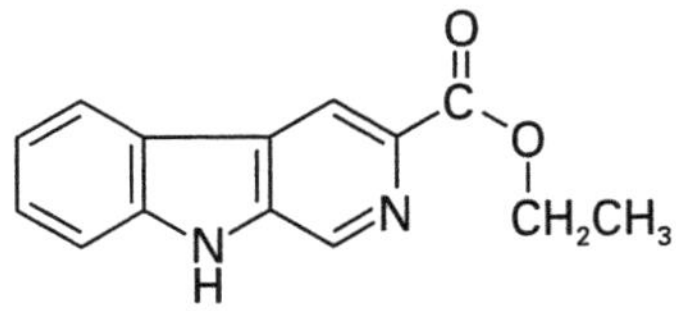

38

pyridine ring **38**. The displacement of this group by two atoms from this position causes a marked decrease in the potency (**39** vs **38**). Further, it was found [78] that the BZR recognizes preferentially the s-cis conformation of the 3-carbonyl group **40**.

Some recent QSAR studies [50, 79] described the effects of physico-chemical properties of substituents at the 3- and various other positions of β-carbolines on their-potency. For a small set of esters studied by Cain et al. [75], Gupta et al. [50] had derived eq. (4) that exhibited the roles of both the hydrophobic and electronic characters of 3-substituents (ester

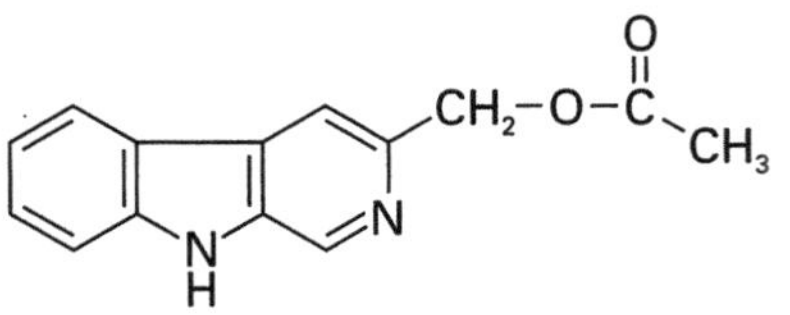

39

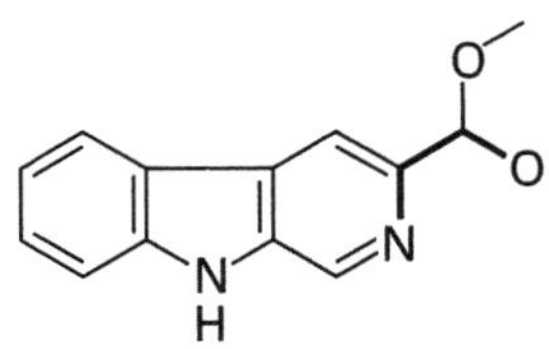

40

groups) and only the hydrophobic effect of the substituents present at the 1-position (alkyl or phenyl). The parabolic correlation in π_1 suggests that only highly hydrophobic (essentially large) groups at the 1-position will be effective. Using the data of Allen et al. [42] for β-carbolines that had a variety of substituents at the 3-position, Sharma et al. [79] derived eq. (5) which exhibited the importance of only the hydrophobic character of the substituents. In the derivation of this equation, however, the most active compound with an ester group at the 3-position (the only ester derivative in the series) was excluded. Allen et al. [42] indicated that a carbonyl moiety at 3-position is not essential. The β-carbolines substituted with electron-withdrawing groups (notwithstanding eq. 5) were also found to have high affinity for the BZR. The binding constant K_i in eq. (4) as well as the IC_{50} in eq. (5) were against the [^{3}H]diazepam binding to the BZR.

$$\log(1/K_i) = 6.457 + 0.974\ (\pm 0.611)\pi_3 + 4.793\ (\pm 1.840)\sigma_3 - 4.282\ (\pm 1.442)\pi_1 + 1.438\ (\pm 0.863)(\pi_1)^2$$
$$n = 14,\ r = 0.98,\ s = 0.47,\ F(4,9) = 39.38 \quad (4)$$

$$\log(1/IC_{50}) = 1.425\ (\pm 0.221)\pi_3 + 6.564$$
$$n = 9,\ r = 0.93,\ s = 0.49,\ F(1,7) = 41.54 \quad (5)$$

The role of the substitution at the 6-position of β-carbolines in the BZR binding affinity was also studied [80, 81]. In a series of 6-benzylamino derivatives **41**, the benzylamino nitrogen was found to be important for the binding [80]. Similarly, in a series of 6-benzyloxy derivatives **42**, the benzyl oxygen was found to be important [81]. In both series, the large phenyl group is supposed to have its hydrophobic importance.

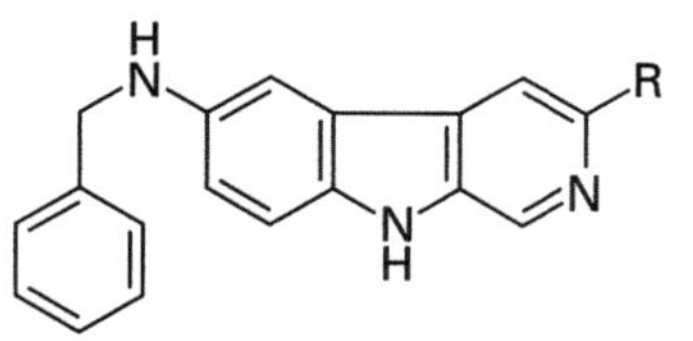

41

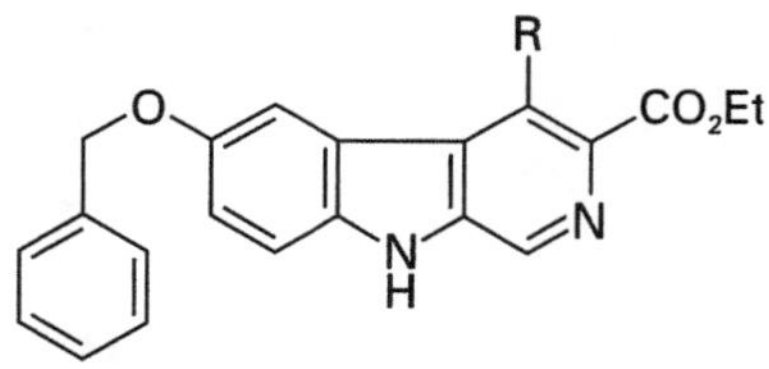

42

For a series of analogues of 6-benzyloxy-β-carbolines, where all the 6-substituents were not necessarily a benzyloxy group [81], Sharma et al. [79] showed the importance of the hydrophobic property of the whole 6-substituent by obtaining the equation,

$$\log(1/IC_{50}) = -2.617\ (\pm 0.274)\pi_{4,6} - 0.334\ (\pm 0.090)I + 8.739$$
$$n = 9,\ r = 0.98,\ s = 0.35,\ F(2,6) = 85.91 \quad (6)$$

where the negative coefficient of $\pi_{4,6}$, representing the combined hydrophobic property of 4- and 6-substituents, indicates that this combination should have the minimum value for an efficient binding at BZR. The indicator parameter I in the equation, used to account for the effect of a methyl group at N(9)-position with a value of unity, denotes that this group will not be advantageous at this position. In fact the presence of hydrogen at this position is supposed to be crucial for the binding, as it may form the hydrogen bond with the receptor; but Villar and Loew [82] suggested that this hydrogen bond may not be very stable. These authors rather paid particular atten-

tion to two most favorable proton-accepting sites, the βN and the substituent at the 3-position [82–84].
A hybridization of 3-carboxy-β-carbolines and 1,4-BZs was also studied [85] to find that the hybrid molecules **43**, incorporating pharmacologically important structural features of both systems, closely satisfy the structural requirements that generally ensure a high affinity of both β-carbolines and benzodiazepines for BZR (e.g. aromaticity of the β-carboline, a carbonyl group at its 3-position, and a π_2-region on BZ, i.e., 5-phenyl).

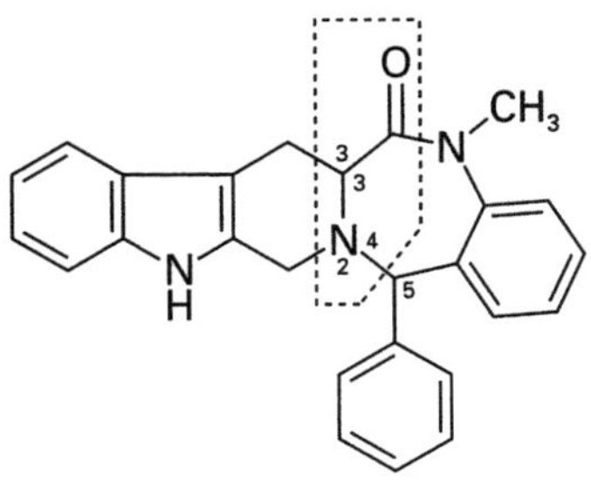

43

(Numbers outside the rings refer to those in β-carbolines and the ones inside the rings to those in BZs. The region enclosed by the dotted line represents the common feature of the two).

5.3 Pyridodiindoles

Pyridodiindoles **5** represent an extended version of β-carbolines but their mode of interaction with BZRs was not found to be much different from that of β-carbolines [40, 86]. The N(7)-H of pyridodiindole (which is N(9)-H of β-carboline) appears to be a necessary structural feature for high binding affinity of its derivatives [86]. Like N(9)-H of β-carbolines, it may also be involved in the hydrogen bonding with the receptor [81]. The substitution effect at various positions of pyridodiindole was also studied [86] but only the substituents at the 2-position were found to augment the activity. At this position, both electron-withdrawing and electron-releasing substituents, provided they were not very large, could be tolerated by the binding site, while the substituents of any nature at any other position could not be tolerated at all [86]. In fact, of crucial importance for the binding of pyridodiindoles with the BZRs is their rigid planar nature [40], which has no degree of conformational freedom. This leads to the strong binding of the compounds with the receptor, resulting in different pharmacological profiles.

5.4 Pyrazoloquinolines and [1]benzopyranopyrazolines, -pyrroles, and -triazoles

Pyrazoloquinolines **6–8**, [1]benzopyranopyrazolines **9**, **10**, [1]benzopyranopyrroles **11**, and [1]benzopyranotriazoles **12** have also been found to interact with the BZRs, of which the first two kinds of ligands have been extensively studied for their structure-activity relationships [87–102]. The SAR studies on pyrazoloquinolin-4-ones **7**, **8**, bearing an aryl ring at position 1 or 2, revealed the following [88–92] concerning their *in vitro* activity (displacement of [^{3}H]flunitrazepam):

(a) The 1-aryl analogues were much more active than the corresponding 2-aryl ones.
(b) The 1-meta-aryl derivatives were the compounds that bound with the highest affinity within this class.
(c) A replacement of the hydrogen at N(5) with a methyl group led to an increase in the activity.
(d) The replacement of the carbonyl group with other substituents and the resulting aromatization of the pyridine moiety greatly decreased the binding affinity.
(e) A bulkier phenyl group at 3-position was of more advantage than a small methyl group.
(f) The position of the nitrogens in the heterocyclic system was very crucial. The shifting of the nitrogen from position 1 to position 3 **8** led to a complete loss in binding affinity.

Such detailed structure-activity relationship could not be discussed in the case of pyrazoloquinolin-3-ones **6**, though they were found to possess high affinity for the BZRs either as agonists, antagonists, or inverse agonists [87, 93–98]. A preliminary study on a series of 2-arylpyrazolo[4,3-c]quinolin-3-ones **6** suggested that the different pharmacological profiles of these compounds were related only to the nature of the substituent at the para position of the 2-aryl ring. Further studies indicated that the lipophilic and electronic characters of the substituted 2-aryl ring may be important for their activities [93] and that the substituent at this ring nearer to its axis of rotation may produce the steric effects [98]. However, in a recent study, Fryer et al. [96] observed that the consideration of any one substituent effect (i.e. lipophilic, electronic, or steric) without concomitant consideration of the others is inadequate as a predictor of biological activity for this class of ligands.

Regarding the substituent effect on other positions of pyrazoloquinolin-3-ones, it was suggested that an electron-withdrawing group at the 8-position may be favorable for an increase in DI subtype receptor affinity [94]. Above all, however, the planarity of the molecules was found to be an essential requirement for the receptor binding of this class of ligands [97].

[1]Benzopyranopyrazolines **9**, **10** are isoesters of pyrazoloquinolines **6**, **7** when the quinoline NH has been replaced by the oxygen of the benzopyrano moiety. It was observed that the benzopyranopyrazol-3-ones **9** were less active than the corresponding pyrazoloquinolin-3-ones **6** [101], while the benzopyranopyrazol-4-ones **10** were reported to have better activity than the corresponding pyrazoloquinolin-4-ones **7** [100]. This observation regarding the latter two isoesters and several other SAR findings about them were well substantiated by a series of QSAR studies [103–106].

For a common structure **44** representing both the isoesters (**7** and **10**), a QSAR analysis on a large set of data compiled from various studies [88–91, 99–102] for the BZR binding against [^{3}H]flunitrazepam revealed eq. (7) [105], where $\pi_{3',5'}$ represents the hydrophobic effects of the substituents of both the meta positions of 1-aryl ring, and the Taft constant $E^s_{2',6'}$ represents the steric effects of both the ortho-position substituents. The indicator parameter I_X accounts for the effect of X(5) and takes the value of 1 if X(5) = NH and zero if X(5) = O or NCH_3. The other indicator parameter I_2 has been used to describe the effect of the replacement of N(2)

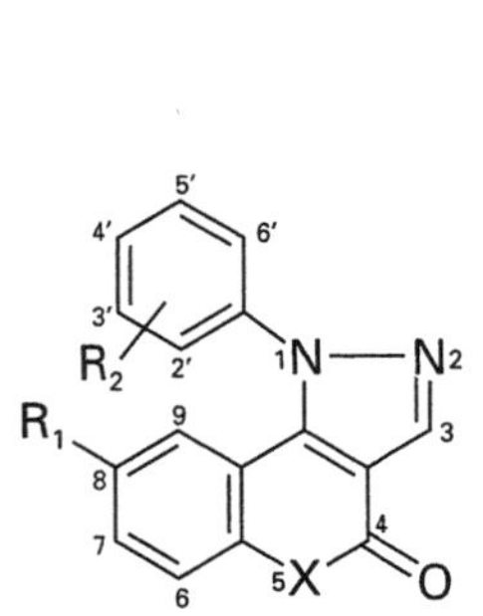

X = O; 1-aryl[1]benzopyrano[3,4-d]pyrazol-4-ones

X = NH; 1-arylpyrazolo[4, 5-c]quinolin-4-ones

44

in certain compounds by CH. It has the value of 1 for N(2) and zero for CH(2). The compounds with CH(2) are in fact called pyrroles **11**.

$$\log(1/IC_{50}) = 1.021(\pm 0.104)\pi_{3',5'} + 0.615\ (\pm 0.086)E^{s}_{2',6'} \\ -1.298\ (\pm 0.098)I_X - 1.090\ (\pm 0.146)I_2 + 7.141 \\ n = 69, r = 0.95, s = 0.37, F(4,64) = 144.16 \quad (7)$$

Now eq. (7) suggests that the substituents at the meta positions will increase the binding affinity through their hydrophobic character but at the ortho positions they will reduce the activity through the steric effects. The negative coefficient of I_X indicates a negative effect of NH(5) in comparison to O(5) or N(5)-CH_3 meaning thereby that [1]benzopyranopyrazolines or 5-substituted pyrazoloquinolines would be better than simple pyrazoloquinolines. Similarly, the negative coefficient of I_2 suggests that replacing N(2) by CH will lead to the better ligands, i.e., pyrroles would have better receptor affinity than the pyrazolines. This was experimentally observed by Colotta et al. [107], who also found that, if instead of replacing N(2) in pyrazole moiety, another nitrogen is inserted in the 3-position, resulting in triazoles **12**, there occurs a complete loss of the activity. Similarly, an isoesteric replacement of CH from position 6 in pyrazoloquinolines by a nitrogen, producing pyrazolonaphthyridines **13**, was found to be detrimental to the binding affinity [108], suggesting that the fused phenyl moiety of pyrazoloquinolines was important in binding with the BZRs. Likewise, the importance of NH in the 5-position of pyrazoloquinolines was noted, when some series of pyrazoloisoquinolines **14** were studied for BZR binding and found to have no activity [109, 110].

In all the above-mentioned classes of ligands, the substitution at position 3 also, in addition to that at position 1, was found to be important, but there was a size limitation. An optimum size was provided by a phenyl group which gave the better anchoring at the receptor site than the methyl group, while the benzyl or rather parasubstituted phenyl groups were detrimental to the binding activity [111]. In fact, it was suggested [107, 111] that the BZR recognition site has several lipophilic areas whose occupancy may lead to different receptor affinities. One of these lipophilic areas, which is occupied by 1-aryl substituent, is crucial to the binding and seems to be a large lipophilic area. The other lipophilic area, which is occupied by the 3-substituent, seems instead to be a small one, having a limited bulk tolerance. Since the substitution of a lipophilic group at the 3-position seems to be important, it was suggested that, if the substitution at this position in triazoles **12** had not been forbidden, the triazoles probably would have had some activity [107]. But if they bear a 3-substituent, the triazole ring would no longer be aromatic and coplanar to the benzopyrano ring, resulting in the loss of compounds' activity as the coplanarity is a prerequisite for the receptor affinity [93].

5.5 Triazoloquinazolines and -quinoxalines

Studies on [1,2,4]triazolo[1,5-c]quinazolin-5-ones **15** [112] and [1,2, 4]triazolo[1,5-a]quinoxalin-4-ones **16** [113–115] suggested that in both systems, the substitution of a highly lipophilic group at the 2-position is very important for their receptor affinity but that, unlike in pyrazoloquinolines, the alkylation of their identically situated N(6) and N(5) nitrogens, respectively, would be detrimental to the activity. However, in both triazoloquinazolines and triazoloquinoxalines the proton acceptor carbonyl group was found to be as important as in the pyrazoloquinolines. It was further found that if the aromatic or heteroaromatic substituent at the 2-position also had a proton accepting atom such as furan oxygen, thiophene sulfur, or, most importantly, an ortho-fluoro group, it provided an additional advantage to the binding. The substitution of a halogen at position 9 in quinazolines or at the equivalent position 8 in quinoxalines was observed to further increase the activity.

5.6 Triazolophthalazines and imidazophthalazines

The two series of phthalazines, the triazolophthalazines **17** [116] and imidazophthalazines **18** [117], were also found to bind with the BZRs. It was observed in both the series that the replacement of the hydrogen at the 6-position by a bulky lipophilic group leads to a decrease in the receptor binding affinity, but while the hydrophilic NH_2 group at this position was found to be favorable in the imidazophthalazines [117], a bulkier tertiary amino group was found to be more favorable at this position in the triazolophthalazines [116]. Since in the latter the substitution at the triazolo ring is allowed only at the 3-position, a phenyl ring there with a substituent at its para position was suggested to be conducive to high receptor affinity [116], but no consistent structure-activity relationship was observed for the substituents at the imidazo ring in imidazophthalazines [117].

5.7 Dipyrazolopyridines and triazolopyrimidines

Dipyrazolopyridin-3-ones **19** are very similar to pyrazoloquinolin-3-ones **6**, except that they have another pyrazole moiety in place of the fused benzo ring of the latter. An SAR study showed that this replacement was not advantageous and there was a loss in the binding affinity [118]. However, this loss could be compensated by a phenyl group at the 8-position and a methyl group at the 6-position of the pyrazole moiety, which probably occupied the corresponding large and small hydrophobic areas at the receptor.

As regards the substitution at the 2-phenyl ring in the pyridine series, the highest binding affinity was observed when either there was no substituent or the substituent was at the para position [118]. This observation was in agreement with that of the corresponding quinoline series **6**. Regarding all the substituent effects in the pyridines, a QSAR study [105] had revealed the following equation which exhibits the predominance of the highly lipophilic 8-phenyl group but suggests that a highly lipophilic group at the 2-phenyl ring would be detrimental to the activity.

$$\log(1/IC_{50}) = 0.992\ (\pm 0.181) I(R_1) - 1.573\ (\pm 0.295)\pi_Y + 5.713$$
$$n = 13, r = 0.92, s = 0.33, F(2,10) = 28.03 \qquad (8)$$

In this equation, the effect of 8-phenyl group is expressed by the dummy parameter $I(R_1)$, which has the value of 1 for this group and zero for CH_3, or H. The π_Y stands for the hydrophobic effect of the substituents at the 2-phenyl ring and, having the negative coefficient, indicates that a highly hydrophobic substituent would not be preferred.

Modifications in 2-aryl[1,2–4]triazoloquinazolin-5-ones **15** by the replacement of the annelated benzene ring with various alicyclic and heterocyclic moieties led to novel structures with potent BZR affinity [119]. Of them, the annelated [1,2,4]triazolopyrimidin-5-ones **20** were found to possess high affinity and the degree of activity was observed to strongly depend upon the N-substituent in the 9-position [119]. Further, as in quinazolines, the N(6) alkylation in pyrimidines too was detrimental to the activity. The best analogue in the derivatives of **20** was the one which had a benzyl group at N(9). Attempts to further improve the situation by replacing the ortho-fluorophenyl at the 2-position with another aryl or any heteroaryl moiety were not found to be encouraging.

5.8 9-Benzyl-9H-purines

Several series of substituted-9-benzyl-9H-purines **21** were studied for their binding to BZRs [120–123]. Among all the compounds studied, the highest affinity was found to be associated with 8-bramo-9-(3'-formamidobenzyl)-6-(dimethylamino) analogue **45**. Replacement of any of the substituents of positions 6, 8, or the 3'-position of the benzyl ring drastically lowered

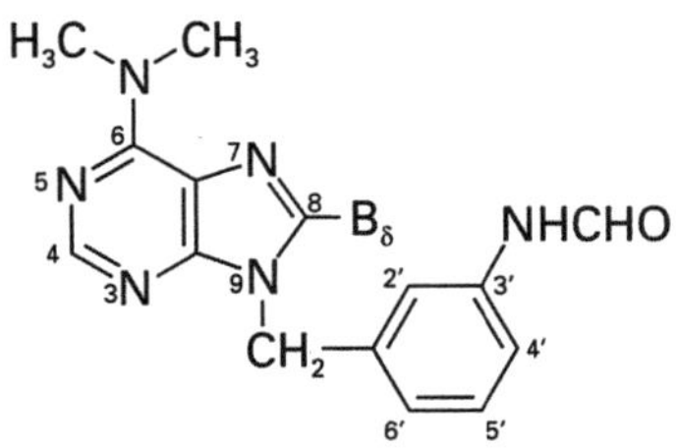

45

the activity. Dropping the bromine from the 8-position led to a 3-fold decrease in the activity, and the removal of the 3'-formamido group resulted in about a 300-fold loss in activity [121]. Increasing the size of the formamido group by substituting the formyl hydrogen with methyl, phenyl, or methoxy resulted in a 80- to 800-fold loss in receptor affinity. However, decreasing its size by replacing the whole CHO moiety with the hydrogen led to a less drastic effect, i.e., there was only a 10-fold decrease in the activity [121].Regarding the 6-substituents, it was observed that there was an insignificant difference in receptor binding affinity if the dimethylamino group was replaced with groups ranging in size from amino to cyclopentylmethylamino [120, 123]. Thus 6-dimethylamino, 8-bromo, and 3'-formamido groups appear to be the optimal requirements for the binding of the benzylpurines with the BZRs. An additional attempt to introduce an alkyl group on the benzylic methylene was of no use [122].

A few QSAR studies were recently performed on these 9-benzyl purines to find out the physico-chemical and electronic effects of the substituents [124, 125]. For a series of 6-dimethyl analogues, the binding affinity data (against [^{3}H]diazepam) of Kelley et al. [120, 121] were found to be correlated with the electron-withdrawing effect of 8-substituent (σ_8) and the electron-withdrawing as well as the hydrophobic effects of the benzyl ring substituents (σ_X and π_X) (eq. 9) [124]. The negative coefficient of π_X in the correlation suggests that a large hydrophobic substituent at the benzyl ring would not be tolerated. Similarly, another correlation obtained [125] for a new set of data [122] on the variation in 6-substituents and the effect of alkylation of benzylic methylene exhibited the size limitation of the substituents at the benzyl ring along with their electronic influence (eq. 10).

$$\log(1/IC_{50}) = 5.078 + 1.441\ (\pm 0.854)\ \sigma_8 - 1.157\ (\pm 0.303)\ \pi_X + 2.719\ (\pm 1.140)\ \sigma_X$$
$$n = 29, r = 0.87, s = 0.48, F(3{,}25) = 25.13 \qquad (9)$$

$$\log(1/IC_{50}) = 0.632\ (\pm 0.256)\ (MR_X) - 0.038\ (\pm 0.019)\ (MR_X)^2 - 0.840\ (\pm 0.714)\ I_s + 4.416$$
$$n = 18, r = 0.88, s = 0.47, F(3{,}14) = 15.59 \qquad (10)$$

The molar refractivity index MR describes the dispersion interaction but a parabolic equation, as eq. 10, shows the size limitation of the substituents. The dummy parameter I_s has been used to account for the configurational effect of the alkyl group (CH_3) at the benzylic methylene. It was given a value of 1 for the R-configuration, –1 for the S-configuration, and zero for the RS-configuration. Its negative coefficient in the equation shows that a methyl group with an S-configuration may be useful, provided the optimal requirements have not been acquired by the ligands. No physico-chemical or electronic parameters used for the 6-substituents were found to be significant in the correlation, indicating that the change in size or nature of the 6-substituent was immaterial.

5.9 N-(Indol-3-ylglyoxylyl)amino acid and amine derivatives

A few SAR studies first performed on N-(indol-3-ylglyoxylyl) amino acid derivatives **22** suggested primarily that the BZR binding of these compounds was dependent upon the amino acid molecular size as well as the hydrophobic and electronic properties of the molecules [126, 127]. It was also observed that esters were more active than the corresponding acids [126, 127] and that both esters and acids exhibited stereoselectivity [127]. The D form of the amino acid moiety was more potent than the L form or the racemic form [127]. Also the study of Primofiore et al. [127] revealed that the most active compounds inhibiting [^{3}H]flunitrazepam binding were those that had a Cl, Br, or NO_2 group at the 5-position. The hydrogen or methoxy substitution at this position resulted in the decrease of the inhibiting potency. All these observations were quantified by the QSAR analysis [124] that revealed eq. 11, suggesting that the 5-substituents may be involved in the dispersion interaction with the receptor but that highly hydrophobic and large substituents are not tolerated by the receptor site. Further, in the equation, the indicator parameter I_2, which is equal to 1 for esters (**22**; R_2 = Et) and zero for acids (R_2 = H), indicates that the esters would be over a 6-fold more active than the corresponding acids. Similarly, the I_s parameter, which has been used for the stereoselectivity with the values of 1, 0, and –1 for D, racemic, and L isomers, respectively, accounts for the positive effect of the D isomers. The additional parameter I_1, used for the R_1 substituent in the amino acid moiety with a value of 1 for R_1 = $CH_2C_6H_5$ and zero for R_1 = CH_3, suggests that a bulky group would not be tolerated at the R_1-position. The data analyzed by QSAR were those obtained by Primofiore et al. [127].

$$\begin{aligned}\log(1/IC_{50}) = {} & 5.218 + 19.769\,(\pm 5.792)V_{w,5} - 72.679\,(\pm 24.286)(V_{w,5})^2 \\ & - 0.974\,(\pm 0.318)\pi_5 - 0.452\,(\pm 0.320)I_1 + 0.800\,(\pm 0.284)I_2 \\ & + 0.546\,(\pm 0.164)I_s \\ & n = 40,\ r = 0.907,\ s = 0.44,\ F(6,33) = 23.28 \qquad (11)\end{aligned}$$

Primofiore et al. [128] also studied the BZR binding affinity of a series of N-(indol-3-ylglyoxylyl)amine derivatives **23**, where the 3-glyoxylyl indole moiety was linked to a biogenic amine such as tryptamine, tyramine, and dopamine. In this kind of ligand too, it was found that the most potent derivatives were those bearing an electron-withdrawing group at the 5-position. They also observed that the methylation at the 1-position of the indole nucleus was detrimental to the binding affinity.

6 An overview of SARs

Now from all these discussions of SAR studies for different kinds of BZR ligands, there have surfaced certain crucial features in each kind of ligand, without which they would not be able to interact with the receptor at all. These features are summarized in Table 1. The similarities and the differences in these crucial features for different classes of ligands make it possible to define the unique nature of the BZRs, which enables the latter to accommodate compounds of different chemical structures.

Table 1
The crucial features in different kinds of BZR ligands

Ligand	Crucial features
Benzodiazepines **1**	fused benzo ring A, C(2)=O, and 5-phenyl
β-Carbolines **4**	3-ester group in s-cis conformation, N(9)–H,N(2), and planarity
Pyridodiindoles **5**	N(7)–H,2-substituent of electronic nature, and rigid planar structure
Pyrazoloquinolin-3-ones **6**	p-substituted-2-aryl-ring, N(5)–H, and C(3)=O
Pyrazoloquinolin-4-ones **7**	m-substituted-1-aryl ring, N(5)–H, C(4)=O, and 3-phenyl
[1]Benzopyranopyrazolines **9**, **10**	as in corresponding pyrazoloquinolines. But O(5) in [1]benzopyranopyrazol-3-ones(**9**) gives less activity than N(5)–H in corresponding pyrazoloquinolines(**6**), while the situation is completely reversed in the case of -4-one analogues (**10**) relative to corresponding pyrazoloquinolines(**7**).
[1,2,4]Triazoloquinazolines and -quinoxalines **15**, **16**	highly lipophilic group at the 2-position, unsubstituted NH and CO of the adjacent positions para to NH, and preferably a proton-accepting atom in the 2-substituent.
[1,2,4]Triazolophthalazines **17**	unsubstituted 6-position and para-substituted 3-phenyl
Imidazophthalazines **18**	unsubstituted 6-position, no detailed SAR
Dipyrazolopyridines **19**	6-methyl, 8-phenyl, and unsubstituted or para-substituted 2-phenyl.
[1,2,4]Triazolopyrimidines **20**	substituted N(9), N(6)–H, and 2–(ortho-fluorophenyl)
9-Benzylpurines **21**	6-dimethylamino,8–Br, and m–NHCHO at the benzyl ring
N-(Indol-3-ylglyoxylyl) amino acids **22**	molecular size of amino acid moiety, its D form, hydrophobic and electronic nature of molecules, Cl, Br, or NO_2 at 5-position, esterification of acid, and N(1)–H
N-(Indol-3-ylglyoxylyl) amines **23**	amine moiety, N(1)–H, and electron-withdrawing group at 5-position.

7 Ligand-BZR interaction models

Table 1 suggests that the BZRs possess certain essential features which may be commonly useful for the binding of all kinds of structurally different ligands. These features may comprise one or two hydrogen-bond donor sites, one or two hydrogen-bond acceptor sites, some lipophilic areas, and a few polar sites. Using the binding data for a set of 29 compounds comprising BZs and molecules from other structural classes, Crippen [129] deduced, with the help of his distance geometry approach, a binding site model for a subset of 18 compounds that consisted of 15 site points and 5 adjustable energy parameters, and concluded that 5 atoms of each ligand can occupy corresponding points in the site and thus constitute a possible BZR pharmacophore. A binding model proposed by Codding and Muir had seven conformationally mobile binding sites [130]. This finding led to the suggestion that the mobility of the sites within the receptor would allow for the differentiation of ligands of different biological activities. This suggestion supported the view, once held by Fryer et al. [22, 24] that the antagonist activity was due to a conformational shift within the receptor.

The SAR studies and the advent of computer modeling studies (alignment rule) led, however, a number of other authors to develop the models for the BZR pharmacophore. Of them, the most important ones have been discussed in the references [36, 42, 55, 56, 65, 81, 106, 110, 115, 127, 128, and 131–139] and summarized recently by Villar et al. [140] and Gupta [141]. Figures 4–15 represent the two-dimensional models for the drug-receptor interactions for the representatives of a few important classes of BZR ligands. The three-dimensional QSARs and the interactive computer graphics have well supported these models [55, 65, 131, 133, 135, 136, 138].

In all the models represented by Figures 4–15, the predominant interactions were the hydrogen bonding and the lipophilic interactions. In certain cases, as in Figures 5, 6, 10, and 12, the ligands were able to form three-center hydrogen bonds with the receptor, acquiring the greater stability. The fused aromatic rings and the planarity of the molecules seem to be of primary importance for all kinds of ligands.

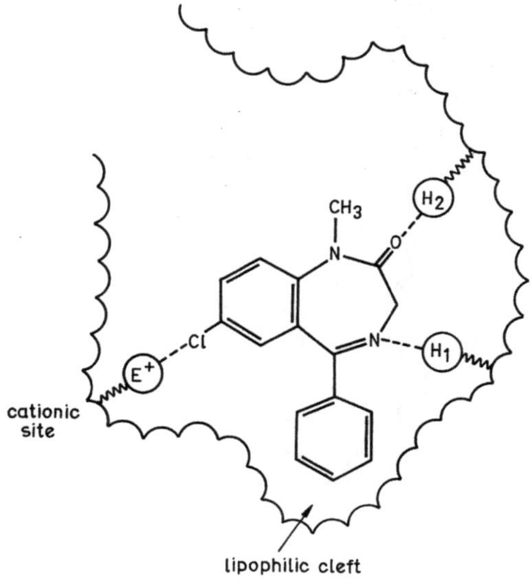

Fig. 4
Interactions of benzodiazepines with agonist pharmacophore of the BZR [81]. The H's associated with the receptor (in all figures) represent the hydrogen-bond donor sites. The hydrogen-bond acceptor site, if any, will be represented by A's.

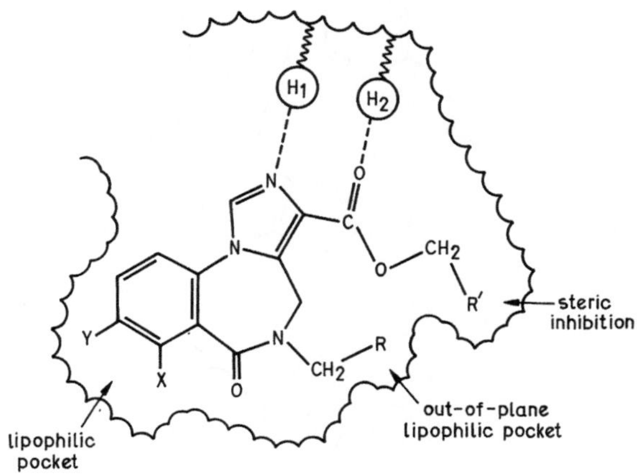

Fig. 5
A model for the interaction of imidazobenzodiazepinone carboxylic esters at the BZR agonist site [53].

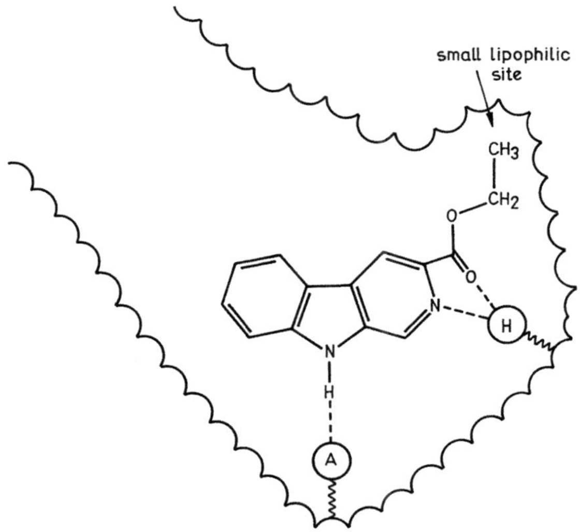

Fig. 6
A model for the interaction of an ester of β-carboline-3-carboxylic acid with inverse agonist site of BZR [131].

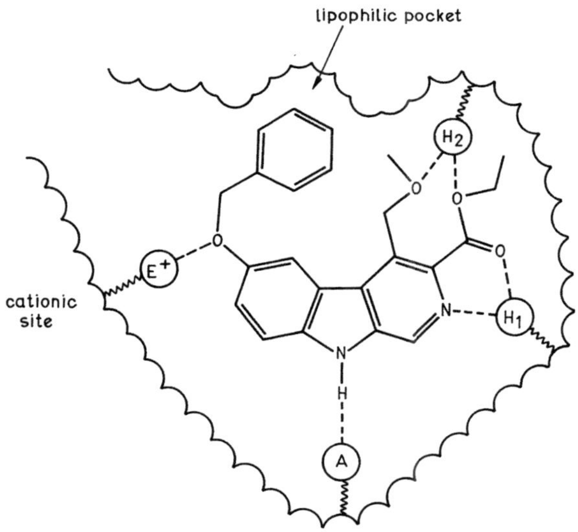

Fig. 7
Interaction of a most important derivative of β-carboline, i.e., 6-(benzyloxy)-4-(methoxymethyl)-β-carboline-3-carboxylic acid ethyl ester, exhibiting full agonist activity, with the BZR [81]. Here the molecule forms 2 three-center hydrogen bonds with the donor sites of the receptor, giving extra stability to the bonding.

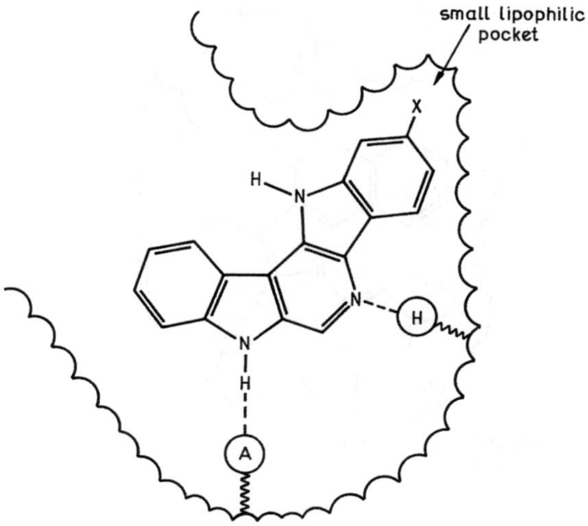

Fig. 8
A model for the interaction of 7,12-dihydro-pyrido[3,2-b: 5,4-b']diindole with inverse agonist/antagonist site of the BZR [110, 133].

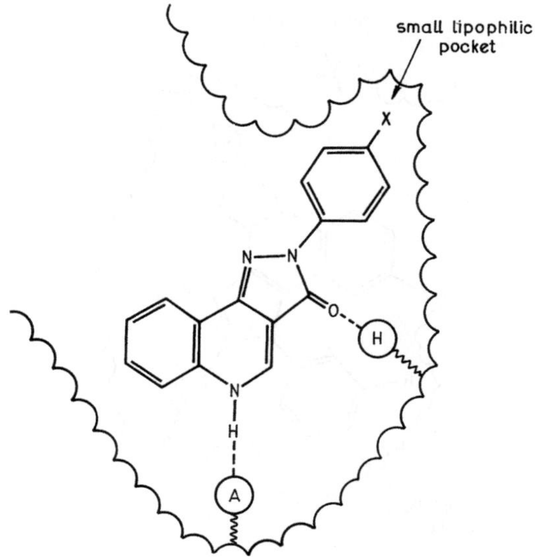

Fig. 9
Interactions at the proposed inverse agonist/antagonist BZR pharmacophore for 2-aryl-pyrazoloquinolin-3-ones [110]. According to Martin et al. [134], N(1) may also participate in the H-bonding.

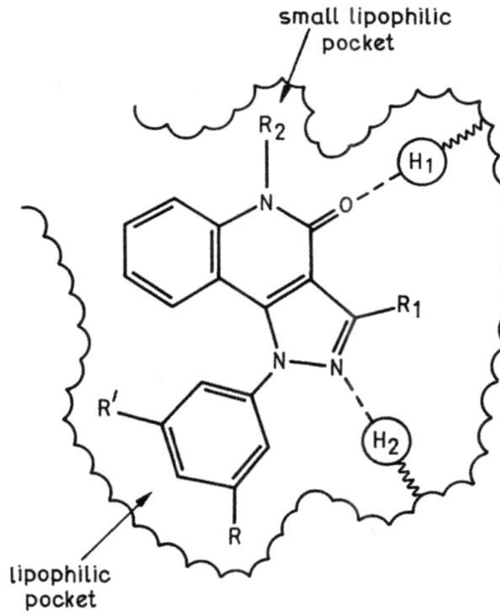

Fig. 10
A model proposed for the interaction of N(5)-substituted-1-arylpyrazoloquinolin-4-ones with inverse agonist/antagonist pharmacophore of the receptor [106].

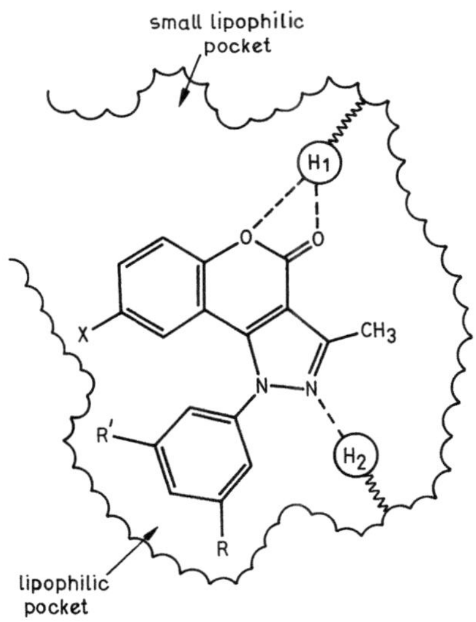

Fig. 11
A model proposed for the interaction of 1-aryl[1]benzopyranopyrazol-4-ones with inverse agonist/antagonist pharmacophore of the BZR [106]. The participation of O(4) in the three-center hydrogen bonding makes these compounds more active than the corresponding pyrazoloquinolines.

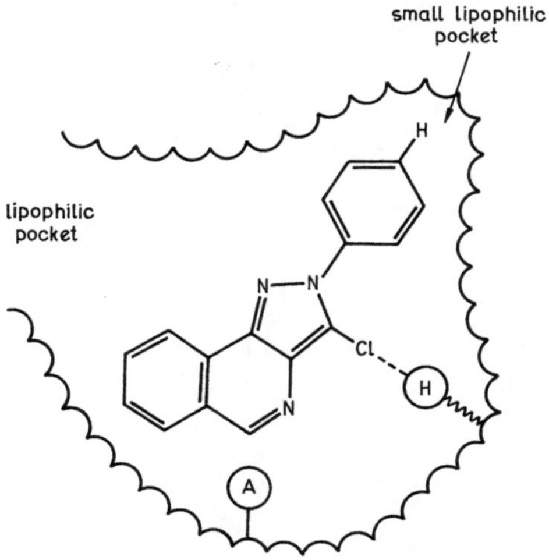

Fig. 12
Interaction of a 2-phenyl-3-chloropyrazoloisoquinoline with inverse agonist/antagonist BZR pharmacophore [110].

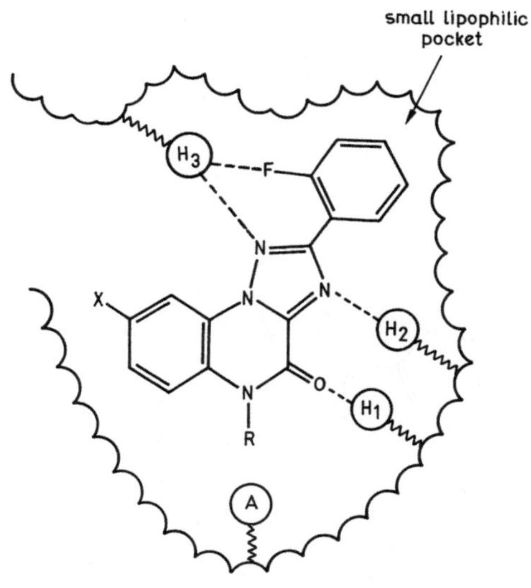

Fig. 13
A proposed model for the interaction of 2-(ortho-fluorophenyl)[1,2,4]triazoloquinoxalin-4-ones [115]. Due to the free rotation of the 2-phenyl ring around the σ-bond, the fluorine may participate in three-center hydrogen bonding with either of H_2 and H_3 sites.

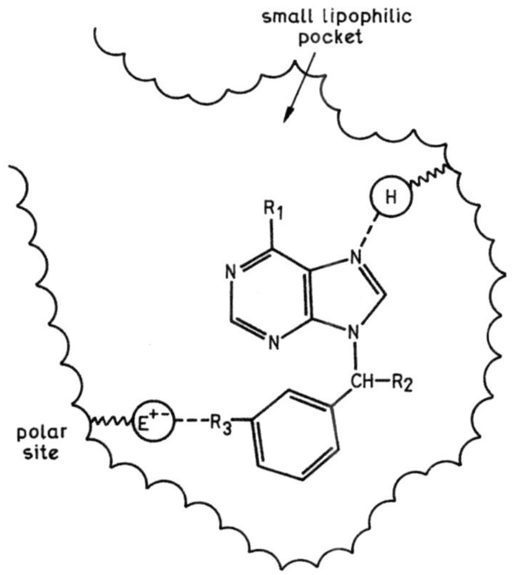

Fig. 14
The interactions of 9-benzylpurines with inverse agonist/antagonist pharmacophore of the BZR [125].

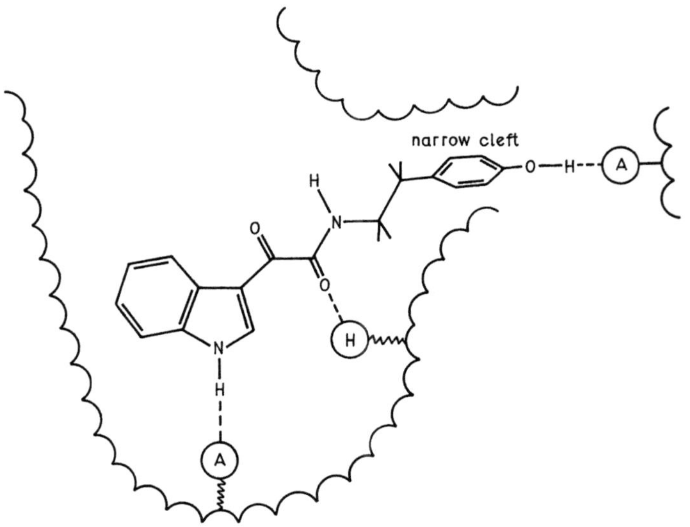

Fig. 15
The binding of an N-(indol-3-ylglyoxylyl)amine derivative with inverse agonist/antagonist site of the BZR [128].

Acknowledgement

The financial assistance provided by the University Grants Commission, New Delhi, is gratefully acknowledged.

References

1 (a) L.H. Sternbach: Medicinal Chemistry Award Address presented at the 16th Medicinal Chemistry Symposium in Kalamazoo, Mich., June 20, 1978;
(b) L.H. Sternbach: J. Med. Chem. *22*, 1 (1978);
(c) L.H. Sternbach: Agents Actions *2*, 193 (1972);
(d) L. H. Sternbach and E. Reeder: J. Org. Chem. *26*, 1111 (1961).

2 (a) L.O. Randall: Dis. Nerv. Syst., Suppl. 7, *22*, Sect. 2 (1961);
(b) L.O. Randall, W. Schallek, G.A. Heise, E.F. Keith, and R.E. Bagdon: J. Pharm. Exp. Ther. *129*, 163 (1960).

3 (a) L.H. Sternbach, E. Reeder, O.Keller, and W. Metlesics: J. Org. Chem. *26*, 4488 (1961), and additional unpublished results;
(b) L.H. Sternbach and E. Reeder: J. Org. Chem. *26*, 4936 (1961);
(c) L.H. Sternbach and L.O. Randall: CNS Drugs, Symp., Hyderabad, India, 53 (1966);
(d) L.H. Sternbach, R.I. Fryer, W. Metlesics, E. Reeder, G. Sach, C. Saucy, and A. Stempel: J. Org. Chem. *27*, 3788 (1962);
(e) L.H. Sternbach, L.O. Randall, R. Banziger, and H. Lehr, in: Medicinal Research Series, Vol. 2, Ed. A. Burger, Marcel Dekker, New York, N.Y. (1968), p. 237;
(f) N.W. Gilman and L.H. Sternbach: J. Heterocycl. Chem. *8*, 297(1971);
(g) R.I. Fryer, R.A. Schmidt, and L.H. Sternbach: J. Pharm. Sci. *53*, 264 (1964);
(h) R. Kalish, E. Broger, G.F. Field, T. Anton, T.V. Steppe, and L.H. Sternbach: J. Heterocycl. Chem. *12*, 49 (1975);
(l) G.A. Archer, R.I. Kalish, R.Y. Ning, B.C. Sluboski, A. Stempel, T.V. Steppe, and L.H. Sternbach: J. Med. Chem. *20*, 1312 (1977).

4 L.E. Hollister, in: Pharmacology of Benzodiazepines. Ed. E. Usdin, Verlag Chemie, Weinheim (1983), p. 29.

5 (a) H. Möhler and T. Okada: Science *198*, 849 (1977);
(b) R.F. Squires and C. Braestrup: Nature *266*, 732 (1977).

6 (a) H. Möhler and J. Okada: Life Sci. *20*, 2101 (1977);
(b) C. Braesttup, and R.F. Squires: Proc. Natl. Acad. Sci., USA *74*, 3805 (1977).

7 W. Haefely, L. Pieri, P. Polc and R. Schaffner, in: Handbook of Experimental Pharmacology, Vol. 55/II, Eds. F. Hoffmeister and Stille, Springer Verlag, Berlin (1981), p. 13.

8 W. Haefely and P. Polc, in : Benzodiazepine-GABA Receptor and Chloride Channels: Structure and Functional Properties. Eds. R.W. Olson and J.C. Venter, Lis, New York (1986), p. 97.

9 A. Nistri and A. Constani : Neuropharmacology *17*, 127 (1978).

10 M.A. Simmonds: Trends. Neurosci. *6*, 279 (1983).

11 M A. Simmonds, in : Actions and Interactions of GABA and Benzodiazepines. Ed. N.G. Bowery, Raven Press, New York (1984), p. 27.

12 N.G. Bowery, D.R. Hill, and A.L. Hudson: Br. J. Pharmacol. *78*, 191 (1983).
13 N.G. Bowery, D.R. Hill, A.L. Hudson, G.W. Price, M.J. Turnbull, and G. P. Wilkin, in: Actions and Interactions of GABA and Benzodiazepines. Ed. N.G. Bowery, Raven Press, New York (1984), p. 81.
14 R. Sherman-Gold and Y. Dudai: FEBS letters *131*, 313 (1981).
15 T.P. Bürch and M.K. Ticku: Proc. Natl. Acad. Sci., USA *78*, 3945 (1981).
16 R. Sherman-Gold and Y. Dudai: Neurochem. Res. *8*, 853 (1983).
17 W. Haefely, E. Kyburz, M. Gerecke, and H. Möhler, in: Advances in Drug Research, Vol. 14, Ed. B. Testa, Academic Press, London (1985), p. 165.
18 D. Römer, H.H. Büscher, R.C. Hill, R. Maurer, I.J. Zeugner, W. Benzon, E.Finner, W. Milkowski, and P.W. Thies: Life Sci. *31*, 1217 (1982).
19 D. Römer, H.H. Büscher, R.C. Hill, R. Maurer, T.F. Petscher, H. Zeugner, W. Benson, E. Finner, W. Milkowski, and P.W. Thies: Nature *298*, 759 (1982).
20 H. Kley, U.Scheidemantel, B. Bering, and W. Müller: Eur. J. Pharmacol. *87*, 503 (1983).
21 W.H. Haefely: Chimia *41*, 389 (1987).
22 R.I. Fryer, in: Comprehensive Medicinal Chemistry, Vol. 3, Eds. C. Hansch, P.G. Sammes, and J.B. Taylor, Pergamon Press, New York (1990), p. 539.
23 P. Pole, E. Bonetti, R. Schaffner, and W. Haefely: Arch. Pharmacol. *321*, 260 (1982).
24 R.I. Fryer, N.W. Gilman, V. Madison, and A. Walser, in: Proceedings of the VIIIth International Symposium on Medicinal Chemistry, Vol. 2, Eds. R. Dahlbom and J.L. Nilsson, Swedish Pharmaceutical Press, Stockholm (1985), p. 265.
25 C. Braestrup, M. Nielsen, and T. Honore, in: CNS Receptors: From Molecular Pharmacology to Behaviour. Eds. P. Mandel and F.V. DeFeudis, Raven Press, New York (1983), p. 237.
26 E. Kyburz: Pharm. Weekl. *121*, 893 (1986).
27 M. Cain, R. Weber, F. Guzman, J. Cook, J. Barker, K. Rice, J. Crawley, S. Paul, and P. Skolnick: J. Med. Chem. *25*, 1081 (1982).
28 S. Cooper: Trends Pharmacol. Sci. *7*, 210 (1986).
29 C. Braestrup, T. Honore, M. Nielsen, E. Petersen and L. Jensen: Biochem. Pharmacol. *33*, 859 (1984).
30 P. Wood, P. Loo, A. Braunwalder, and N. Yokoyama: J. Pharmacol. Exp. Ther. *231*, 572 (1984).
31 N. Yokohama, B. Ritter, and A.D. Neubert: J. Med. Chem. *12*, 337 (1982).
32 C. Boast, E. Snowhill, and J. Smike: J. Pharmacol. Biochem. Behav. *23*, 639 (1985).
33 A.J. Czernik, B. Tetrack, H. Kalinsky, S. Psychoyos, W. Cash, C. Tsai, R. Rinehart, F. Granat, R. Lovell, D. Brundish, and R.Wade: Life Sci. *30*, 363 (1982).
34 J. Albright, D. Moran, W. Wright, Jr., J. Collins, B. Beer, A. Lippa, and E. Greenblatt: J. Med. Chem. *4*, 592 (1981).
35 K. Biziere, J. Bourguignon, J. Chambon, M. Heaulme, A. Perio, S. Tebib, and C.G. Wermuth: Br. J. Pharmacol. *90*, 1983 (1987).
36 S. Tebib, J.-J. Bourguignon, and C.-G. Wermuth: J. Computer-Aided Mol. Design *1*, 153 (1987).
37 R.I. Fryer, in: The Benzodiazepines: From Molecular Biology to Clinical Practice. Ed. E. Costa, Raven Press, New York (1983), p. 7.
38 R.I. Fryer, C. Cook, N.W. Gilman, and A. Walsher: Life Sci. *39*, 1947 (1986).
39 J.C. Fong, K. Okada, and M. Goldstein: Eur. J. Pharmacol. 77, 57 (1982).
40 M. Trudell, A. Basile, H. Shannon, P. Skolnick, and J.M. Cook: J. Med. Chem. *30*, 456 (1987).

41 H. Takeda, H. Shindo, T. Sasatani, N. Chomei, A. Matsushita, M. Eigyo, K. Kawasaki, S. Murata, Y. Takahara, and H. Shintaku: J. Med. Chem. *31*, 1738 (1988).
42 M. Allen, T. Hagen, M. Trudell, P. Codding, P. Skolnick, and J.M. Cook: J. Med. Chem. *31*, 1854 (1988).
43 L.H. Sternbach, L.O. Randall, and S.R. Gustavson: Psychopharmacological Agents *1*, 137 (1964).
44 L.H. Sternbach, L.O. Randall, R. Banziger, and H. Lehr, in: Drugs Affecting the Nervous System. Ed. A. Burger, Dekker, New York (1968), p. 237.
45 L.H. Sternbach, in: The Benzodiazepines. Eds. S. Garatlini, E. Mussini, and L.O. Randall, Raven Press, New York (1973), p. 1.
46 L.H. Sternbach: Prog. Drug Res. *22*, 229 (1978).
47 R.I. Fryer, W. Leimgruber, and Trybulski: J. Med. Chem. *25*, 1050 (1982).
48 P.A. Borea, G. Gilli, and V. Bertolasi: Il Farmaco, Ed. Sci. *34*, 1073 (1979).
49 P.G. Baraldi, S. Manfredini, V. Periotto, D. Simino, M.Guarneri, and P.A. Borea: J. Med. Chem. *28*, 683 (1985).
50 S.P. Gupta, R.N. Saha, and V. Mulchandani: J. Molec. Recog. *5*, 75 (1992).
51 F. Watjen, R. Baker, M. Engelstoff, R. Herbert, A. MacLeod, A. Knight, K. Merchant, J. Moseley, J. Saunders, C.J. Swain, E. Wong, and J.P. Springer: J. Med. Chem. *32*, 2282 (1989).
52 Z-Q. Gu, B.R. de Costa, G. Wong, K.C. Rice, and P. Skolnick: J. Label. Compd. Radiopharm. *31*, 1049 (1992).
53 S. Ananthan, S.D. Clayton, S.E. Ealick, G. Wong, G.E. Evoniuk, and P. Skolnick: J. Med. Chem. *36*, 479 (1993).
54 Z.-Q. Gu, G. Wong, C. Dominguez, B.R. de Costa, K.C. Rice, and P. Skolnick: J. Med. Chem. *36*, 1001 (1993).
55 G. Wong, K.E. Koehler, P. Skolnick, Z.-Q. Gu, S. Ananthan, P. Schönholzer, W.Hunkler, W. Zhang, and J.M. Cook: J. Med. Chem. *36*, 1820 (1993).
56 R.I. Fryer, P. Zhang, K.-Y. Lin, R.B. Upasani, G. Wong, and P. Skolnick: Med. Chem. Res. *3*, 183 (1993).
57 D.M. Turner, D.W. Sapp, and R.W. Olsen: J. Pharmacol. Exp. Ther. *247*, 1236 (1991).
58 G. Wong and P. Skolnick: Eur. J. Pharm. Mol. Pharm. Sec. *225*, 63 (1992).
59 G. Wong, P. Skolnick, J. Katz, and J. Witkin: J. Pharm. Ex. Ther., in press. (1994).
60 E.R. Korpi, M. Uusi-Oukari, and K. Wegeluis: Eur. J. Pharm. *213*, 323 (1992).
61 R.C. Sharma, P. Singh, and T.N. Ojha: Res. Commun. Chem. Pathol. Pharmacol. 80, 357(1993).
62 V. Nacci and I. Fiorini: Il Farmaco, Ed. Sci. *38*, 112 (1983).
63 V. Nacci, I. Fiorini, S. Vomero, I. Taddei, and E. Taddei: Il Farmaco, Ed. Sci. *39*, 289 (1984).
64 V. Nacci, I. Fiorini, A. Garofalo, and A. Cagnotto: Il Farmaco, Ed. Sci. *45*, 545 (1990).
65 I. Fiorini, V. Nacci, S.M. Ciani, A. Garofalo, G. Campiani, L. Savini, E. Novellino, G. Greco, P. Bernasconi, and T. Mennini: J. Med. Chem. *37*, 1427 (1994).
66 H. Rommelspacher, C. Nanz, H.O. Borbe, K.J. Feshske, W.E. Müller, and U. Wollert: Naunyn-Schmiedeberg's Arch. Pharmacol. *314*, 97 (1980).
67 H. Rommelspacher, C. Nanz. H.O. Borbe, K.J. Feshske, W.E. Müller, and U. Wollert: Eur. J. Pharmacol. *70*, 409 (1981).
68 W.E. Müller, K.J. Fehske, H.O. Borbe, U. Wollert, C. Nanz, and H. Rommelspacher: Pharmacol. Biochem. Behav. *14*, 693 (1981).
69 H. A. Robertson, G.B. Baker, R.T. Coutts, A. Benderly, R.A. Locock, and I.L. Martin: Eur. J. Pharmacol. *76*, 281 (1981).

70 C. Braestrup, M. Nielsen, and C.E. Olsen: Proc. Natl. Acad. Sci., USA *77*, 2288 (1980).
71 C. Braestrup and M. Nielsen: J. Neurochem. *37*, 333 (1981).
72 K.J. Fenske, I. Zube, H.O. Borbe, U. Wollert, and W.E. Müller: Naunyn-Schmiedeberg's Arch. Pharmacol. *319*, 172 (1982).
73 F.J. Ehlert, W.R. Roeske, and H.I. Yamamura: Life Sci. *29*, 235 (1981).
74 J.D. Hirsch, R.L. Kochman, and P R. Sumner: Mol. Pharmacol. *21*, 618 (1982).
75 M. Cain, R.W. Weber, F. Guzman, J.M. Cook, S.A. Barker, K.C. Rice, J.N. Crawley, S.M. Paul, and P. Skolnick: J. Med. Chem. *25*, 1081 (1982).
76 K.P. Lippke, W.G. Schunack, W. Wenning, and W.E. Müller: J. Med. Chem. *26*, 499 (1983).
77 F. Guzman, M. Cain, P. Larscheid, T. Hagen, J.M. Cook, M. Schweri, P. Skolnick, and S.M. Paul: J. Med. Chem. *27*, 564 (1984).
78 G. Dorey, G. Poissonnet, M.-C. Potier, L.P. de Carvalho, P. Venault, G. Chapouthier, J. Rossier, P. Potier, and R.H. Dodd: J. Med. Chem. *32*, 1799 (1989).
79 R.C. Sharma, T.N. Ojha, S. Tiwari, and P. Singh: Drug Des. Discov. *9*, 135 (1992).
80 T.H. Hagen, P. Skolnick, and J.M. Cook: J. Med. Chem. *30*, 750 (1987).
81 S.P. Hollinshead, M.L. Trudell, P. Skolnick, and J.M. Cook: J. Med. Chem. *33*, 1062 (1990).
82 H.O. Villar and G.H. Loew: Int. J.Quantum Chem., Quantum Biol. Symp. *16*, 261 (1989).
83 G.H. Loew, J.R. Nienow, J.A. Lawson, L. Toll, and E.T. Uyeno: Mol. Pharmacol. *28*, 17 (1985).
84 G.H. Loew, J.R. Nienow, and M. Poulsen: Mol. Pharmacol. *26*, 19 (1984).
85 R.H. Dodd, C. Ouannès, M.-C. Potier, L.P. de Carvalho, J. Rossier, and P. Potier: J. Med. Chem. *30*, 1248 (1987).
86 M.L. Trudell, S.L. Lifer, Y.-C. Tan, M.J. Martin, L. Deng, P. Skolnick, and J.M. Cook: J. Med. Chem. *33*, 2412 (1990).
87 N. Yokoyama, B. Ritter, and A.D. Neubert: J. Med. Chem. *25*, 337 (1982).
88 L. Cecchi, F. Melani, G. Palazzino, G. Filacchioni, C. Martini, E. Pennacchi, and A. Lucacchini: Il Farmaco, Ed. Sci. *40*, 509 (1985).
89 F. Melani, L. Cecchi, G. Palazzino, G. Filacchioni, C. Martini, E. Pennacchi, and A. Lucacchini: J. Med. Chem. *29*, 291 (1986).
90 F. Melani, L. Cecchi, G. Palazzino, G. Filacchioni, C. Martini, E. Penacchi, and A. Lucacchini: J. Pharm. Sci. *75*, 1175 (1986).
91 G. Palazzino, L. Cecchi, F. Melani, V. Colotta, G. Filacchioni, C. Martini, and A. Lucacchini: J. Med. Chem. *30*, 1737 (1987).
92 V. Colotta, L. Cecchi, F. Melani, D. Catarzi, G. Filacchioni, C. Martini, G. Gianaccini, M. Tonelli, and A.Lucacchini: Drug Des. Deliv. *8*, 325 (1992).
93 H.O. Villar, E.T. Uyeno, L. Toll, W. Polgar, M.F. Davies, and G.H. Loew: Mol. Pharmacol. *36*, 589 (1989).
94 G. Wong, Z.-Q. Gu, R.I. Fryer, and P. Skolnick: Med. Chem. Res. *2*, 217 (1992).
95 R.I. Fryer, R. Rios, P. Zhang, Z.-Q. Gu, G. Wong, A.S. Basile, and P. Skolnick: Med. Chem. Res. *3*, 122 (1993).
96 R.I. Fryer, P. Zhang, R. Rios, Z.-Q. Gu, A.S. Basile, and P. Skolnick: J. Med. Chem. *36*, 1669 (1993).
97 S. Takada, H. Shinde, T. Sasatani, N. Chomei, A. Matsushita, M. Eigyo, K. Kawasaki, S.Murata, Y. Takahara, and H. Shintaku: J. Med. Chem. *31*, 1738 (1988).

98 S. Shindo, S. Takada, S. Murata, M. Eigyo, and A. Matsushita: J. Med. Chem. *32*, 1213 (1989).

99 V. Colotta, L. Cecchi, F. Melani, G. Palazzino, and G. Filacchioni: Tetrahedron Letters *28*, 5165 (1987).

100 V. Colotta, L. Cecchi, G. Filacchioni, F. Melani, G. Palazzino, C. Martini, G. Giannaccini, and A. Lucacchini: J. Med. Chem. *31*, 1 (1988).

101 V. Colotta, L. Cecchi, F. Melani, G. Palazzino, G. Filacchioni, C. Martini, G. Giannaccini, and A. Lucacchini: J. Pharm. Sci. *78*, 239 (1989).

102 V. Colotta, L. Cecchi, F. Melani, G. Filacchioni, C. Martini, S. Gelli, and A. Lucacchini: J. Pharm. Sci. *80*, 276 (1991).

103 S.P. Gupta, R.N. Saha, J.K. Gupta, and P. Singh: Res. Commun. Chem. Pathol. Pharmacol. *65*, 119 (1989).

104 P. Singh, T.N. Ojha, and R.C. Sharma: Res. Commun. Chem. Pathol. Pharmacol. *67*, 151 (1990).

105 P. Singh, T.N. Ojha, R.C. Sharma, and S. Tiwari: Indian J. Chem. *32B*, 555 (1993).

106 S.P. Gupta and Anitha Paleti: Communicated.

107 V. Colotta, L. Cecchi, F. Melani, G. Filacchioni, C. Martini, G. Giannaccini, and A. Lucacchini: J. Med. Chem. *33*, 2646 (1990).

108 L. Cecchi, V. Colotta, G. Filaccchioni, F. Melani, G. Palazzino, and A. Galli: Il Farmaco, Ed., Sci. *42*, 671 (1987).

109 L. Cecchi, V. Colotta, F. Melani, G. Palazzino, G. Filacchioni, C. Martini, G. Giannaccini, and A. Lucacchini: J. Pharm. Sci. *78*, 437 (1989).

110 M.S. Allen, P. Skolnick, and J.M. Cook: J. Med. Chem. *35*, 368 (1992).

111 V. Colotta, L. Cecchi, F. Melani, G. Filacchioni, C. Martini, S. Gelli, and A. Lucacchini: Il Farmaco, Ed. Sci. *46*, 1139 (1991).

112 J.E. Francis, W.D. Cash, B.S. Barbaz, P.S. Bernard, R.A. Lovell, G.C. Mazzenga, R.C. Friedman, J.L. Hyun, A.F. Braunwalder, P.S. Loo, and D.A. Bennett: J. Med. Chem. *34*, 281 (1991).

113 V.Colotta, L. Cecchi, D.Catarzi, G. Conti, G. Filacchioni, C. Martini, L. Giusti, and A. Lucacchini: Il Farmaco, Ed. Sci. *48*, 1051 (1993).

114 D. Catarzi, L. Cecchi, V. Colotta, F. Melani, G. Filacchioni, C. Martini, L. Giusti, and A. Lucacchini: Il Farmaco, Ed. Sci. *48*, 1065 (1993).

115 D. Catarzi, L. Cecchi, V. Colotta, F. Melani, G. Filacchioni, C. Martini, L. Giusti, and A. Lucacchini: J. Med. Chem. *37*, 2846 (1994).

116 G. Targia, E. Occelli, E. Toja, D. Barone, N. Corsico, L. Gallico, and F. Luzzani: J. Med. Chem. *31*, 1115 (1988).

117 D. Catarzi, L. Cecchi, V. Colotta, G. Conti, F. Melani, G. Filacchioni, C. Martini, L. Giusti, and A. Lucacchini: Il Farmaco, Ed.Sci. *48*, 447 (1993).

118 F. Melani, L. Cecchi, V. Colotta, G. Filacchioni, C. Martini, G. Giannaccini, and A. Lucacchini: Il Farmaco, Ed. Sci. *44*, 585 (1989).

119 J.E. Francis, D.A. Bennett, J.L. Hyun, S.L. Rovinski, C.L. Amrick, P.S. Loo, D. Murphy, R.F. Neale, and D.E. Wilson: J. Med. Chem. *34*, 2899 (1991).

120 J.L. Kelley, E.W. McLean, R.M. Ferris, and J.L. Howard: J. Med. Chem. *32*, 1020 (1989).

121 J.L. Kelley, E.W. McLean, J.A. Linn, M.P Krochmal, R.M. Ferris, and J.L. Howard: J. Med. Chem. *33*, 196 (1990).

122 J.L. Kelley, E.W. McLean, R.M. Ferris, and J.L. Howard: J. Med. Chem. *33*, 1910 (1990).

123 J.L. Kelley, E.W. McLean, R.M. Ferris, and J.L. Howard: J. Heterocyclic Chem. *28*, 1099 (1991).

124 R.N. Saha, J. Meera, N. Agrawal, and S.P. Gupta: Drug Des. Deliv. *7*, 219 (1991).
125 S.P. Gupta and V. Mulchandani: Indian J. Biochem. Biophys. *30*, 181 (1993).
126 C. Martini, T. Gervasio, A. Lucacchini, A.D. Settimo, G. Primofiore, and A.M. Martini: J. Med. Chem. *28*, 506 (1985).
127 G. Primofiore, A.M. Marini, F.D. Settimo, C. Martini, A. Bardellini, G. Giannaccini, and A. Lucacchini: J. Med. Chem. *32*, 2514 (1989).
128 A.M. Bianucci, A.D. Settimo, F.D. Settimo, G. Primofiore, C. Martini, G. Giannaccini, and A. Lucacchini: J. Med. Chem. *35*, 2214 (1992).
129 G.M. Crippen: Mol. Pharmacol. *22*, 11 (1982).
130 P.W. Codding and A.K. Muir: Mol. Pharmacol. *28*, 178 (1985).
131 M.S. Allen, Y.-C. Tan., M.L. Trudell, K. Narayanan, L.R. Schindler, M.J. Martin, C. Schultz, T.J. Hagen, K.F. Koehler, P.W. Codding, P. Skolnick, and J.M. Cook: J. Med. Chem. *33*, 2343 (1990).
132 P.A. Borea, G. Gilli, V. Bertolasi, and V. Ferretti: Mol. Pharmacol. *31*, 334 (1987).
133 M.S. Allen., A.J. LaLoggia, L.J. Dorn, M.J. Martin, G. Costantino, T.J. Hagen, K.F. Koehler, P. Skolnick, and J.M. Cook: J. Med. Chem. *35*, 4001 (1992).
134 M.J. Martin, M.L. Trudell, H.D. Araúzo, M.S. Allen, A.J. LaLoggia, L. Deng, C.A. Schultz, Y.-C. Tan, Y. Bi, K. Narayanan, L.J. Dorn, K.F. Koehler, P. Skolnick, and J.M. Cook: J. Med. Chem. *35*, 4105 (1992).
135 W. Zhang, K.F. Koehler, B. Harris, P. Skolnick, and J.M. Cook: J. Med. Chem. *37*, 745 (1994).
136 H. Diaz-Araúzo, G.E. Evoniuk, P. Skolnick, and J.M. Cook: J. Med. Chem. *34*, 1754 (1991).
137 A. Yliniemelä, J. Gynther, K. Konschin, H. Tylli, and J. Rouvinen: Int. J. Quantum. Chem.,Quantum Biol. Symp. *16*, 273 (1989).
138 G. Georges, D.P. Vercauteren, D.J. Vanderveken, R. Horion, G. Evrard, J.G. Fripiat, J.-M. Andre, and F. Durant: Int. J. Quantum Chem., Quantum Biol. Symp. *17*, 1 (1990).
139 H.O. Villar and G. H. Loew: Int. J. Quantum Chem., Quantum Biol. Symp. *18*, 131 (1991).
140 H.O. Villar, M.F. Davies, G.H. Loew, and P.A. Maguire: Life Sci, *48*, 593 (1991).
141 S.P. Gupta: Indian J. Chem. *33B*, 105 (1994).

Progress in Drug Research, Vol. 45 (E. Jucker, Ed.)

The medicinal chemistry and therapeutic potentials of ligands of the histamine H_3 receptor

By R. Leurs#, R.C. Vollinga and H. Timmerman
Leiden/Amsterdam Center for Drug Research, Department of Pharmacochemistry, Vrije Universiteit, De Boelelaan 1083, 1081 HV Amsterdam, The Netherlands
Author for correspondence

1 Introduction

The monoamine histamine is one of the several chemical messengers involved in the concerted regulation of (patho)physiological processes. In rat brain, histamine can be found in a restricted population of neurons originating from the tuberomammillary nucleus of the hypothalamus [1, 2]. These histaminergic neurons project diffusely to several brain areas and are involved in the regulation of physiological functions (e.g. sleep/wakefullness, feeding, cardiovascular control, neuroendocrine control) [1, 2]. In the periphery histamine is mainly found in mast cells, basophils and enterochrommafin cells. Mast cell degranulation after IgG-allergen interactions results in a massive release of histamine, which is responsible for many of the well-known symptoms of allergic conditions [3, 4]. In gastric mucosa histamine is especially stored in enterochromaffin cells, from which it can be release upon stimulation with gastrin or acetylcholine [5]. In turn, histamine stimulates the parietal cell, resulting in gastric acid secretion [5].

The various actions of histamine are currently thought to be mediated by three pharmacologically different receptor subtypes [1, 6, 7]. It was already in 1966 that Ash and Schild [8] recognized the differences in actions of histamine on the guinea-pig ileum and the stomach and heart. Since only the actions on the ileum could be blocked by the "anti-histamines" they proposed the existence of two receptor subtypes [8]. It lasted until 1972 for the final acceptation of this subclassification. A rational synthesis program led Black and co-workers to introduce burimamide that was able to block the actions of histamine on the heart and the stomach [9]. From then on the "anti-histamines" were recognized as H_1 receptor antagonist, wheras the new blockers were named H_2 antagonists.

It lasted until 1983 for the first description of the histamine H_3 receptor [10]. Although evidence for a role of histamine as a neurotransmitter in the brain had been accumulating, the observation of a selective regulation of histamine release [10] and synthesis [11] in rat brain cortex by so-called H_3 autoreceptors was a major contribution to our understanding of the role of histamine in brain neurotransmission. Arrang et al. [10] observed that [^{3}H]-histamine was released from rat brain cortex slices, preloaded with [^{3}H]-histidine, after a potassium depolarization. Yet, this [^{3}H]-histamine release was subjected to a negative feedback by histamine itself and this effect was antagonized by several H_2 antagonists [10]. The potency order for these H_2 antagonists did not correlate with their activities at the histamine H_2 receptor, whereas also the H_2 agonist impromidine appeared to be a competitive antagonist in the [^{3}H]-histamine release assay in the brain [10]. Thus, the pharmacological profile of this receptor-mediated effect was completely different from the known pharmacology of the histamine H_1- and the H_2-receptor. These observations led Arrang and co-workers to suggest the presence of a third histamine H_3 receptor subtype in various rat brain areas [10]. Using microdialysis [12–14], push-pull canula superfusion [15] or *ex vivo* histamine determination [16–22] several authors were able to show *in vivo* effects of H_3 receptor stimulation in both rat and mouse brain. Histamine levels measured with microdialysis in e.g. the rat anterior hypothalamus can be effectively reduced after peripheral H_3 agonist application (Fig 1). Moreover, the administration of H_3 antagonists leads to an increase in the histamine levels (Fig. 1), indicating the presence of a basal *in vivo* activation of the H_3 receptor by endogenously released histamine. Besides the regulation of the histamine release, both *in vitro* and *in vivo*, the H_3 receptor also exerts an inhibitory effect on the synthesis of histamine in histaminergic neurons in the rat cortex and hypothalamus [11]. Although a relationship between the inhibitory effects on the histamine release and synthesis is likely, no information on the molecular mechanisms of these two regulatory pathways is currently available.

In recent years it was found that the H_3 receptor not only regulates the release of histamine, but also acts as an heteroreceptor on many neurons in the CNS. H_3 heteroreceptors were shown to be involved in the *in vitro* and *in vivo* regulation of the release of acetylcholine [15, 23, 24], dopamine [25, 26], noradrenaline [27, 28] and serotonin [25, 29] in brain tissue of several species. H_3 heteroreceptors have in recent years also been identified in several peripheral tissues, like the airways [3] and the GI tract [30]. In peripheral tissues, H_3 receptors have been reported to regulate the release of e.g acetylcholine [31–34] noradrenaline [35, 36], serotonin [37] and probably various neuropeptides [38–42]. Based on these findings the H_3 receptor should be considered as an important general regulatory mechanism, which affects a variety of brain functions, but also influences various physiological processes in peripheral tissues.

In view of these considerations the H_3 receptor has been the target for a successful development of selective H_3 receptor agonists and antagonists. In the present paper we will describe in full detail the medicinal chemistry of selective agonists and antagonists and the various molecular pharmacological properties of the target protein. Finally, we will briefly discuss the current therapeutic potential of selective H_3 agonists and antagonists.

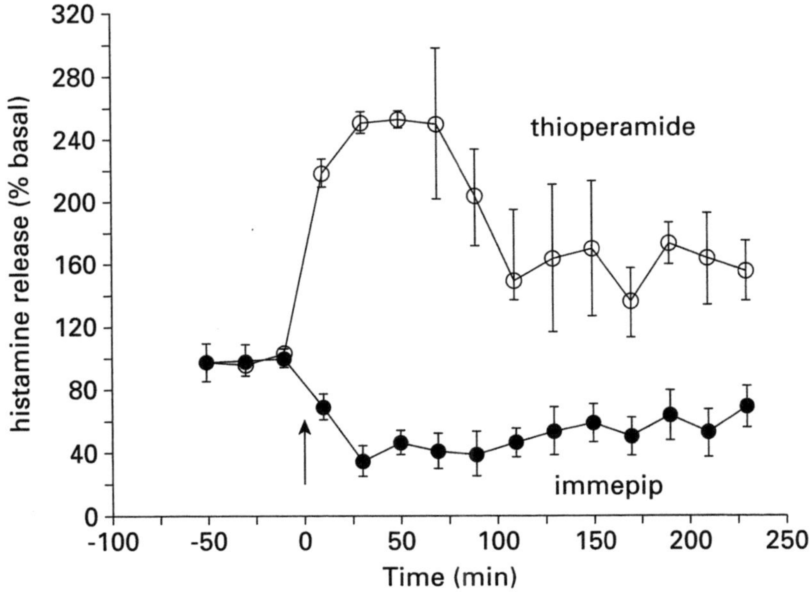

Fig. 1
In vivo effects of the H_3 agonist immepip and the H_3 antagonist thioperamide on the histamine levels in the rat anterior hypothalamus as determined by microdialysis. After the measurement of basal histamine release immepip (5 mg/kg) or thioperamide (5 mg/kg) was injected i.p at timepoint 0 min (indicated by the arrow). Subsequently 20 min-fractions were collected and assayed for histamine by HPLC [13].

2 Medicinal chemistry of H_3 receptor ligands

Since the first description of the H_3 receptor in 1983 by Arrang et al. [10] many potent and selective compounds have been found. In this section we present in detail the development of various potent agonists and antagonists, but we will also focuss on moderately active or inactive compounds, since these ligands are often very useful for structure-activity relationship studies.

2.1 Histamine H_3 agonists

2.1.1 Derivatives of histamine as H3 agonists

Since histamine (**1**) itself is already remarkably active on the histamine H_3 receptor at very low concentrations, it is not surprising that most potent H_3 agonists, have been derived from its structure. The 4(5)-alkyl-imidazole moiety in the structure of histamine (**1**), has proven to be essential

Table 1.
Histamine H_3 receptor activity of some histamine analogues, in which the imidazole ring is replaced by other heterocycles

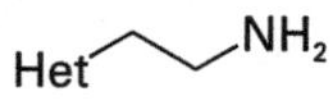

No.	Compound	Het	pD_2 value[a]	Ref.
1	histamine	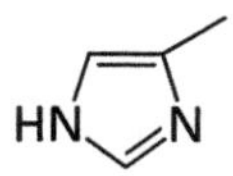	7.4 (7.3)[b]	[10,42,43,]
2	amthamine	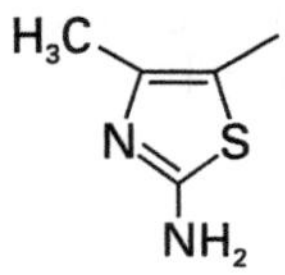	4.7[c]	[44]
3	2-(2-aminoethyl)-thiazole	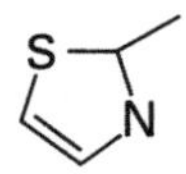	< 3.0	[10]
3	3(5)-(2-aminoethyl)-pyrazole	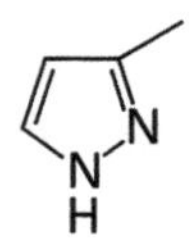	< 4.0	[45]
3	3-(2-aminoethyl)-isoxazole	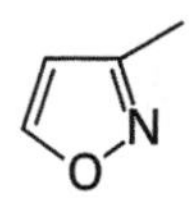	< 4.0	[45]
3	2-(2-aminoethyl)-pyridine	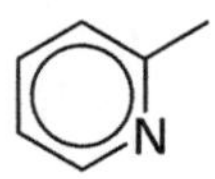	< 4.0	[45]

[a] Determined by evaluation of the influence of the compound on K^+-stimulated [^{3}H]-histamine release on rat cortex, as described by Arrang et al. [10].

[b] Determined by evaluation of the influence of the compound on electrically evoked, NANC contractions of guinea pig intestine preparations, as described by Menkveld et al. [42].

[c] Determined by evaluation of the influence of the compound on electrically evoked, cholinergic contractions of guinea pig intestine preparations, as described by Vollinga et al. [31].

Table 2.
Histamine H_3 activity of some 2-substituted ω-aminoalkyl imidazoles

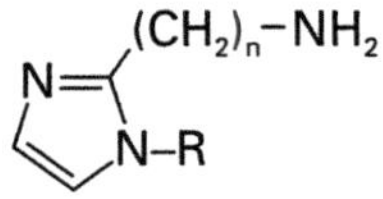

No.	Compound	n	R	pD_2 value[a]	Ref.
7	2-(2-aminoethyl)imidazole	2	H	< 4.0	[45]
8	2-(3-aminopropyl)imidazole	3	H	< 4.0	[45]
9	2-(4-aminobutyl)imidazole	4	H	< 4.0	[45]
10	1-methyl-2-(2-aminoethyl)imidazole	2	CH_3	< 4.0	[45]
11	1-methyl-2-(3-aminopropyl)imidazole	3	CH_3	< 4.0	[45]

[a] Determined by evaluation of the influence of the compound on K^+-stimulated [^{3}H]-histamine release on rat cortex, as described by Arrang et al. [10].

Table 3.
Histamine H_3 receptor activity of several ring substituted histamine analogues

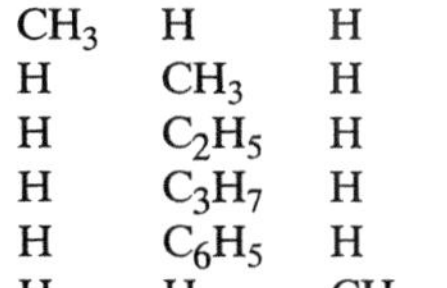

No.	Compound	R_1	R_2	R_3	R_4	R_5	pD_2 value[a]	Ref.
1	histamine	H	H	H	H	H	7.4	[10]
12	N^τ-methylhistamine	CH_3	H	H	H	H	< 6.0	[10]
13	2-methylhistamine	H	CH_3	H	H	H	< 4.3	[10]
14	2-ethylhistamine	H	C_2H_5	H	H	H	< 4.0	[45]
15	2-*n*-propylhistamine	H	C_3H_7	H	H	H	< 4.0	[45]
16	2-phenylhistamine	H	C_6H_5	H	H	H	< 4.0	[45]
17	N^π-methylhistamine	H	H	CH_3	H	H	< 6.0	[10]
18	4(5)-methylhistamine	H	H	H	CH_3	H	< 3.0	[10]
19	(R)-α,N^τ-dimethylhistamine	CH_3	H	H	H	(R)-CH_3	4.3	[45]
20	(±)-5(4),α-dimethylhistamine	H	H	H	CH_3	CH_3	< 4.0	[45]

[a] Determined by evaluation of the influence of the compound on K^+-stimulated [^{3}H]-histamine release on rat cortex, as described by Arrang et al. [10].

for H_3 agonism. Replacement of the imidazole ring by other heterocycles, resulted in compounds without agonistic activity on the histamine H_3 receptor, although the H_2 agonist amthamine (**2**) has been described to be a very weak, but full H_3 agonist (see Table 1). Besides the imidazole ring, also the 2-aminoethylene chain is of great importance. If the 2-aminoethylene chain of histamine is connected to the 2-position of the imidazole ring instead of the 4(5)-position, all activity is lost (see Table 2).

Substituents on the imidazole ring are not allowed for agonistic activity. From Table 3 it is obvious that alkylation of the imidazole ring of histamine in any position, leads to a strong decrease in agonistic activity. This emphasizes the distinct structural demands of this particular histamine receptor, since methylation of the 2-position of histamine (2-methylhistamine, **13**) leads to a rather selective H_1 agonist and 4(5)methylhistamine (**18**) is an H_2 agonist.

Whereas for agonistic activity on the H_3 receptor the imidazole ring may not be replaced by other ring systems or substituted, modifications of the side chain of histamine have resulted in some very potent and selective H_3 agonists (Table 4 and Table 5). Especially the introduction of a methyl group on the ethylene chain of histamine resulted in compounds that are highly potent on the H_3 receptor. Upon methylation, the stereoselective character of the H_3 receptor becomes apparent, since the (R)-enantiomer of α-methylhistamine **21** is about 100 times more potent than its (S)-enantiomer **22** (rat cortex). Because of its potency and selectivity (about 20,000 times more potent on the H_3 receptor than on the H_1- and H_2 receptors),[16] (R)-α-methylhistamine is often used as the standard agonist for pharmacological assays related to histamine H_3 receptors.

Replacement of the methyl group by a chloromethyl- or a hydroxymethyl group leads to a reduction of activity, which might be the result of steric hindrance (**23–26**). However, also these compounds display a large difference in activity between the (R)- and the (S)-enantiomer (compare **23** and **25** with **24** and **26**, respectively). The eutomer (most active enantiomer) has the same absolute configuration as (R)-α-methylhistamine (**21**). The reported weak antagonistic activity of (±)-α-aminomethylhistamine (**30**) may be explained in a different manner, since this compound can also be regarded as an analogue of the H_3 antagonist homohistamine (**109**) (see histamine H_3 antagonists, Table 14).

The introduction of a methyl group on the β-position of the ethylene chain of histamine results in a potent H_3 agonist as well ((±)-β-methylhistamine, **31**) and also here an increase of the van der Waals volume of the substituent leads to a decrease of activity, since (±)-β-ethylhistamine (**32**) is a very weak agonist.

Table 4.
Agonistic activity of several optically pure substituted histamine analogues at the H_3 receptor

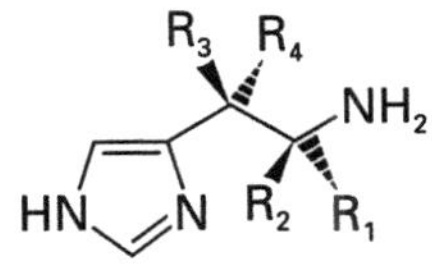

No.	Compound (HA = histamine)	R_1	R_2	R_3	R_4	pD_2 value[a]	Ref.
1	HA	H	H	H	H	7.4	[10]
21	(R)-α-methylHA	CH_3	H	H	H	8.4, 7.8[b]	[16, 31]
22	(S)-α-methylHA	H	CH_3	H	H	6.3	[16]
23	(S)-α-chloromethylHA	CH_2Cl	H	H	H	5.9	[45]
24	(R)-α-chloromethylHA	H	CH_2Cl	H	H	4.7	[45[
25	(S)-α-hydroxymethylHA	CH_2OH	H	H	H	5.7	[45]
26	(R)-α-hydroxymethylHA	H	CH_2OH	H	H	4.2	[45]
27	(R)α,(S)β-dimethylHA	CH_3	H	CH_3	H	8.5	[47]
28	(S)α,(R)β-dimethylHA	H	CH_3	H	CH_3	6.5	[47]

[a] Determined by evaluation of the influence of the compound on K^+-stimulated [^{3}H]-histamine release on rat cortex, as described by Arrang et al. [10].
[b] Determined by evaluation of the influence of the compound on electrically evoked, cholinergic contractions of guinea pig intestine preparations, as described by Vollinga et al. [31].

Whereas large substituents on the ethylene chain of histamine are not allowed (see also the cyclohexylhistamines **39** and **40**), the histamine derivative with two methyl groups on the α-position **33** is still a good agonist. β,β-Dimethylhistamine (**37**) however, is a very weak agonist, suggesting that there is not enough space in the 'active site' of the receptor, to accommodate two methyl groups on the β-position. If both the α- and the β-position are methylated, (R)α,(S)β-dimethylhistamine (**27**) is the active diastereoisomer. This compound is equipotent to (R)-α-methylhistamine (**21**) on the rat cortex and (S)α,(R)β-dimethylhistamine (**28**) is equipotent to (S)-α-methylhistamine (**22**), indicating that the stereochemistry of the α-methyl group largely determines the activation of the receptor. In addition to its high potency, (R)α,(S)β-dimethylhistamine (**27**) is also highly selective, displaying an activity that is about 100,000-fold higher at the H_3 receptor than at the H_1- and H_2 receptors [46].
Another interesting reported histamine analogue with good H_3 agonistic activity is 'cyclopropylhistamine' (4(5)-(2-aminocyclopropyl)-1*H*-imidazole) (**38**) [52]. This molecule has been reported in a Patent Application [49] as a full H_3 agonist and for its small and rigid structure might be very useful for structure-activity relationship and molecular modelling stud-

Table 5.
Agonistic activity of several substituted histamine analogues at the H_3 receptor (unresolved mixture of enantiomers)

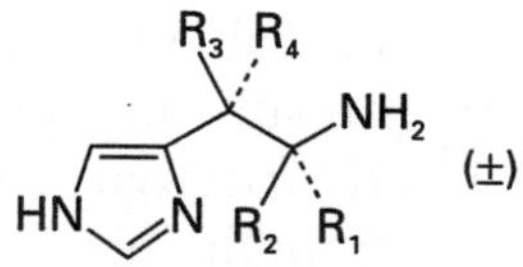

No.	Compound (HA = histamine)	R_1	R_2	R_3	R_4	pD_2 value[a]	Ref.
29	(±)-α-ethylHA	C_2H_5	H	H	H	5.0	[47]
30	(±)-α-aminomethylHA	CH_2NH_2	H	H	H	pA_2=5.3	[45]
31	(±)-β-methylHA	H	H	CH_3	H	7.7	[47]
32	(±)-β-ethylHA	H	H	C_2H_5	H	5.0	[47]
33	α,α-dimethylHA	CH_3	CH_3	H	H	7.6	[47]
34	(±)-α-methylhistidine	CH_3	CO_2H	H	H	5.8	[45]
35	erythro-α,β-dimethylHA	CH_3	H	CH_3	H	8.2	[46, 47]
36	threo-α,β-dimethylHA	H	CH_3	CH_3	H	6.7	[46, 47]
37	β,β-dimethylHA	H	H	CH_3	CH_3	5.8	[48]
38	(±)-cyclopropylHA	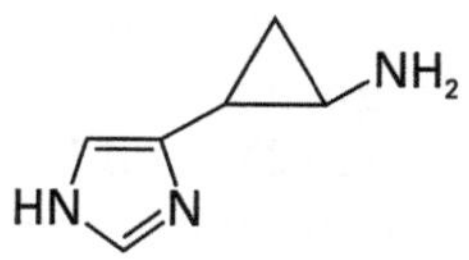				8.0	[49]
39	(±)-*trans*-α-methyl-cyclohexylHA	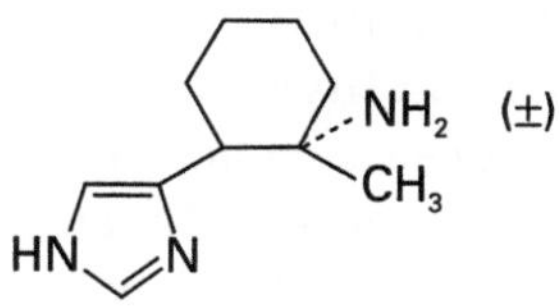				pK_i < 5.7b	[50]
40	(±)-*cis*-α-methyl-cyclohexylHA	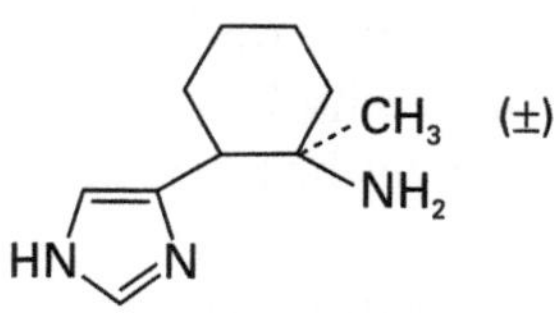				pK_i < 5.7b	[50]

[a] Determined by evaluation of the influence of the compound on K^+-stimulated [^{3}H]-histamine release on rat cortex, as described by Arrang et al. [10].
[b] Determined on guinea pig brain tissue, measuring the displacement of [^{3}H]N^α-methylhistamine, as described by Korte et al. [51]

ies. Unfortunately nothing more has been reported in the literature about this compound. It is likely that the sample as described in the Patent Application consisted of a mixture of all four possible stereoisomers of cyclopropylhistamine (**38**), because a non-stereoselective synthesis route was used for its preparation. For the use of cyclopropylhistamine (**38**) in fur-

ther SAR or molecular modelling studies, the determination of the eutomer of this compound is obligatory.
In addition to alkylations on the side chain of histamine the β-amino group has also been alkylated (see Table 6). The introduction of one methyl group on the amino group results in a potent H_3 agonist and even two methyl groups are tolerated for activity (although there is a large difference in activity between N^{α}-methylhistamine (**41**) and N^{α},N^{α}-dimethylhistamine (**42**) on the electrically stimulated [^{3}H]-histamine release assay). The introduction of larger substituents on the amino group leads to a decrease in activity. Whereas N^{α}-ethylhistamine (**43**) is still a full agonist, the incorporation of the amino group in a pyrrolidine ring results in a partial agonist (compound **44**) and introduction of a n-propyl group leads to a complete loss of activity (N^{α}-n-propylhistamine, **45**).
Intriguing is the observation that (R)-α-methylhistamine (**21**) and N^{α}-methylhistamine (**41**) are both potent H_3 agonists, but that (R)α,N^{α}-dimethylhistamine (**46**) is a weak agonist. This could mean that there is not enough space at the receptor to tolerate substituents on both the α-position and the amino group. Another possible explanation may be that (R)-α-methylhistamine (**21**) and N^{α}-methylhistamine (**41**) are in a different conformation when binding to the receptor or that (R)α,N^{α}–dimethylhistamine (**46**) is in another conformation than (R)-α-methylhistamine (**21**) and Nα-methylhistamine (**41**). However it must be noted that the trend of a decrease in activity, going from (R)-α-methylhistamine (**21**) to its (S)-enantiomer **22**, can also be observed between the enantiomers of α,N^{α}-dimethylhistamine (**46** and **47**), as well as between the enantiomers of α-chloromethyl-N^{α}-methylhistamine (**48** and **49**). Introduction of the more hydrophilic α-hydroxymethyl group to N^{α}-methylhistamine is clearly not tolerated as both enantiomers (**50** and **51**) are inactive.
Recently a new series of histamine analogues has been described, in which the structure of histamine is partly incorporated in a ring structure (see Table 7 and Table 8). In this series, variations in ring size and substituents were performed. SCH 49648 (**52**), which can be regarded as a rigid analogue of (R)-α-methylhistamine (**21**) is still quite active, although less potent than (R)-α-methylhistamine itself. It has been reported that SCH 49648 (**52**) and SCH 50971 (**54**) were both as effective as (R)-α-methylhistamine (**21**), measured as the *in vivo* inhibition of an electrically induced CNS hypertensive response [50].
When comparing affinities, SCH 49648 (**52**) (same absolute configuration as (R)-α-methylhistamine) (**21**) can be regarded as the eutomer and SCH 49647 (**53**) as the distomer.

Table 6.
H_3 Agonistic activity of several N^{α}-alkyl substituted histamine analogues

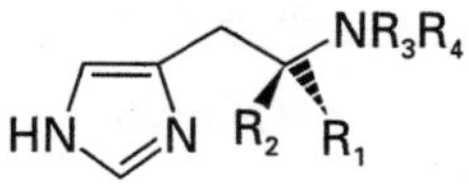

No.	Compound	R_1	R_2	R_3	R_4	pD_2 value[a]	Ref.
41	N^{α}-methylhistamine	H	H	CH_3	H	7.8 (8.7[b])	[10, 31, 43]
42	N^{α},N^{α}-dimethylhistamine	H	H	CH_3	CH_3	7.6 (7.3[b])	[10, 43]
43	N^{α}-ethylhistamine	H	H	C_2H_5	H	7.1	[53]
44	4(5)-(2-pyrrolidin-ethyl) imidazole	H	H	$-(CH_2)_4-$		6.0[c]	[16]
45	N^{α}-n-propylhistamine	H	H	C_3H_7	H	< 5.2	[53]
46	(R)α,N^{α}-dimethylhistamine	CH_3	H	CH_3	H	5.8	[54]
47	(S)α,N^{α}-dimethylhistamine	H	CH_3	CH_3	H	4.3	[54]
48	(S)α-chloromethyl-N^{α}-methylhistamine	CH_2Cl	H	CH_3	H	5.3	[54]
49	(R)α-chloromethyl-N^{α}-methylhistamine	H	CH_2Cl	CH_3	H	3.0	[54]
50	(S)α-hydroxymethyl-N^{α}-methylhistamine	CH_2OH	H	CH_3	H	3.2	[45]
51	(R)α-hydroxymethyl-N^{α}-methylhistamine	H	CH_2OH	CH_3	H	3.0	[45]

[a] Determined by evaluation of the influence of the compound on K^+-stimulated [^{3}H]-histamine release on rat cortex, as described by Arrang et al. [10].
[b] Determined by evaluation of the influence of the compound on electrically-stimulated [^{3}H]-histamine release on rat cortex, as described by Van der Werf et al. [55].
[c] Partial agonist (α = 0.6).

Whereas large substituents on the β-position of the ethylene chain of histamine were not tolerated (see Table 5), it is remarkable that SCH 50971 (**54**), which can also be regarded as an analogue of β-ethylhistamine (**32**) is even slightly more active than SCH 49648 (**52**). This means that large substituents on the β-position are tolerated, but that the stereochemistry on this position is very critical for H_3 agonism.
Another intriguing observation is that the absolute configurations of the 3-position of the pyrrolidine ring of SCH 49648 (**52**) and SCH 50971 (**54**) are different, but that the affinities of both compounds for the H_3 receptor are alike. This would indicate totally different orientations of both compounds when binding to the receptor.
When comparing the affinities of the unresolved (mixture of enantiomers) ring-closed histamine analogues (Table 8), an increase of the ring size from a five membered ring to a six-membered ring (**73**, **74**) results in a

Table 7.
Histamine H_3 activity of some optically pure ring-closed histamine analogues

No.	Compound		Structure	pD_2 value[a]	pK_i value[b]	Ref.
52	SCH 49648	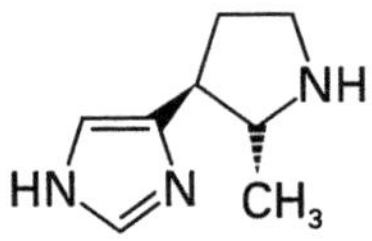	(+)-[2R,3S]	7.1	8.5	[50]
53	SCH 49647	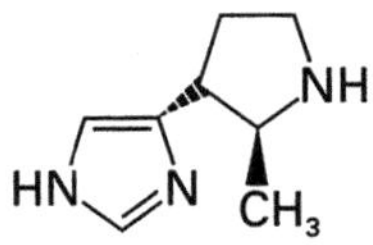	(–)-[2S,3R]	-[c]	7.5	[50]
54	SCH 50971	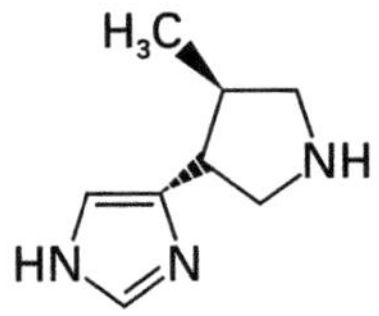	(+)-[3R,4R]	7.5	8.6	[50]
55	SCH 50972	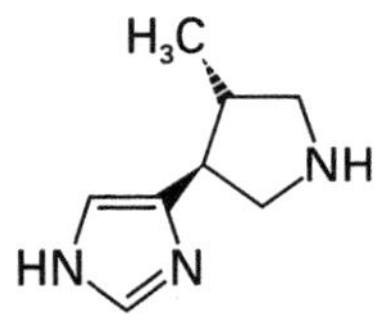	(–)-[3S,4S]	-[c]	7.5	[50]

[a] Determined by evaluation of the influence of the compound on electrically evoked, cholinergic contractions of guinea pig intestine preparations, as described by Vollinga et al. [31].
[b] Determined on guinea pig brain tissue, measuring the displacement of [^{3}H]N$^{\alpha}$-methylhistamine, as described by Korte et al. [51].
[c] Not reported.

large decrease in affinity (compare **57** with **73**). A decrease of ring size to a four- membered ring (**72**) leads to a compound with a high affinity for the H_3 receptor, but less selectivity, since H_1 activity has been reported for **72** [50]. Also for the large series of five-membered rings, the introduction of methyl substituents seems to be essential for selectivity, since the nor-methyl analogue (**56**) exhibits H_1 activity as well [50].
The introduction of larger substituents on the pyrrolidine ring results in a strong decrease in activity. The compounds with the highest affinities carry a methyl group on the 2-position (**57**) or at the 4-position (**62**), *trans* (not on the same site of the pyrrolidine ring) to the imidazole ring. However the introduction of two methyl groups, one on the 2-position and the other at the 4-position, both *trans*-orientated, relatively to the imid-

Table 8.
Histamine H_3 activity of some ring-closed histamine analogues (enantiomers unresolved)

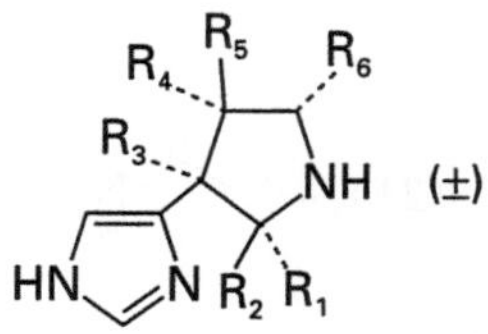

No.	R_1	R_2	R_3	R_4	R_5	R_6	pK_i value[a]	Ref.
56	H	H	H	H	H	H	8.5; 8.7	[50, 56]
57	CH_3	H	H	H	H	H	8.2; 8.5	[50, 56]
58	$CH_2C_6H_5$	H	H	H	H	H	< 5.8	[50, 56]
59	H	CH_3	H	H	H	H	6.8	[50, 56]
60	H	$(CH_2)_2C_6H_5$	H	H	H	H	6.2	[56]
61	H	H	CH_3	H	H	H	6.8	[50, 56]
62	H	H	H	CH_3	H	H	8.1; 8.3	[50, 56]
63	H	H	H	C_2H_5	H	H	6.8; 6.4	[50, 56]
64	H	H	H	C_5H_{11}	H	H	6.3	[50, 56]
65	H	H	H	H	CH_3	H	8.5	[50]
66	H	H	H	H	C_5H_{11}	H	7.1	[50, 56]
67	H	H	H	H	H	CH_3	7.2; 7.1	[50, 56]
68	CH_3	CH_3	H	H	H	H	7.2; 6.2	[50, 56]
69	CH_3	H	H	CH_3	H	H	< 5.7	[50]
70	CH_3	H	H	H	CH_3	H	6.7	[50]
71	H	H	H	CH_3	CH_3	H	7.0	[50]
72				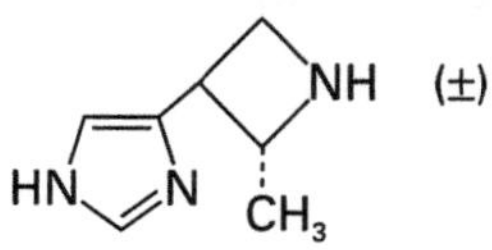			8.2	[50, 56]

No.	Structure	pK_i value[a]	Ref.
73	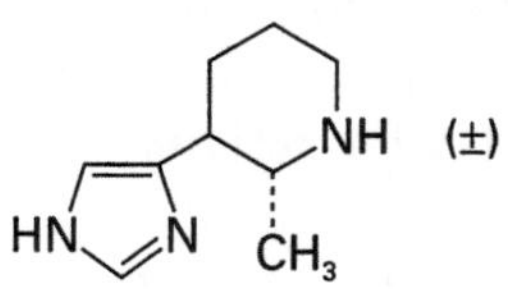	< 5.7	[50]
74	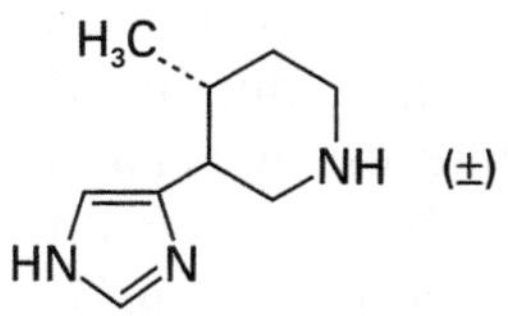	6.4	[50]

[a] Determined on guinea pig brain tissue, measuring the displacement of $[^3H]N^{\alpha}$-methylhistamine, as described by Korte et al. [51].

Table 9.
Histamine H_3 activities of some analogues of imetit

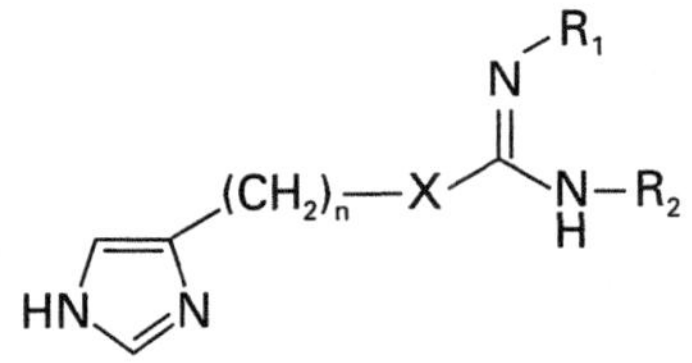

No.	Compound	n	X	R_1	R_2	pD_2 value	Ref.
75	imetit	2	S	H	H	8.1[a,b] (9.0[c])	[17, 57–59]
76	SKF 91606	2	CH_2	H	H	9.0[b]	[58]
77	VUF 83100	2	NH	H	H	6.3[a] (7.4[d,e])	[57, 60]
78	VUF 8621	2	S	CH_3	H	7.3[a] (7.8[c])	[57, 59]
79	VUF 8973	2	S	CH_3	CH_3	pA_2 = 6.6[a] (7.3[c])	[57, 59]
80	VUF 8321	1	S	H	H	5.2[a]	[57]
81	VUF 8328	3	S	H	H	pA_2 = 8.0[a]	[57]

[a] Determined by evaluation of the influence of the compound on electrically evoked, NANC contractions of guinea pig intestine preparations, as described by Menkveld et al. [42].
[b] Determined by evaluation of the influence of the compound on electrically evoked, cholinergic contractions of guinea pig intestine preparations, as described by Vollinga et al. [31].
[c] Determined by evaluation of the influence of the compound on K^+-stimulated [^{3}H]-histamine release on rat cortex, as described by Arrang et al. [10].
[d] Determined by evaluation of the influence of the compound on electrically-stimulated [^{3}H]-histamine release on rat cortex, as described by Van der Werf et al. [55].
[e] Partial agonist ($\alpha = 0.5$).

azole ring (compound, **69**), is not tolerated, suggesting a different binding orientation between the 2-methyl- (**57**) and the 4-methyl derivative (**62**). The derivative with a *cis*-orientated methyl group relatively to the imidazole ring on the 4-position (**65**) has a high affinity as well, but has again been described to display H_1 activity [50].

2.1.2 *Derivatives of imetit as H3 agonists*

So far only substitution of the sidechain of histamine has been discussed. Yet, the replacement of the amino group by other protonated groups has recently resulted in several interesting H_3 agonists. The replacement of the amino group of histamine by e.g. an isothiourea group leads to the very potent and selective H_3 agonist imetit (**75**, Table 9).
Several analogues of imetit have been prepared (see Table 9). The sulphur atom of the isothiourea group of imetit (**75**) is not involved in an interaction with the H_3 receptor, since SKF 91606 (**76**) is even more potent. SKF 91606 (**76**) is the most potent H_3 agonist so far, but its activity has

only be reported once [58]. Replacement of the isothiourea group of imetit by a guanidine group (VUF 83100, **77**) results in a drastic decrease of activity. The introduction of substituents on the isothiourea group of imetit (**75**) is not well tolerated for agonism, since the monomethylated imetit derivative VUF 8621 (**78**) is less active and the introduction of two methyl groups results in a moderately active antagonist VUF 8973 (**79**). Variation in the length of the alkyl chain is also not allowed for H_3 agonistic activity and VUF 8328 (**81**) is even a potent H_3 antagonist. Apparently the distance between the amidine system and the imidazole ring is very strict for H_3 agonism. Interestingly, the distance between the hydrogen donating protonated imino nitrogen and the imidazole ring is much longer (ca. 8Å) than the two methylene groups in histamine (ca. 4.5 Å) (see also section 2.1.3).
The introduction of a methyl group on the 5-position of the imidazole ring of imetit leads to a weak agonist (VUF 9032, **82**) and a methyl group on the 2-position results even in a very weak antagonist (VUF 8974, **83**). Replacement of the imidazole ring with other heterocycles results in inactive compounds (see Table 10). Only VUF 8863 (**85**) has been reported to be a very weak partial agonist. These results indicate again the importance of the 4(5)-alkyl-imidazole moiety for H_3 agonism and the intolerance (probably sterical hindrance) for additional substituents on this ring.

2.1.3 Derivatives of immepip as H_3 agonists

Following the observation that imetit (**75**) is a potent agonist, despite the different distance between the protonated nitrogen of the isothiourea and the imidazole ring compared to histamine (see section 2.1.2), the length of the sidechain of histamine was varied. As a result agonistic activity at the guinea-pig jejunum was lost; suprisingly potent H_3 antagonists were obtained. These compounds will be described in full detail in section 2.2.1. Yet, cyclization of a lengthened sidechain is allowed for agonistic activity. The compound, immepip (**88**) has a pD_2 value of 8.0 on the guinea pig intestine and is therefore equipotent with (R)-α-methylhistamine (**21**) and imetit (**75**) on the same assay [31, 61], but immepip has quite a distinct structure (Table 11). For immepip the proton-donating ammonium group of the piperidine ring is located at a distance of four methylene groups (ca. 7.5 Å) from the imidazole ring. These observations make immepip (in combination with histamine and imetit) a very interesting structure for SAR- and molecular modelling studies.
The affinities of immepip (**88**) and some of its analogues as determined on guinea pig brain tissue (see Table 11), have also been reported independently in a Patent Application [62]. From Table 11 it can be seen that

Table 10
Histamine activities of analogues of imetit, in which the imidazole has been replaced by other heterocycles

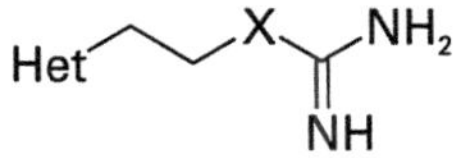

No.	Compound	Het	X	pD_2 value	Ref.
82	VUF 9032	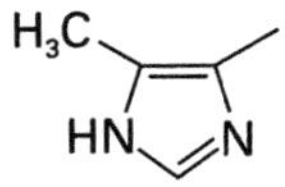	S	6.0 ($\alpha = 0.9$)[a]	[57]
83	VUF 8974	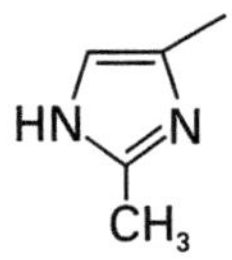	S	$pA_2 = 5.4$[a]	[57]
84	VUF 8844	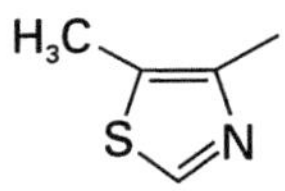	S	inactive[b]	[60]
85	VUF 8863	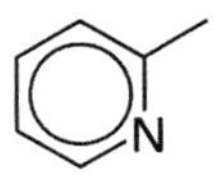	S	6.0 ($\alpha = 0.5$)[b]	[60]
86	VUF 8848	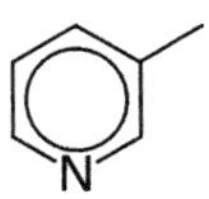	S	inactive[b]	[60]
87	VUF 8862	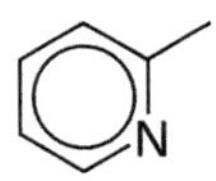	NH	inactive[b]	[60]

[a] Determined by evaluation of the influence of the compound on electrically evoked, NANC contractions of guinea pig intestine preparations, as described by Menkveld et al. [42].
[b] Determined by evaluation of the influence of the compound on electrically-stimulated [^{3}H]-histamine release on rat cortex, as described by Van der Werf et al. [55].

Table 11
Affinities of some analogues of immepip (**88**), determined on guinea pig brain tissue (entantiomers unresolved)

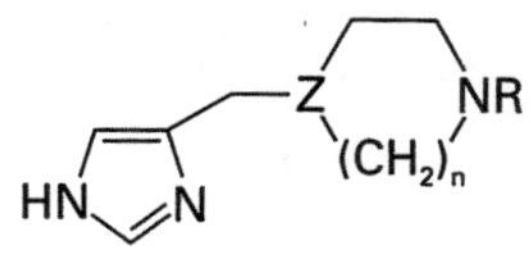

No.	Z	n	R	pK_i value[a]	Ref.
88[b]	CH	2	H	9.5	[62]
89	CH	1	H	7.0	[56]
90	CH	1	CH_3	8.5	[56]
91	CH	2	CH_3	9.1	[62]
92	N	2	H	8.3	[63]
93	N	3	H	7.1	[56]
94		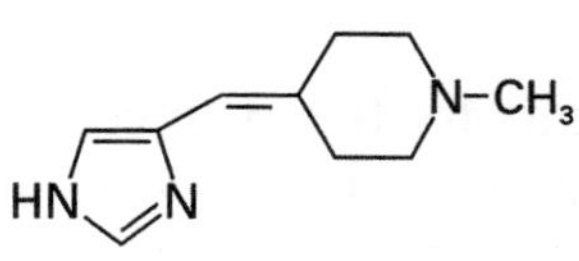		7.9	[62]
95		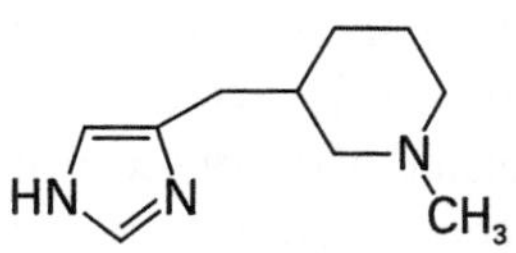		6.7	[62]
96		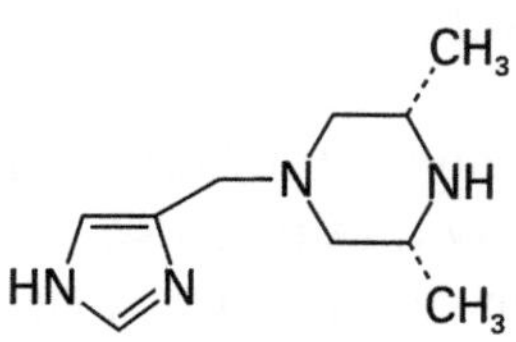		< 5.2	[63]
97		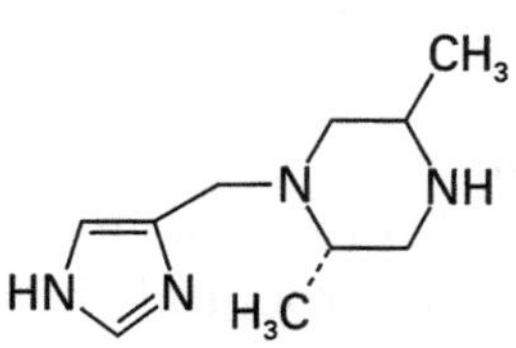		< 5.2	[63]

[a] Determined on guinea pig brain tissue, measuring the displacement of [^{3}H] N$^\alpha$-methylhistamine, as described by Korte et al. [51].

[b] Immepip; $pD_2 = 8.0$ as determined by evaluation of the influence of the compound on electrically evoked, cholinergic contractions of guinea pig intestine preparations, as described by Vollinga et al. [31].

Table 12.
Histamine H_3 activity of some bifunctional amidine derivatives

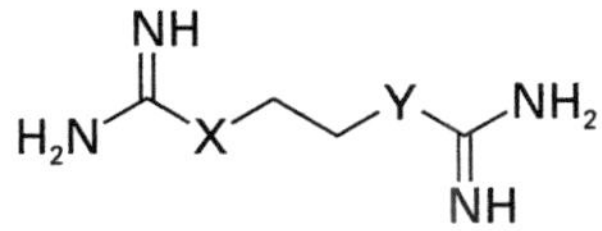

No.	Compound	X	Y	H_3 activity[a]	Ref.
98	VUF 8430	S	NH	$pD_2 = 5.9$ ($\alpha = 0.5$)	[60]
99	VUF 8332	S	S	$pA_2 = 6.0$	[60]
100	VUF 8309	NH	NH	inactive	[60]

[a] Determined by evaluation of the influence of the compound on electrically stimulated [^{3}H]-histamine release on rat cortex, as described by Van der Werf et al. [55].

immepip (**88**) has a high affinity for the H_3 receptor. Methylation of the amino group leads to a slight decrease in affinity (compound **91**). Replacement of the piperidine ring of immepip by a pyrrolidine ring however, results in a drastic reduction of affinity (compound **89**). It must be noticed that this compound has not been resolved in its enantiomers. Surprisingly, methylation of the amino group of this pyrrolidine derivative **89**, yields a compound with a strongly increased affinity (compound **90**). The replacement of the piperidine ring by the synthetically more convenient piperazine ring (compound **92**), results in a ten-fold decrease of affinity, and the introduction of methyl substituents on the piperazine ring leads to a drastic loss of affinity.

Because immepip (**88**) has the highest affinity of the compounds mentioned in Table 11, it seems likely that it is also the most active H_3 agonist from Table 11. However, in order to draw definite conclusions for structure-activity relationship studies it is necessary to determine the functional H_3 activities of the analogues represented in Table 11.

2.1.4 *Miscellaneous H_3 agonists*

Obviously, the 4(5)-alkyl-imidazole moiety seems to be essential for activation of the H_3 receptor, since this structural element is apparent in all potent H_3 agonists known at this time. The only non-imidazole derivatives known so far, which have been reported to be weakly and partially active at the H_3 receptor are VUF 8863 (**85**) (see Table 10) and VUF 8430 (**98**) (see Table 12). When an interaction of either the isothiourea group or the guanidine group of VUF 8430 (**98**) is assumed, it is interesting to see that the compound with two guanidine groups **100** is inactive and that

Table 13.
Histamine H_3 antagonistic activity of some N^{α}- substituted histamine analogues

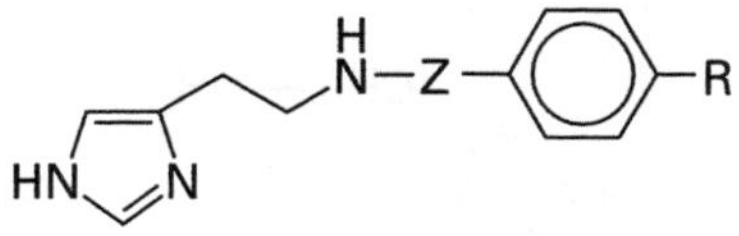

No.	Z	R	pA_2 value[a]	Ref.
101	$(CH_2)_2$	H	5.5	[64]
102	$(CH_2)_3$	H	6.2	[64]
103	$(CH_2)_4$	H	6.2	[64]
104	$(CH_2)_5$	H	5.7	[64]
105	$(CH_2)_2O$	H	6.4	[64]
106	$(CH_2)_2S$	H	5.6	[64]
107	$(CH_2)_2S$	Cl	6.6	[64]

[a] Determined by evaluation of the influence of the compound on K^+-stimulated [^{3}H]-histamine release on rat cortex, as described by Arrang et al. [10].

the bis-isothiourea derivative **99** is a weak antagonist. Apparently both functions are required for (partial) activation of the H_3 receptor by VUF 8430 (**98**). Based on these results it might be speculated that the guanidine group is capable of activating the receptor (although weakly), but that the isothiourea group of VUF 8430 (**98**) is required for the binding to the receptor. This could also explain why the guanidine derivative of imetit (VUF 83100, **77**) is less active (see Table 9), since the guanidine group is less capable of binding to the receptor.

2.2 Histamine H_3 antagonists

2.2.1 Derivatives of histamine as H_3 antagonists

From Table 6 it is clear that large substituents on the amino group of histamine diminish the H_3 agonistic activity. Moreover, in Table 13 some other N^{α}-substituted histamine derivatives are presented, which have been reported as weak H_3 antagonists. In this series of compounds only a minor effect of the length of the alkyl chain, separating the phenyl ring from the amino group, is noticed. Apparently the position of this phenyl ring is not very important for antagonistic activity. However a ten-fold increase in antagonistic activity is observed when a 4-chloro group is introduced on the phenyl ring of **106**, indicating that lipophilicity plays a role in the binding of these compounds to the H_3 receptor (compound **107**).

Table 14.
Histamine H_3 antagonistic activity of some homologues of histamine, in which the length of the ω-aminoalkyl chain is varied.

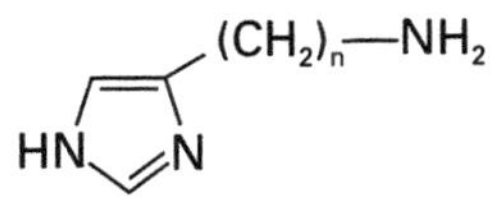

No.	Compound	n	pA_2 value[a]	Ref.
108	VUF 8319	1	inactive	[65]
1	histamine	2	$pD_2 = 7.3$[b]	[10]
109	homohistamine	3	5.9	[65]
110	VUF 4701	4	7.7	[65]
111	impentamine (VUF 4702)	5	8.4	[65]
112	VUF 4732	6	7.8	[65]
113	VUF 4733	8	6.0	[65]
114	VUF 4734	10	6.0	[65]
30	(±)-α-aminomethyl-histamine	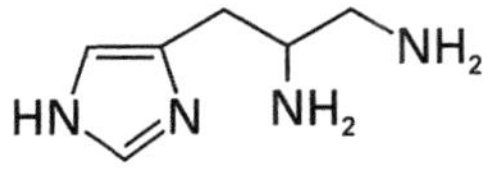	5.3[c]	[45]
115	(±)-α-methyl-homohistamine	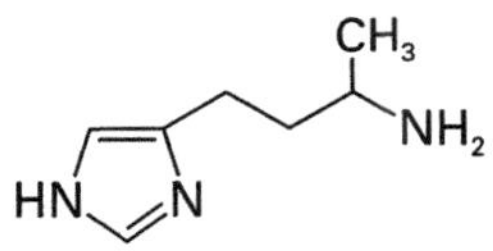	$pD_2 < 4.0$[c]	[45]

[a] Determined by evaluation of the influence of the compound on electrically evoked, cholinergic contractions of guinea pig intestine preparations, as described by Vollinga et al. [31].
[b] Determined by evaluation of the influence of the compound on electrically evoked, NANC contractions of guinea pig intestine preparations, as described by Menkveld et al. [42].
[c] Determined by evaluation of the influence of the compound on K^+-stimulated [^{3}H]-histamine release on rat cortex, as described by Arrang et al. [10].

As already described in section 2.1.3, elongation of the side chain of histamine (**1**) resulted in compounds with H_3 antagonistic properties (see Table 14), with impentamine (**111**) as the most potent and selective H_3 antagonist from this series. Both the H_1 and H_2 affinities for this compound are more than 1000-fold lower than its H_3 affinity [65].
The fact that homohistamine (**109**) is a weak antagonist, might explain why α-aminomethylhistamine (**30**, already mentioned in Table 5) is a weak antagonist, since this compound can also be regarded as an analogue of homohistamine. For the same reason, α-methylhomohistamine (**115**), which has been reported to show no H_3 agonistic activity, might be a weak antagonist as well. So far no H_3 receptor affinity has been reported.

Table 15.
Histamine H_3 antagonistic activity of some analogues of histamine with an aminopropylene chain, enclosed in a piperidine ring

No.	Structure	pA_2 value[a]	Ref.
116	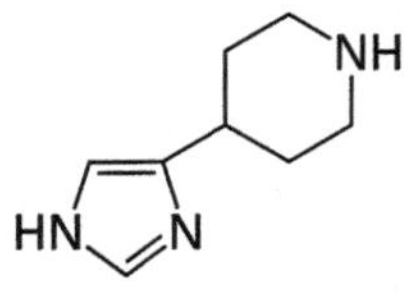	5.7 (6.2[b])	[45, 66]
117	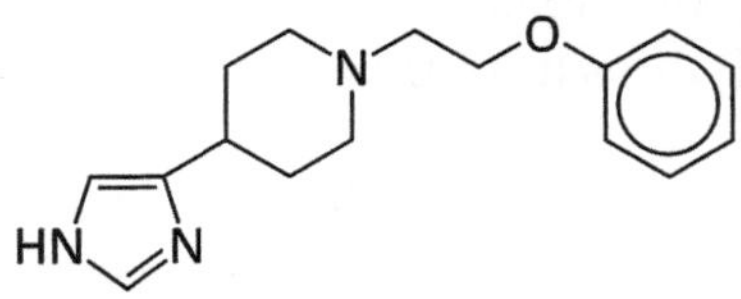	7.2	[67]
118	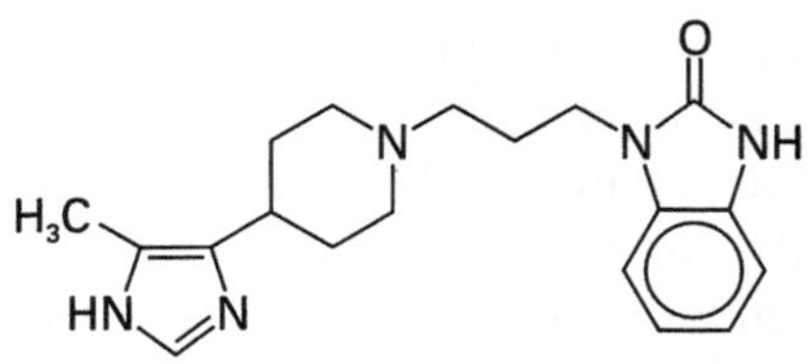	6.3	[67]
119	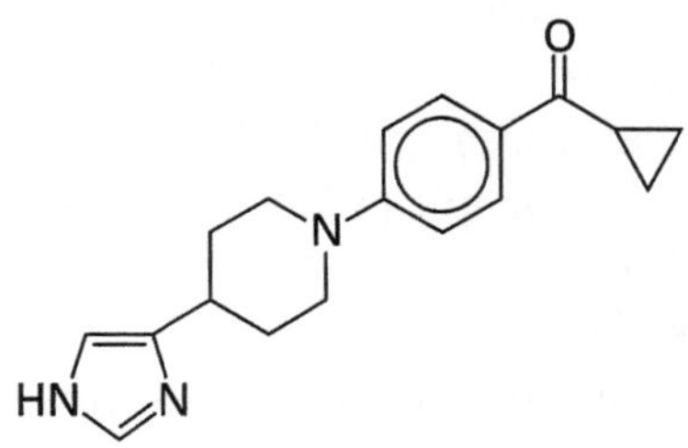	7.4	[67]

[a] Determined by evaluation of the influence of the compound on K^+-stimulated [^{3}H]-histamine release on rat cortex, as described by Arrang et al. [10].
[b] Determined by evaluation of the influence of the compound on electrically evoked, cholinergic contractions of guinea pig intestine preparations, as described by Vollinga et al. [31].

The rigid piperidine analogue of homohistamine, **116**, is still a weak antagonist; coupling of a lipophilic moiety to the amino group leads to an increase of antagonistic activity (see Table 15). Introduction of a methyl group on the 5-position of the imidazole ring presumably results in a decrease of affinity, although compound **118** is slightly more potent than **116** on the rat cortex.

2.2.2 Derivatives of imetit asH_3 antagonists

Derivatization of the potent H_3 agonist imetit (**75**) also resulted in antagonists (see Table 10 and 16). Methylation of the 2-position of the imidazole ring of imetit results in a moderately active antagonist (VUF 8974, **83**), whereas 5-methylimetit (**82**, see Table 10) is a weak agonist. Substitution of the isothiourea group with more than one methyl group leads to moderately active H_3 antagonists. The introduction of a phenyl group, separated from the isothiourea group by an alkyl chain leads to good antagonists. The length of this alkyl spacer does not seem to be very strict. The introduction of a methyl group on the isothiourea group of the phenylethyl derivative VUF 9029 (**125**) does not influence the activity (see VUF 9051 (**126**)).

Elongation of the ethylene chain of imetit (**75**) however, has a drastic effect on the activity. VUF 8328 (**81**) is already a potent antagonist and the introduction of a phenyl group to the isothiourea group, separated by an alkyl spacer, leads to more potent H_3 antagonists. Replacement of a phenyl group by a non-aromatic cyclohexyl group (VUF 9163, **132**) has no effect on the H_3 antagonistic activity, suggesting that receptor binding by this part of the molecule is through a hydrophobic interaction and not a π-π interaction. This is verified by the introduction of a chloro group in the para position of the benzyl group, resulting in clobenpropit (**131**), the most potent H_3 antagonist reported so far (pA_2 value of 9.9 at guinea pig ileum). This observation led to the development of the first selective, radiolabeled H_3 antagonist [^{125}I]-iodophenpropit (**134**), which is currently used as a radioligand for histamine H_3 receptor binding studies and will be discussed in detail in section 3 [68–70].

It is interesting to note that **138** might also fit in this series. Although the isothiourea group is "reversed", a pA_2 value comparable to the ω-phenylalkyl derivatives of imetit is reported in a patent application. The same is true for compound **139**, which may also be regarded as an analogue of imetit. This could be an indication that binding of this series of compounds depends on the interaction of a nitrogen with the receptor and that the sulphur atom is not important.

The isothiourea group of the imetit analogues has also been replaced by a guanidine group. As previously found for imetit itself (see Table 9), the introduction of the nitrogen leads to a reduction in activity. Although a lower level of actvity is obtained, a pattern comparable to the substituted imetit series (described above) can be observed (see Table 17).

Table 16.
Histamine H_3 antagonistic activity of several substituted analogues of imetit

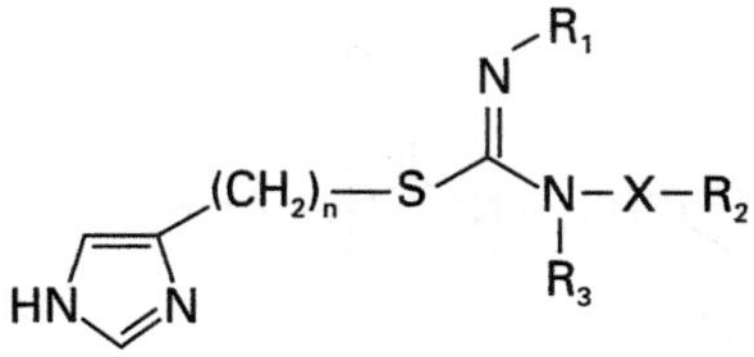

No.	Compound	n	R_1	X	R_2	R_3	pA_2 value[a]	Ref.
120		2	H	–	CH_3	CH_3	6.3[b]	[59]
79	VUF 8973	2	CH_3	–	CH_3	H	6.6 (7.3[b])	[57, 59]
121		2		$-(CH_2)_2-$	–	H	6.6[b]	[59]
122		2	CH_3	–	CH_3	CH_3	6.3[b]	[59]
123	VUF 8397	2	H	–	C_6H_5	H	7.0	[57]
124	VUF 9028	2	H	CH_2	C_6H_5	H	7.8	[57]
125	VUF 9029	2	H	$(CH_2)_2$	C_6H_5	H	8.0	[57]
126	VUF 9051	2	CH_3	$(CH_2)_2$	C_6H_5	H	7.8	[57]
127	VUF 9030	2	H	$(CH_2)_3$	C_6H_5	H	7.6	[57]
128	VUF 9031	2	H	$(CH_2)_4$	C_6H_5	H	7.7	[57]
129	VUF 8404	2	H	$(CH_2)_2SCH_2$	C_6H_5	H	7.5 (<5.3[c])	[43, 57]
81	VUF 8328	3	H	–	H	H	8.0	[57]
130	VUF 9107	3	H	CH_2	C_6H_5	H	8.8	[57]
131	clobenpropit	3	H	CH_2	C_6H_5–4–Cl	H	9.9	[57]
132	VUF 9163	3	H	CH_2	C–C_6H_{11}	H	8.8	[57]
133	VUF 9151	3	H	$(CH_2)_2$	C_6H_5	H	8.8	[57]
134	iodophenpropit	3	H	$(CH_2)_2$	C_6H_5–4–I	H	9.6	[69]
135	VUF 9152	3	H	$(CH_2)_3$	C_6H_5	H	8.3	[57]
136	VUF 4571	3	H	$(CH_2)_4$	C_6H_5	H	8.5	[57]
137	VUF 8414	3	H	$(CH_2)_2SCH_2$	C_6H_5	H	8.6	[57]

No.	Compound	Structure	pA_2 value[a]	Ref.
83	VUF 8974	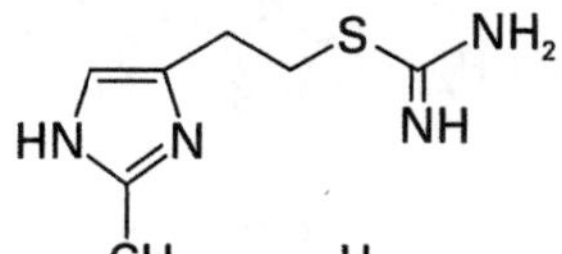	5.4	[57]
138		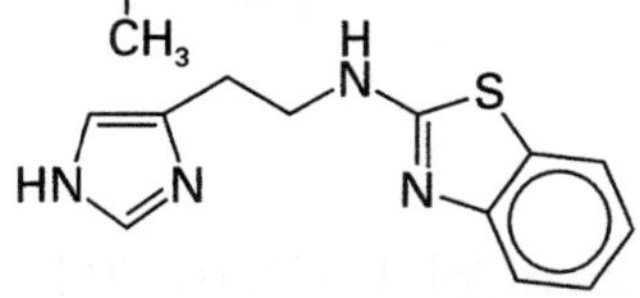	7.4[b]	[71]
139		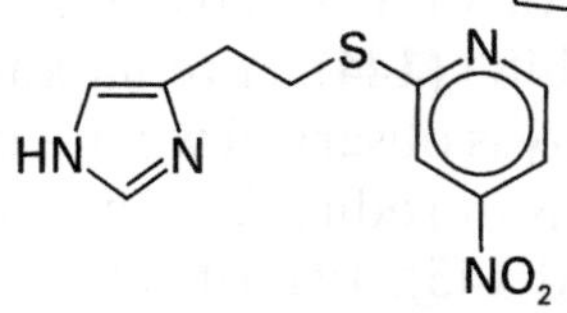	7.5[b]	[71]

[a] Determined by evaluation of the influence of the compound on electrically evoked, NANC contractions of guinea pig intestine preparations, as described by Menkveld et al. [42].
[b] Determined by evaluation of the influence of the compound on K^+-stimulated [^3H]-histamine release on rat cortex, as described by Arrang et al. [10]. Values from patent application.
[c] Determined by evaluation of the influence of the compound on electrically-stimulated [^3H]-histamine release on rat cortex, as described by Van der Werf et al. [55].

Table 17.
Histamine H_3 antagonistic activity of some substituted guanidine analogues of imetit.

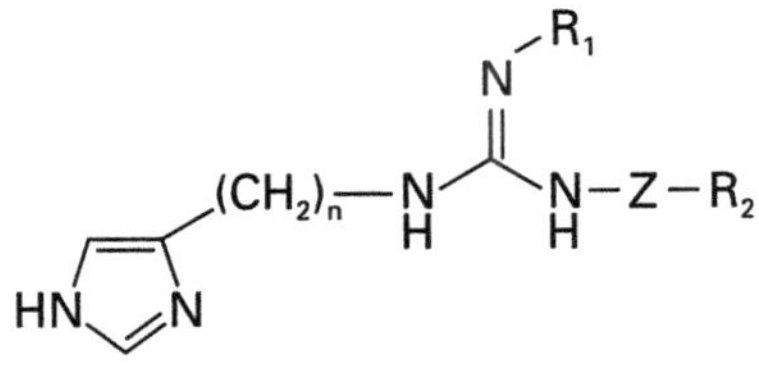

No.	Compound	n	R_1	Z	R_2	pA_2 value	Ref.
77	VUF 83100	2	H	–	H	$pD_2 = 6.3$[a] (7.4)[b,c]	[57, 60]
140	VUF 8845	2	NO_2	–	H	inactive[b]	[60]
141	VUF 9006	2	H	–	phenyl	5.8[a]	[57]
142	VUF 9007	2	H	$(CH_2)_2$	phenyl	6.3[a]	[57]
143	VUF 8411	2	H	$(CH_2)_2SCH_2$	phenyl	> 5.3[b]	[43]
144	SKF 91486	3	H	–	H	7.1[d]	[10]
145		3	H	CH_2	cyclohexyl	9.2[e] (8.8[f])	[72]
146		3	$CO_2C(CH_3)_3$	CH_2	cyclohexyl	8.7[e] (7.4[f])	[72]
147	VUF 8405	3	H	$(CH_2)_2SCH_2$	phenyl	7.9[a]	[57]
148	impromidine	3	H	$(CH_2)_2SCH_2$	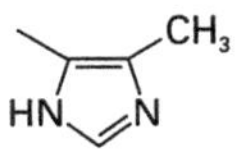	7.2[a]	[10]
149	VUF 8413	3	H	$(CH_2)_2SCH_2$	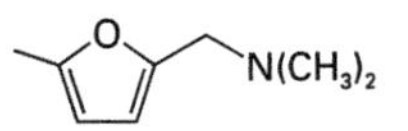	6.9[a]	[60]
150	VUF 8407	3	H	$(CH_2)_2SCH_2$	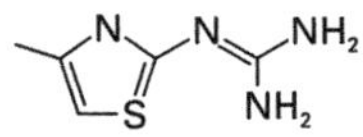	7.4[a]	[60]
151	VUF 8406	3	CN	$(CH_2)_2SCH_2$	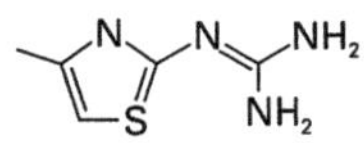	> 5.3[b]	[43]
152		4	$CO_2C(CH_3)_3$	–	cyclohexyl	7.3[e] (6.9[f])	[72]

Elongation of the ethylene chain of VUF 83100 (**77**) leads to the reasonably active H_3 antagonist SKF 91486 (**144**). A remarkable hundred-fold increase of H_3 antagonistic activity is observed when a cyclohexyl group, separated by a methylene group is introduced to the guanidine group of SKF 91486 (**144**) (see compound **145**). Esterification of the guanidine group of **145** reduces the antagonistic activity (compound **146**). It is worth noting that this reduction is more drastic on the guinea pig intestine assay than on the mouse cortex assay. The butylene derivative **152** is less active than its propylene analogues, but the compound is still reasonably active. This might also explain the moderate H_3 antagonistic properties of mifen-

Table 17. (Continued).

No.	Compound	Structure	pA_2 value	Ref.
153		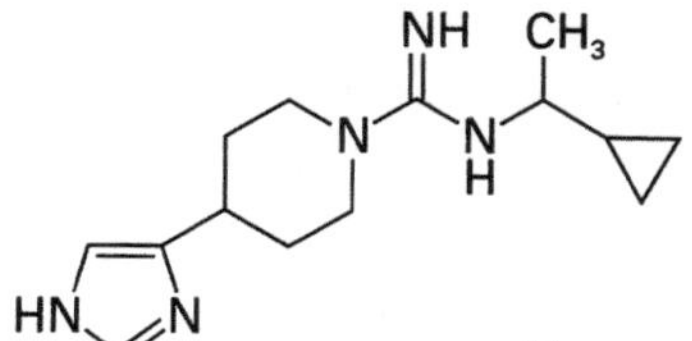	7.9[d]	[67]
154	mifentidine	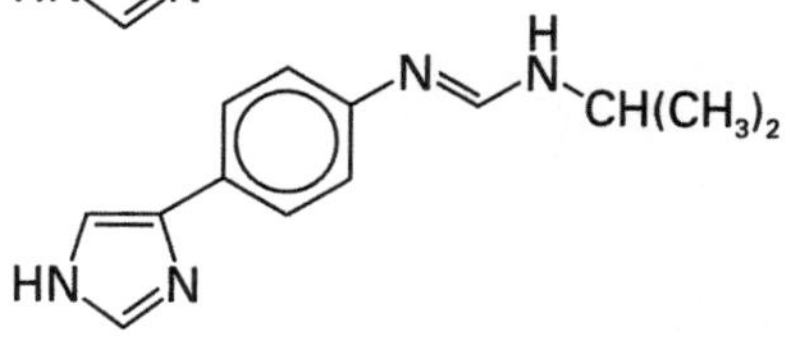	7.0[d]	[73]

[a] Determined by evaluation of the influence of the compound on electrically evoked, NANC contractions of guinea pig intestine preparations, as described by Menkveld et al. [42].
[b] Determined by evaluation of the influence of the compound on electrically-stimulated [^{3}H]-histamine release on rat cortex, as described by Van der Werf et al. [55].
[c] Partial agonist ($\alpha = 0.5$).
[d] Determined by evaluation of the influence of the compound on K^+-stimulated [^{3}H]-histamine release on rat cortex, as described by Arrang et al. [10].
[e] Determined by evalüation of the influence of the compound on electrically stimulated [^{3}H]-noradrenaline release on mouse cortex, as described by Schlicker et al. [28].
[f] Determined by evaluation of the influence of the compound on electrically evoked, cholinergic contractions of guinea pig intestine preparations, as described by Vollinga et al. [31].

tidine (**154**) (comparable distance between the imidazole ring and the amidine system).

The propylene chain between the imidazole ring and the amidine system however is optimal for antagonistic activity for this series of guanidine analogues, which was also observed for the isothiourea analogues, described in Table 16. Since both series of analogues are likely to interact in a comparable manner with the H_3 receptor, it seems that the nitrogen of the guanidine group, connected directly to the 4(5)-alkylimidazole moiety, is not required for binding.

2.2.3 *Derivatives of impromidine as H_3 antagonists*

The H_3 antagonistic activity of the H_2 agonist impromidine (**148**) has been described already in the first paper on the H_3 receptor [10]. The replacement of the propylene chain which separates the unsubstituted imidazole ring and the guanidine group, with an ethylene chain, results in a slight increase of antagonistic activity (see Table 18, compound **155**). Methyl-

Table 18.
Histamine H_3 antagonistic activity of some analogues of impromidine

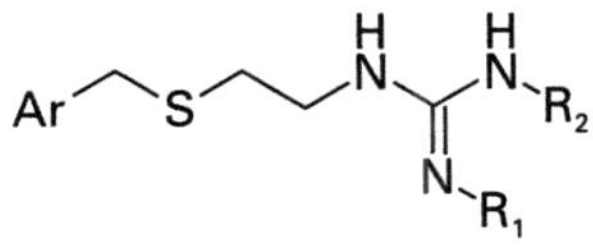

No.	Compound	Ar	R_1	R_2	pA_2 value[a]	Ref.
148	impromidine	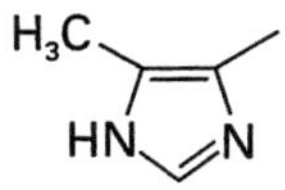	H	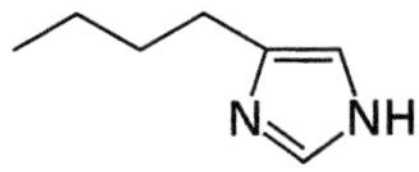	7.2	[10]
155		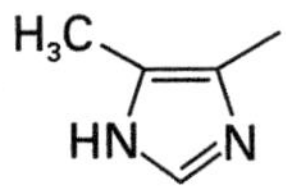	H	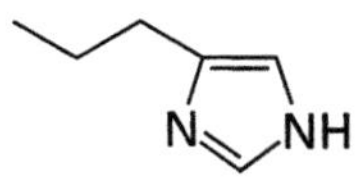	7.7	[45]
156	(S)-sopromidine	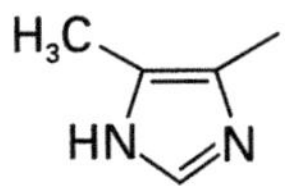	H	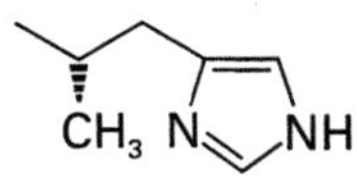	7.4	[54]
157	(R)-sopromidine	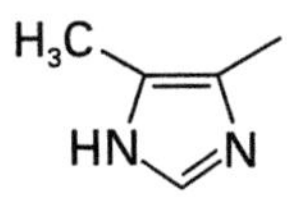	H	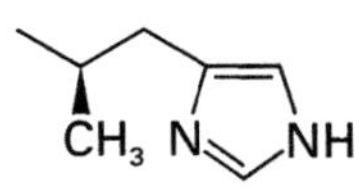	7.2	[54]
147	VUF 8405	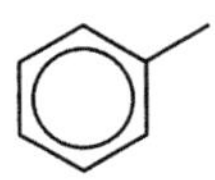	H	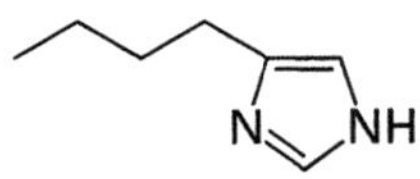	7.9[b]	[57]
150	VUF 8407	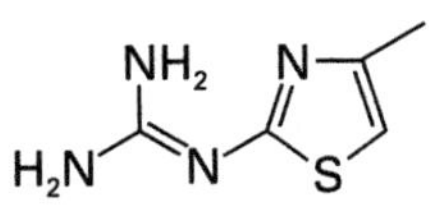	H	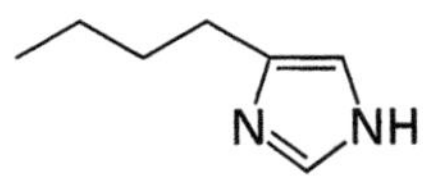	7.4[b]	[60]
149	VUF 8413	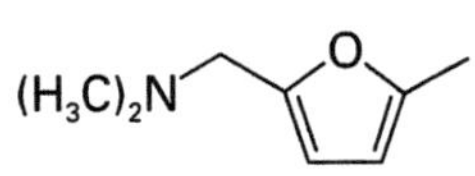	H	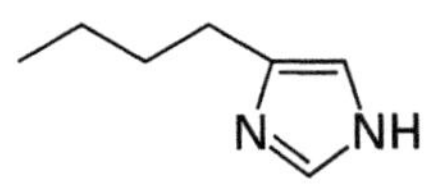	6.9[b]	[60]
158	cimetidine	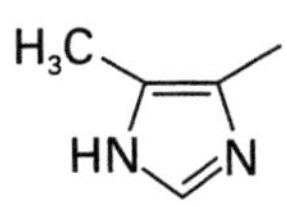	CN	CH_3	4.5	[10]
159	tiotidine	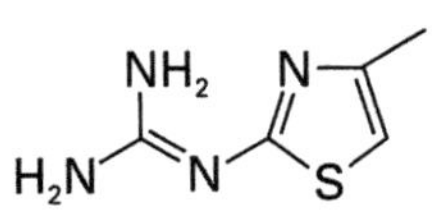	CN	CH_3	4.8	[60]

Table 18. (continued)

No.	Compound	Ar	R_1	R_2	pA_2 value[a]	Ref.
151	VUF 8406	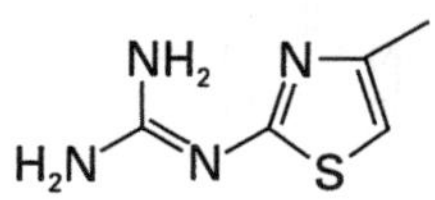	CN	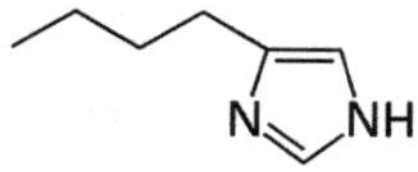	> 5.3[c]	[43]
160	ranitidine	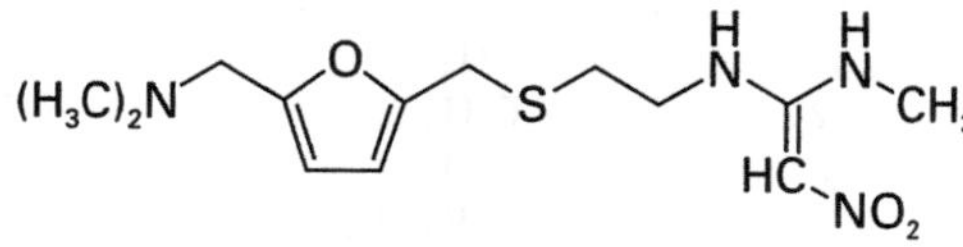			4.3	[60]

[a] Determined by evaluation of the influence of the compound on K+-stimulated [3H]-histamine release on rat cortex, as described by Arrang et al. [10].
[b] Determined by evaluation of the influence of the compound on electrically evoked, NANC contractions of guinea pig intestine preparations, as described by Menkveld et al. [42].
[c] Determined by evaluation of the influence of the compound on electrically-stimulated [3H]-histamine release on rat cortex, as described by Van der Werf et al. [55].

ation of the ethylene chain in a comparable manner to the one for α-methylhistamine, does not have much effect on the antagonistic activity (enantiomers of sopromidine **156** and **157**). Since no stereoselectivity can be observed between these compounds, an interaction of the unsubstituted imidazole ring in the same manner as for agonists does not have to be considered.

Replacement of the 5-methyl-imidazole ring of impromidine (**148**) is allowed. For instance VUF 8405 (**147**), in which the 5-methyl-imidazole ring is replaced by a phenyl group, is an even more potent H_3 antagonist than impromidine (**148**). This indicates that the 5-methyl-imidazole ring is not essential for the antagonistic activity of impromidine. This is confirmed by the observation that cimetidine (**158**) is almost inactive. Although the introduction of a cyano group to the guanidine, as with cimetidine, might have a negative effect on the antagonistic activity of the compound, it must be noted that VUF 8406 (**151**), which still contains the 4(5)-propylimidazole moiety, has been found to be more active as H_3 antagonist than its parent compound tiotidine (**159**). This means that the antagonistic activity of impromidine depends on the unsubstituted imidazole ring and the guanidine system, separated by an alkyl spacer (as described in Table 17) and not on the 5-methyl-imidazole part on the other side of the guanidine group.

Table 19.
Histamine H_3 antagonistic activity of several analogues of burimamide

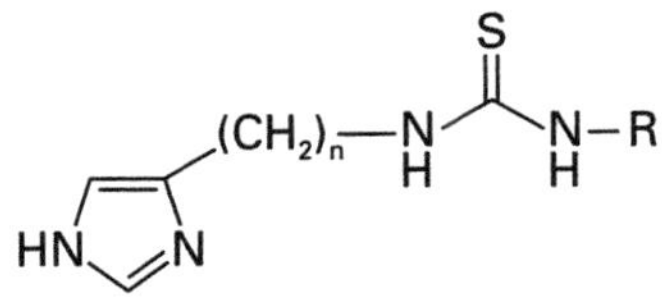

No.	Compound	n	R	pA_2 value[a]	Ref.
161	VUF 4577	2	CH_3	5.5	[74]
162	VUF 4578	2	C_2H_5	5.3	[74]
163	VUF 4579	2	C_3H_7	5.4	[74]
164	VUF 4580	2	$CH(CH_3)_2$	4.8	[74]
165	VUF 4581	2	c-C_6H_{11}	5.9	[74]
166	VUF 4582	2	C_6H_5	5.2	[74]
167	VUF 4583	2	$CH_2C_6H_5$	5.8	[74]
168	VUF 4584	2	$(CH_2)_2C_6H_5$	5.9	[74]
169	norburimamide	3	CH_3	6.1 (6.4[b])	[31, 73, 74]
170	VUF 4631	3	C_2H_5	7.1	[74]
171	VUF 4632	3	C_3H_7	7.0	[74]
172	VUF 4633	3	$CH(CH_3)_2$	7.1	[74]
173	VUF 4634	3	c-C_6H_{11}	6 9	[74]
174	VUF 4635	3	C_6H_5	6.9	[74]
175	VUF 4636	3	$CH_2C_6H_5$	6.7	[74]
176	VUF 4637	3	$(CH_2)_2C_6H_5$	6.7	[74]
177	burimamide	4	CH_3	7.1 (7.2[b])	[10, 31, 74]
178	VUF 4681	4	C_2H_5	7.4	[74]
179	VUF 4682	4	C_3H_7	7.3	[74]
180	VUF 4683	4	$CH(CH_3)_2$	7 5	[74]
181	VUF 4684	4	c-C_6H11	7 1	[741
182	VUF 4685	4	C_6H_5	7.6	[74]
183	VUF 4686	4	CH_2C_6Hs	6.8	[74]

2.2.4 *Derivatives of burimamide as H_3 antagonists*

2.2.4.1 Burimamide derivatives

The good antagonistic activity of the H_2 antagonist burimamide (**177**) for the H_3 receptor led to the development of a large series of burimamide analogues (see Table 19). In this series, the length of the alkyl chain, separating the imidazole ring from the thiourea group, was varied from an ethylene chain to a hexylene chain. Elongation of the alkyl chain clearly results in an increase of the H_3 antagonistic activity. Besides the activity, the selectivity for the H_3 receptor was also increased [74]. The pentylene- and hexylene analogues of burimamide are about ten times more potent

Table 19. (Continued).

No.	Compound	n	R	pA_2 value[a]	Ref.
184	VUF 4687	4	$(CH_2)_2C_6H_5$	7.0	[74]
185	VUF 4613	5	CH_3	8.0	[74]
186	VUF 4614	5	C_2H_5	8.0	[74]
187	VUF 4615	5	C_3H_7	7.7	[74]
188	VUF 4616	5	$CH(CH_3)_2$	7.7	[74]
189	VUF 4617	5	c-C_6H_{11}	7.5	[74]
190	VUF 4618	5	C_6H_5	7.6	[74]
191	VUF 4619	5	$CH_2C_6H_5$	7 7	[74]
192	VUF 4742	5	$CH_2C_6H_5$–(4)–Cl	8.1	[74]
193	VUF 4620	5	$(CH_2)_2C_6H_5$	7.5	[74]
194	VUF 4740	6	CH_3	7.9	[74]
195	VUF 4741	6	C_6H_5	8.0	[74]
196	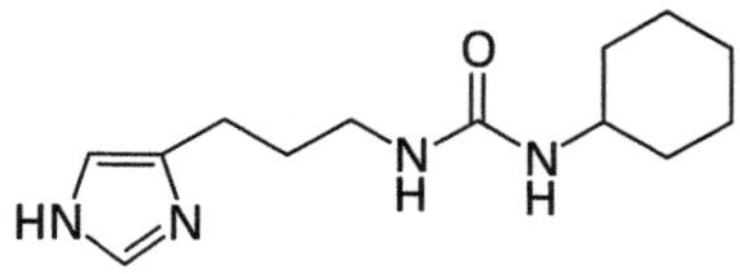			7.3	[72]
197	metiamide 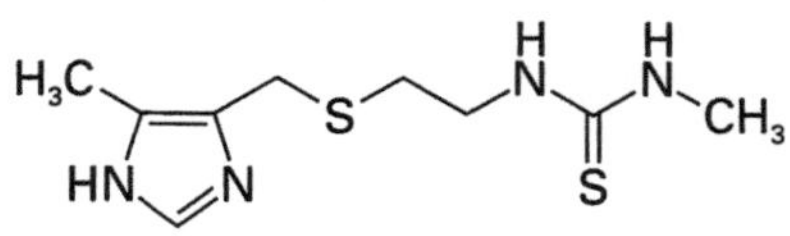			5.6[b]	[10]

[a] Determined by evaluation of the influence of the compound on electrically evoked, cholinergic contractions of guinea pig intestine preparations, as described by Vollinga et al. [31].
[b] Determined by evaluation of the influence of the compound on K^+-stimulated $[^3H]$-histamine release on rat cortex, as described by Arrang et al. [10].

than burimamide (**177**) itself, whereas the affinity for the H_2 receptor for the pentylene series was 100–1000-fold lower. Whereas the length of the alkyl spacer had a large influence on the H_3 antagonistic activity, the N-thiourea substituents hardly influence the activity. This could mean that this series of antagonists bind in a non-lipophilic environment to the receptor, different from e.g. the amidine analogues described in Table 16 and 17. Also in the burimamide series, methylation of the imidazole ring seems to be disastrous, since metiamide (**197**) is only a very weak antagonist. The replacement of the thiourea group of VUF 4634 (**173**) with an urea group (compound **196**) is obviously allowed.

Table 20.
Histamine H_3 antagonistic activity of some analogues of thioperamide

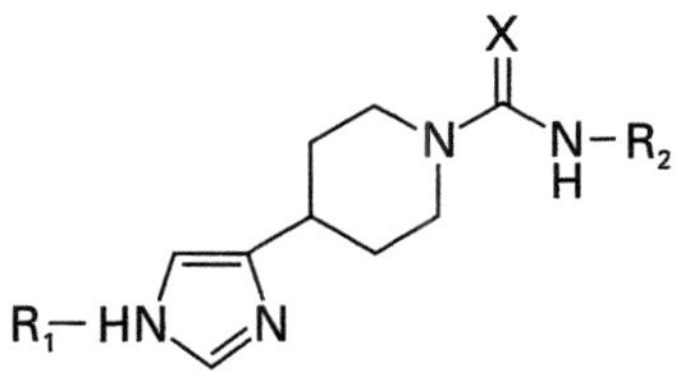

No.	R_1	X	R_2	pA_2 value[a]	Ref.
198	H	S	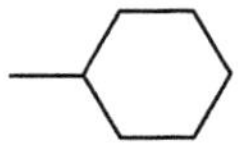	8.9[b]	[10, 31]
199	H	S	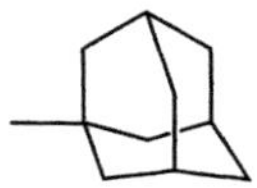	7.5	[67]
200	H	NH	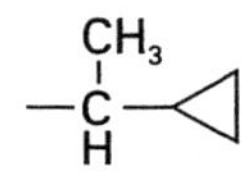	7.9	[67]
201	H	O	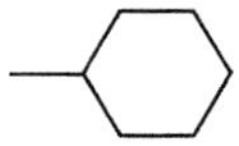	7.4	[67]
202	H	O	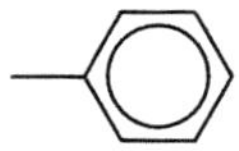	6.8	[67]
203	H	O	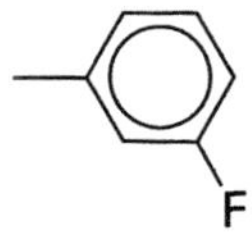	7.6	[67]
204	H	O	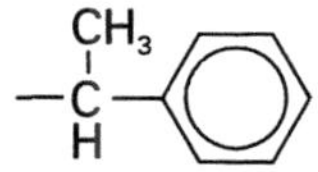	8.0	[67]
205	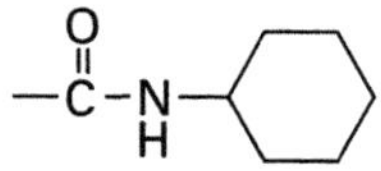	O	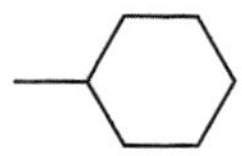	7.6	[67]

Table 20. (Continued)

No.	R_1	X	R_2	pA_2 value[a]	Ref.
206	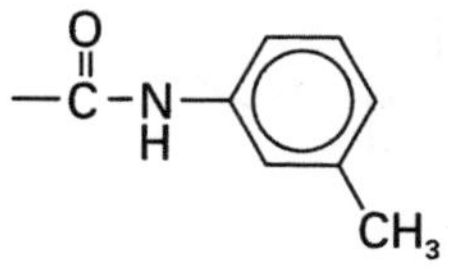	O	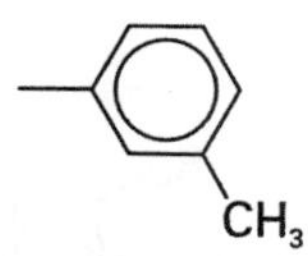	7.1	[67]
207	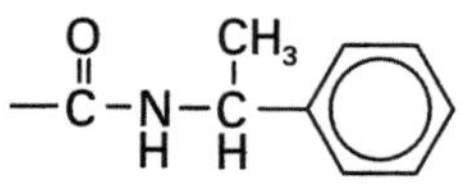	O	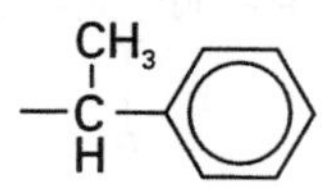	7.7	[67]
208	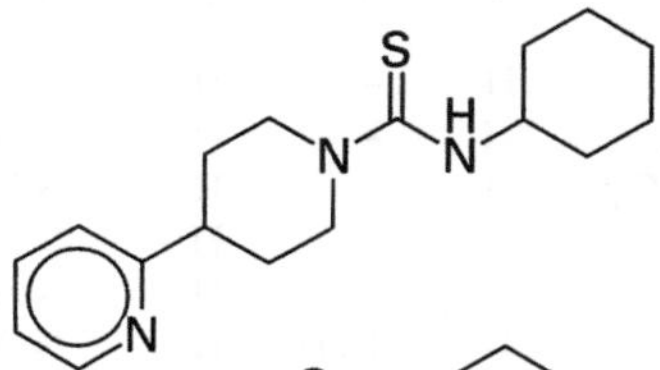			4.9	[45]
209	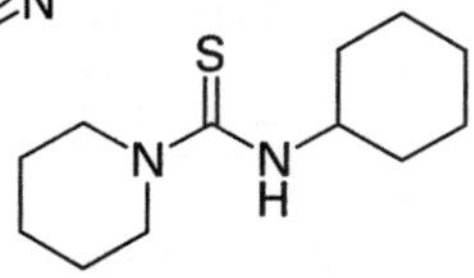			< 5.0	[76]
210	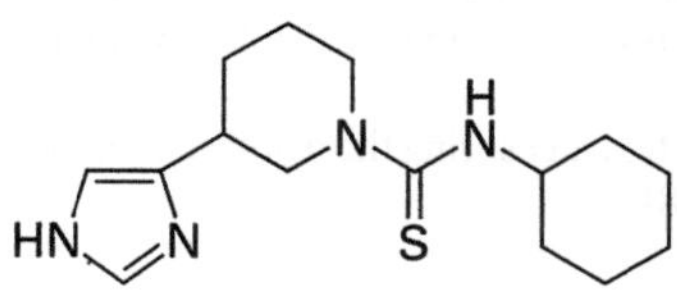			7.4	[67]

[a] Determined by evaluation of the influence of the compound on K^+-stimulated [^{3}H]-histamine release on rat cortex, as described by Arrang et al. [10].
[b] Same value determined by evaluation of the influence of the compound on electrically evoked, cholinergic contractions of guinea pig intestine preparations, as described by Vollinga et al. [31].

2.2.4.2 Thioperamide derivatives

The first potent and selective antagonist for the H_3 receptor was thioperamide (**198**), which in fact can be regarded as a rigid analogue of norburimamide (**169**) and VUF 4634 (**173**). According to patent literature [67], replacement of the cyclohexyl ring with the bulky adamantane group results in a large decrease of antagonistic activity (compound **199**). Moreover the replacement of the thiourea group of thioperamide by an urea group, results in a less active compound (**201**). This is puzzling, since the substitution of a thiourea group of norburimamide (**169**) by an urea group (see Table 19, compound **196**), does not result in a decrease of activity.

Table 21.
Histamine H_3 antagonistic activity of some substituted thioperamide analogues

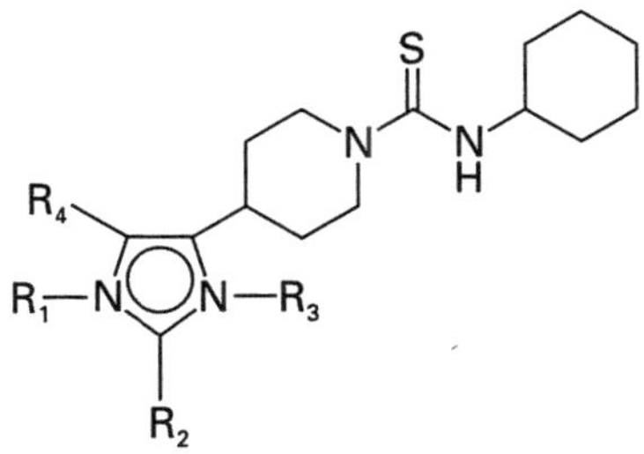

No.	Compound	R_1	R_2	R_2	R_2	pA_2 value[a]	pK_i value	Ref.
198	thioperamide	H	H	–	H	8.9	8.5[b]	[75, 77]
211	N^{τ}-methylthioperamide	CH_3	H	–	H	6.8	6.8[b]	[75, 77, 78]
212	N^{τ}-benzylthioperamide	$CH_2C_6H_5$	H	–	H	N.D.	< 6.0[c]	[78]
213	2-methylthioperamide	H	CH_3	–	H	N.A.	4.5[b]	[75, 77]
214	2-aminothioperamide	H	NH_2	–	H	N.A.	< 4.0[b]	[75, 77]
215	N^{π}-methylthioperamide	—	H	CH_3	H	N.A.	5.6[b]	[75, 77]
216	5-methylthioperamide	H	H	–	CH_3	8.4	6.8[b]	[75, 77]
217	5-aminothioperamide	H	H	–	NH_2	N.A.	< 4.0[b]	[75, 77]

N.D. = Not Determined; N.A. = Not Active

[a] Determined by evaluation of the influence of the compound on electrically evoked, cholinergic contractions of guinea pig intestine preparations, as described by Vollinga et al. [31].

[b] Affinity value, determined on rat cortex, measuring the displacement of $[^3H]$ N^{α}-methylhistamine, as described by Bordi et al. [77].

[c] Affinity value, determined on rat cortex, measuring the displacement of $[^3H]$ N^{α}-methylhistamine, as described by Amin Khan et al. [78].

Apparently norburimamide (**169**) and its rigid analogue thioperamide (**198**), bind in a distinct manner to the receptor. Substituents on the N^{τ}-position of the imidazole ring of some urea-containing thioperamide analogues are allowed (e.g. compound **201** compared to compound **205**). More substitutions on the imidazole ring of thioperamide have been performed (see Table 21). For thioperamide (**198**), methylation of the N^{τ}-position leads to a drastic decrease of activity (N^{τ}-methylthioperamide, **211**), but methylation of the N^{π}-position results in a completely inactive compound **215**.

Whereas substituents on the 2-position are not allowed (2-methylthioperamide, **213**, Table 21), 5-methylthioperamide (**216**) has been reported to be a potent antagonist [75]. There is however a remarkable discrepancy between the antagonistic activity of 5-methylthioperamide (**216**) as determined on the guinea pig intestine assay and the much lower affinity of this compound determined on a rat cortex binding assay (Table 21). At this moment there is still no clear idea about H_3 receptor subtypes, but this compound might be of interest in this respect.

2.2.5 Miscellaneous ω-functionalized 4(5)-alkyl imidazoles

2.2.5.1 Amides

The observation that the most simple N^{α}-acylated derivative of histamine, N^{α}-acetylhistamine (**218**), displayed weak H_3 antagonistic activity, led to the development of a series of acylated analogues of histamine (see Table 22). The introduction of a lipophilic group (e.g. a phenyl- or cycloalkyl group), to the amide group, separated by an alkyl chain results in moderately active antagonists.

It appears that the distance of the lipophilic group relatively to the imidazole ring is determining the activity and not the position of the amide group, since **224** and **226** are as potent as **231** and **234**, respectively. Apparently the polar group in the side chain is less important for this series of analogues. Also the exchange of the amide group by a thioamide group does not influence the activity (if compound **233** and **240** are compared). Whereas the introduction of a lipophilic group enhances the activity, the introduction of a heterocycle does not increase the potency (comparing **226** and **227**). Branching of the side chain of these amide analogues leads to an increased activity (see compound **234** and **242**). Methylation in the α-position of **224** however, with the same stereochemistry as (R)-α-methylhistamine (**21**), results in only a weak antagonist **236**. Methylation or replacement of the imidazole ring is again not allowed.

A remarkable compound is verongamine (**237**), fitting perfectly in this series of compounds. It has been reported as an H_3 antagonist, but only affinity data were provided [80, 82]. Verongamine (**237**) is isolated from the marine sponge *Verongula gigantea* and is therefore probably the first discovered endogenous compound with H_3 antagonistic properties.

2.2.5.2 Carbamates, esters and ketones

Other carbonylic histamine derivatives have also been described as H_3 antagonists, like the carbamates presented in Table 23. All these compounds are good antagonists, with comparable activities. The carbamate group may even be replaced by a ketone and the activity remains (compound **259**), again diminishing the importance of the polar group for this series of antagonists. Replacement of the carbamate group by an ester group has resulted in a marked increase of activity however (if **253** is compared with **245**). Unfortunately, only an extensive series of carbamate derivatives has been reported.

Table 22.
Histamine H_3 antagonistic activity of several N^{α}-acylated histamine analogues

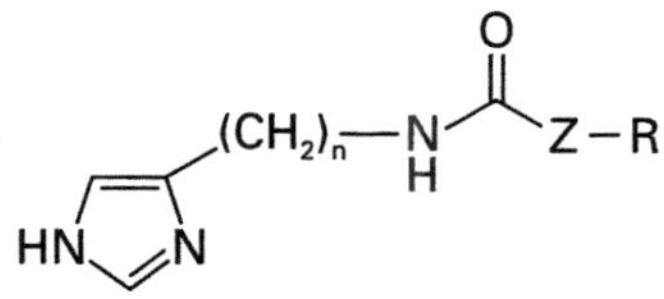

No.	n	Z	R	pA_2 value[a]	Ref.
218	2	–	methyl	5.9	[79]
219	2	CH_2	phenyl	6.0	[64]
220	2	$(CH_2)_2$	phenyl	6.2	[64]
221	2	CH_2O	phenyl	6.1	[64]
222	2	CH_2S	CH(phenyl)$_2$	6.0	[64]
223	2	$(CH_2)_2$	CH(phenyl)$_2$	6.0	[64]
224	2	$(CH_2)_3$	phenyl	7.1	[64]
225	2	CH_2SCH_2	phenyl	6.2	[64]
226	2	$(CH_2)_3$	cyclohexyl	7.3	[64]
227	2	$(CH_2)_3$	4(5)-imidazolyl	6.0	[64]
228	2	$(CH_2)_3$	2-pyridyl	6.0	[64]
229	2	CH_2SCH_2	2-pyridyl	5.7	[64]
230	2	$(CH_2)_4$	phenyl	6.7	[64]
231	3	$(CH_2)_2$	phenyl	7.3	[71]
232	3	CH_2CHCH_3	phenyl	7.5	[71]
233	3	$(CH_2)_2$	cyclopentyl	7.2[b] (7.6[c])	[72]
234	3	$(CH_2)_2$	cyclohexyl	7.3[b] (7.6[c])	[72]
235	3	$(CH_2)_3$	cyclohexyl	7.2	[71]
236		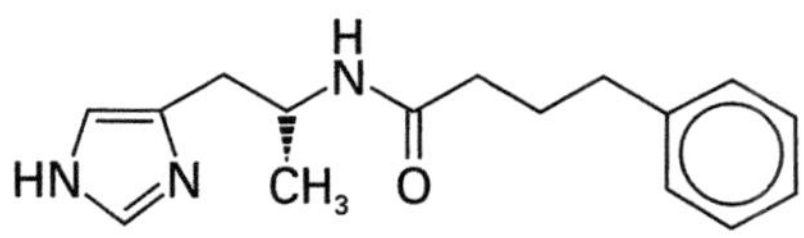		6.0	[79]
237[d]		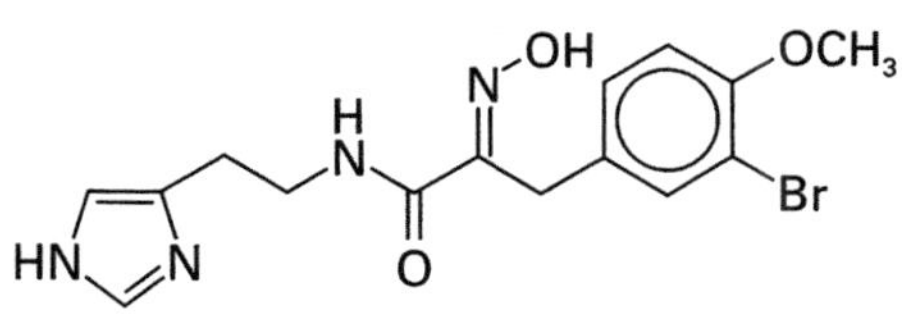		pK_i = 6.3[e]	[80]
238		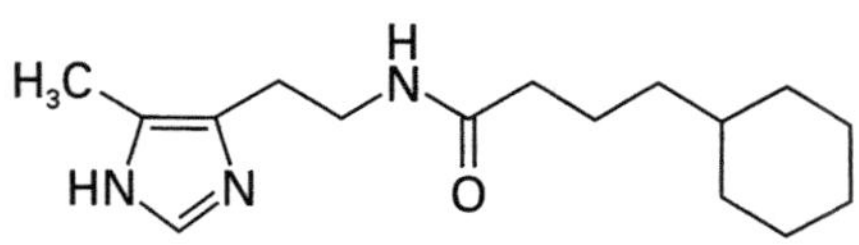		< 5.0	[79]
239		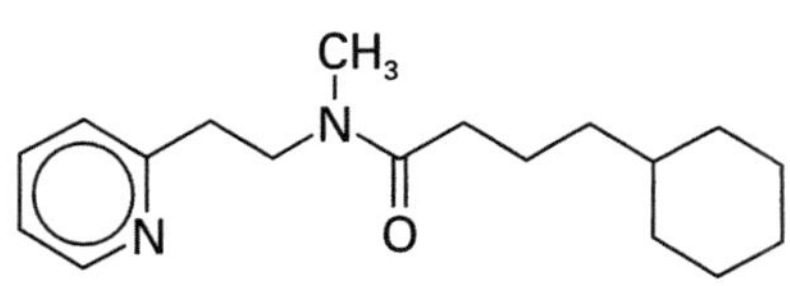		< 5.0	[64]

Table 22. (Continued).

No.	Structure	pA_2 value[a]	Ref.
240	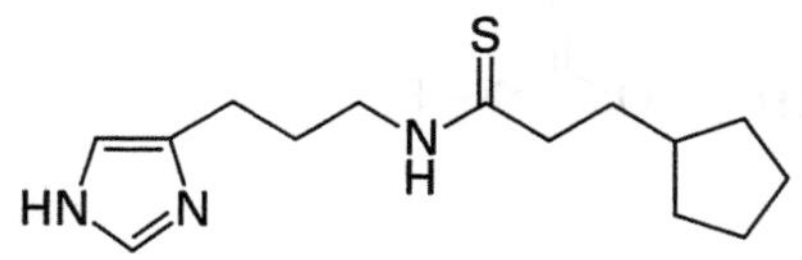	7.4[b] (7.6[c])	[72]
241	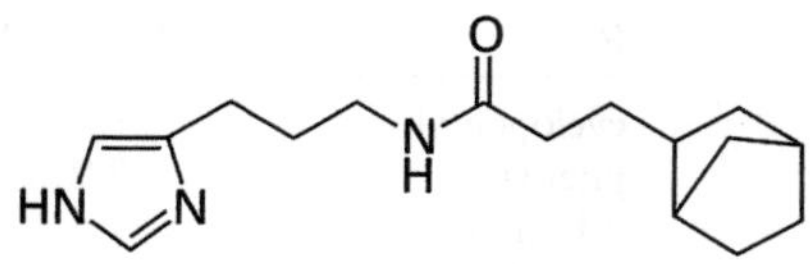	7.5[b] (7.7[c])	[72]
242	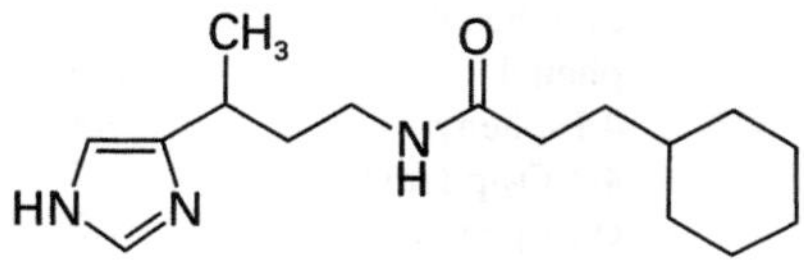	8.0[b] (7.8[c])	[72]
243	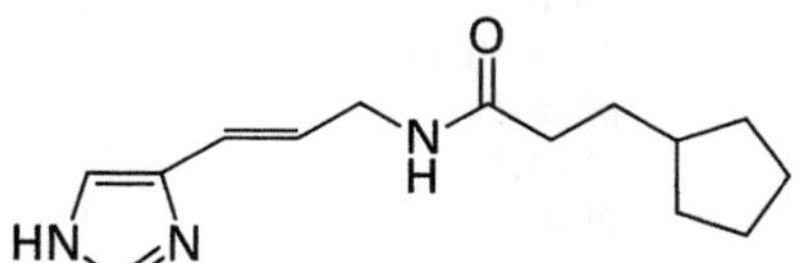	7.4	[71]
244	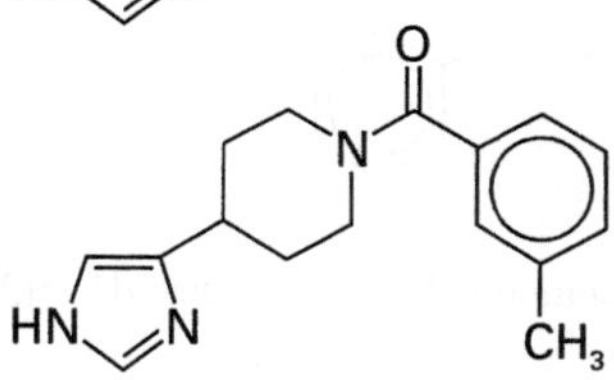	7.3	[67]

[a] Determined by evaluation of the influence of the compound on K^+-stimulated $[^3H]$-histamine release on rat cortex, as described by Arrang et al. [10].
[b] Determined by evaluation of the influence of the compound on the electrically stimulated $[^3H]$-noradrenaline release on mouse cortex, as described by Schlicker et al. [28].
[c] Affinity value (pK_i), determined on rat cortex, measuring the displacement of $[^3H]$ N^{α}-methylhistamine, as described by Kathmann et al. [81].
[d] Verongamine.
[e] Affinity value, determined on guinea pig brain tissue, measuring the displacement of $[^3H]$ N^{α}-methylhistamine, as described by Korte et al. [51].

2.2.5.3 Ethers

The observation that with the carbonylic antagonists, discussed above, there is no great importance of a functional polar group, seems to be confirmed by a series of ether derivatives (see Table 24). In this series, the functional group has been replaced by an oxygen atom and a variety of

Table 23.
Histamine H_3 antagonstic activity of several carbonylic histaminergic imidazole derivatives

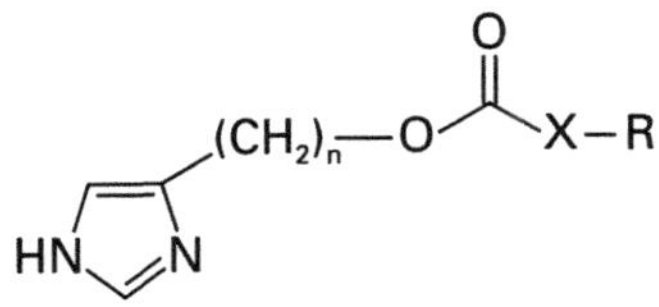

No.	n	X	R	pA_2 value[a]	Ref.
245	3	$(CH_2)_2$	cyclopentyl	8.5	[71]
246	3	NH	phenyl	7.9	[83]
247	3	NH	3-F-phenyl	7.6	[83]
248	3	NH	4-F-phenyl	7.6	[71]
249	3	NH	cyclohexyl	7.2	[83]
250	3	$NHCH_2$	phenyl	8.0	[83]
251	3	$NHCH_2$	4-F-phenyl	7.6	[83]
252	3	$NHCH_2$	4-NO_2-phenyl	7.7	[71]
253	3	$NHCH_2$	cyclopentyl	7.2	[83]
254	3	$NHCH_2$	cyclohexyl	8.0	[83]
255	3	$NHCH_2$	2-thiophenyl	7.7	[83]
256	3	NCH_3CH_2	phenyl	7.7	[71]
257	3	NHCO	phenyl	7.3	[71]
258	3	$NH(CH_2)_2$	phenyl	8.0	[83]
259		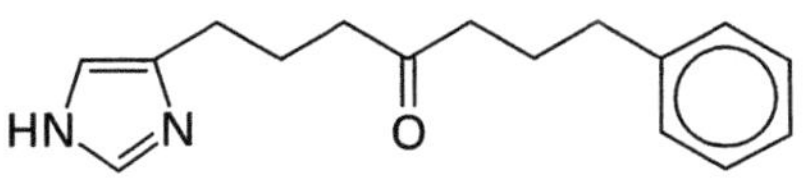		7.7	[71]

[a] Determined by evaluation of the influence of the compound on K^+-stimulated [^{3}H]-histamine release on rat cortex, as described by Arrang et al. [10].

lipophilic groups with different steric and electronic parameters have been introduced, but all the compounds are comparable good antagonists. From this series of compounds, Ligneau et al. [84] recently developed iodoproxyfan (**272**) as a radiolabel for the H_3 receptor. This will be discussed in detail in section 3.1.

2.2.6 *Derivatives of dimaprit as H_3 antagonists*

In addition to impromidine (**148**), another H_2 agonist that has been shown to display H_3 antagonistic activity is dimaprit (**284**) (Table 25).
A few derivatives of dimaprit (**284**) have been investigated; the results are presented in Table 25. Variation in the alkyl chain length results in the compounds nordimaprit (**285**) and homodimaprit (**286**). Whereas shortening of the alkyl chain of dimaprit (**284**) causes a decrease of activ-

Table 24.
Histamine H_3 antagonistic activity of several ether derivatives of histamine

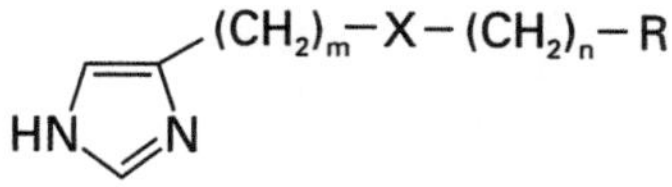

No.	m	n	R	pA_2 value[a]	Ref.
260	2	0	4-CN-phenyl	8.0	[71]
261	2	0	4-C_3H_7-phenyl	7.7	[71]
262	2	0	4-NO_2-phenyl	7.5	[71]
263	2	0	2-naphthyl	7.0	[71]
264	3	0	4-CN-phenyl	7.9	[71]
265	3	0	4-CF_3-phenyl	7.8	[71]
266	3	1	phenyl	7.7	[85]
267	3	1	3-F-phenyl	7.9	[85]
268	3	1	3-I-phenyl	8.2	[86]
269	3	1	4-Br-phenyl	7.9	[85]
270	3	1	4-Cl-phenyl	7.7	[86]
271	3	1	4-F-phenyl	8.0	[85]
272[b]	3	1	4-I-phenyl	8.3	[86]
272[b]	3	1	4-[^{125}I]-phenyl	pK_i = 10.2[c]	[84]
273	3	1	cyclohexyl	8.0	[85]
274	3	1	1-naphthyl	7.7	[85]
275	3	1	2-naphthyl	7.7	[85]
276	3	1	2-quinolyl	7.3	[85]
277	3	1	4-biphenyl	7.2	[85]
278	3	2	phenyl	7.6	[86]
279	3	3	phenyl	7.8	[86]
280	3	3	4-Br-phenyl	7.8	[71]
281	3	3	4-Cl-phenyl	7.9	[71]
282	3	3	4-F-phenyl	8.2	[71]
283	3	3	cyclohexyl	7.7	[71]

[a] Determined by evaluation of the influence of the compound on K^+-stimulated [^{3}H]-histamine release on rat cortex, as described by Arrang et al. [10].
[b] Iodoproxyfan.
[c] Affinity value, determined on rat cortex [84].

ity, elongation does not effect the activity very much. There is no change in activity when the dimethylamino group of dimaprit is replaced by an isothiourea group (as in VUF 8333, **287**). Shortening of the alkyl chain of **287** to two methylene units does not effect the activity (VUF 8332, **99**). This is not unexpected, since the distance between the amino group and the isothiourea group of homodimaprit (**286**) is comparable to the distance of a nitrogen atom from one of the isothiourea groups of VUF 8332 (**99**) to the other isothiourea group.

Table 25.
Histamine H_3 antagonistic activity of some analogues of dimaprit

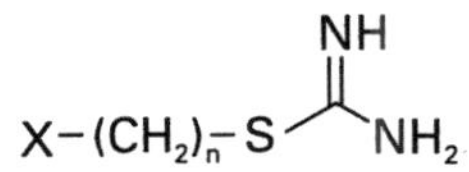

No.	Compound	X	n	pA_2 value	pK_i value[a]	Ref.
284	dimaprit	$(CH_3)_2N$	3	6.2[b] (5.5[c])	6.6	[73, 81]
285	nordimaprit	$(CH_3)_2N$	2	5.6[b,d]	6.0	[81]
286	homodimaprit	$(CH_3)_2N$	4	6.0[b] (5.8[e])	6.4	[60, 81]
99	VUF 8332	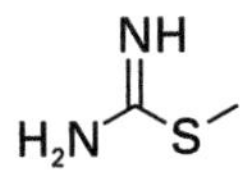	2	6.0[f]		[60]
287	VUF 8333	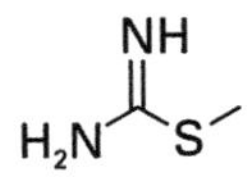	3	6.0[f]		[60]

[a] Affinity value, determined on rat cortex, measuring the displacement of [^{3}H] N$^\alpha$-methylhistamine, as described by Kathmann et al. [81].
[b] Determined by evaluation of the influence of the compound on electrically stimulated [^{3}H]-noradrenaline release on mouse cortex, as described by Schlicker et al. [28].
[c] Determined by evaluation of the influence of the compound on K^+-stimulated [^{3}H]-histamine release on rat cortex, as described by Arrang et al. [10].
[d] Reversible non-competitive antagonism.
[e] Determined by evaluation of the influence of the compound on electrically evoked, NANC contractions of guinea pig intestine preparations, as described by Menkveld et al. [42].
[f] Determined by evaluation of the influence of the compound on electrically-stimulated [^{3}H]-histamine release on rat cortex, as described by Van der Werf et al. [55].

2.2.7 *Miscellaneous H_3 antagonists*

A few other compounds with activity at histaminergic receptors, but lacking an imidazole ring, have been screened for H_3 antagonism. The potent H_1 antagonists chlorpheniramine (**289**) (both enantiomers were tested), mepyramine (**290**) and cyclizine (**291**) do not display any potent antagonistic H_3 activity (see Table 26). Moreover, the H_2 antagonist zolantidine (**292**) is described to be inactive as an H_3 antagonist as well. Betahistine (**288**), which has been described as a weak agonist on the H_1- and the H_2 receptor, displays a very weak antagonistic activity on the H_3 receptor. Finally, two laboratories recently described that the atypical neuroleptic clozapine displays a high affinity for the H_3 receptor and functionally behaves as an antagonist [87, 88]. In view of its semi-rigid structure clozapine might be very useful for molecular modelling studies.

Table 26.
Histamine H_3 antagonistic activity of some miscellaneous comounds.

No.	Compound	Structure	pA_2 value[a]	Ref.
288	betahistine	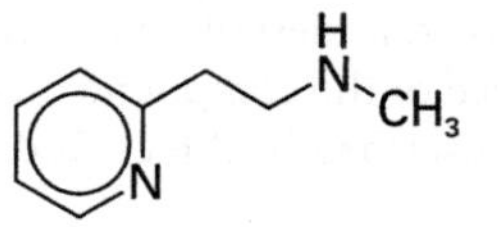	5.2	[89]
289	chlorpheniramine	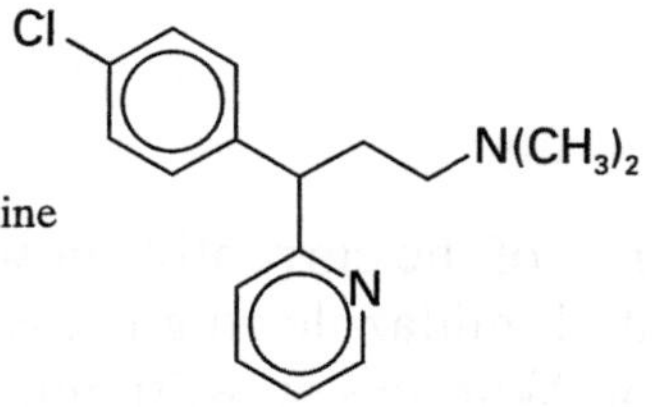	< 7.2[b]	[10]
290	mepyramine	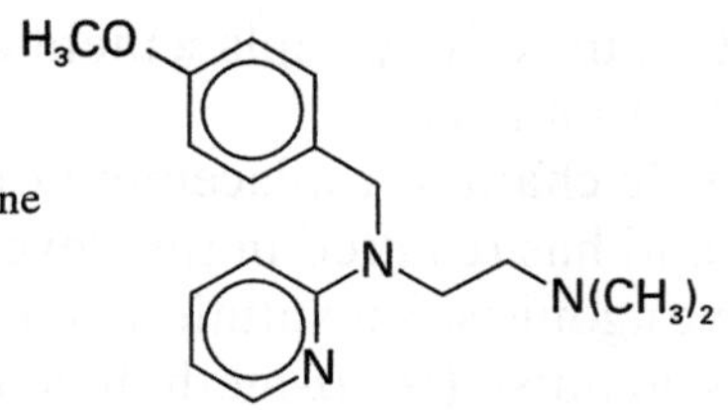	< 5.5	[73]
291	cyclizine	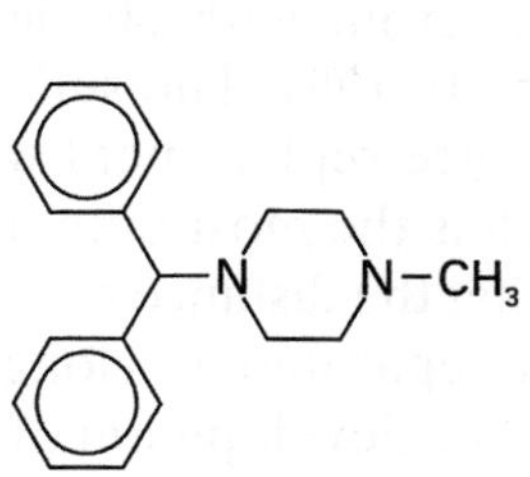	< 6.2	[10]
292	zolantidine	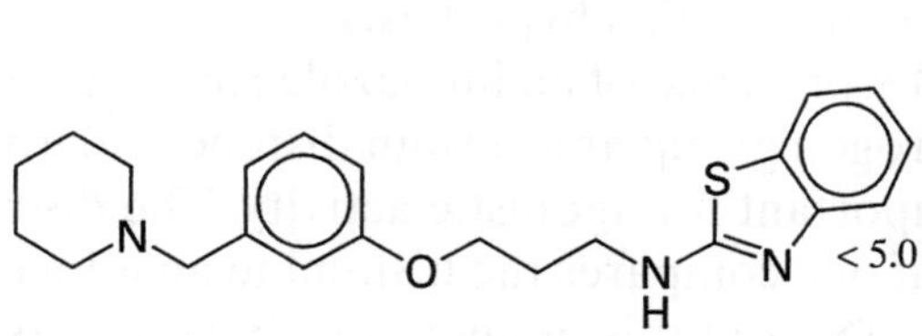	< 5.0	[73]
293	clozapine	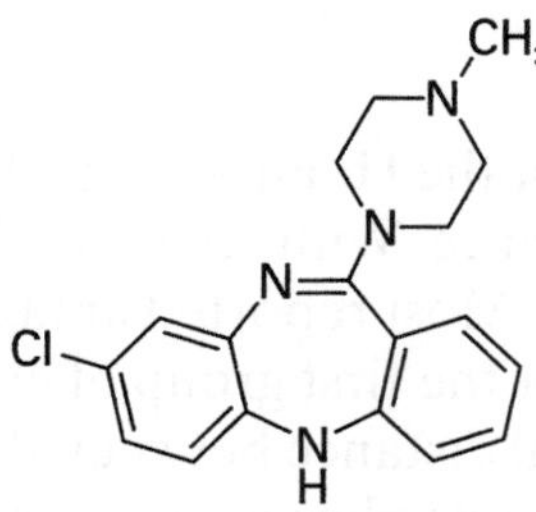	6.3[c] (7.1[d])	[87, 88]

[a] Determined by evaluation of the influence of the compound on K^+-stimulated [^{3}H]-histamine release on rat cortex, as described by Arrang et al. [10].
[b] Both enantiomers; pA_2 value < 7.2.
[c] Determined by evaluation of the influence of the compound on electrically stimulated [^{3}H]-noradrenaline release on mouse cortex, as described by Schlicker et al. [28].
[d] Determined by evaluation of the influence of the compound on electrically stimulated [^{3}H]-serotonin release on rat cortex, as described by Alves Rodrigues et al. [88].

2.3 Conclusions

2.3.1 H_3 agonists

Comparing the different structures of the currently known H_3 agonists, it is clear that the 4(5)-substituted imidazole ring is essential for agonistic activity at the H_3 receptor. Whereas substituents on the imidazole ring lead to a strong reduction in activity, replacement of the imidazole group results in inactive compounds.
Substitution of the ethylamino side chain or replacement of the amino group is in some cases allowed and has resulted in the development of several highly potent and selective agonists. Substitution of the side chain has resulted in the potent H_3 agonist (R)-α-methylhistamine (**21**), whereas replacement of the amino group with a basic isothiourea group resulted in the potent agonist imetit (**75**). The sulfur atom in the isothiourea group is not essential, since replacement with a carbon atom resulted in SKF 91606 (**76**), which is the most potent agonist known so far. This compound also stresses that the distance between the basic function and the imidazole ring can be separated by a longer alkyl chain than the ethylene chain in histamine. The development of the agonist immepip (**88**) fully confirms this hypothesis.
Apparently the presence of an imidazole ring and a basic function with a cationic nitrogen group at a certain distance relative to the heterocyclic ring is important for agonistic activity. The discrepancies between this distance if one compares the histamine anaologues with imetit (**75**) and immepip (**88**) is at this moment not fully understood.

2.3.1 H_3 antagonists

As found for the agonists also for the H_3 antagonist the 4(5)-substituted imidazole ring is of great importance. With regard to the side chain many variations appear to be allowed. Most reported antagonists can be classified into four main groups. For the first group of elongated histamine and imetit analogues the optimal distance between the imidazole group and the cationic nitrogen was found to be around a pentylene chain. This has e.g. resulted in the potent antagonist impentamine (**111**). Substitution of the isothiourea of the elongated imetit analogues with highly lipophilic aralkyl moieties led to very potent antagonists like clobenpropit (**131**). Since it can be hypothesized that the elongated histamine and imetit analogues bind to the same sites in the receptor, it is of great interest to investigate the introduction of lipophilic substituents in impentamine.

The second group of antagonists is formed by the burimamide analogues. These compounds probably bind in a distinct manner to the receptor protein with a nonprotonated (at physiological pH) thiourea group. In contrast to the imetit analogues the introduction of lipophilic substituents does not lead to improvement of the antagonistic potency. Variation of the chain length of the alkyl spacer of the burimamide analogues has a large effect on the H_3 antagonistic activity.

Although thioperamide can be regarded as a rigid analogue of norburimamide, this compound seems to exhibit a different binding behaviour towards the H_3 receptor than the more flexible burimamide analogues. Replacement of the thiourea group of thioperamide by an urea group leads to a strong decrease in activity. Yet, in the burimamide series a similar replacement does not affect the activity (see e.g. VUF 4634 **173** vs **196**). Therefore it seems that the analogues of burimamide and thioperamide interact in different ways with the H_3 receptor.

Finally, there is a large series of compounds in which the functional group is of less importance and is even not protonated. Especially the ether analogues in table 24 show a high potency. Apparently the lipophilic moiety, separated from the imidazole ring by an alkyl spacer is sufficient for H_3 antagonistic activity.

3 Molecular pharmacology of the H_3 receptor

Following the extensive description of the medicinal chemistry of the H_3 receptor ligands, attention will be given to the protein target. In recent years, the availability of highly specific and potent ligands has greatly increased the possibilities for molecular pharmacological research. In turn, only detailed knowlegde of the protein target will finally lead to rational drug design.

3.1 Radioligands for the H_3 receptor

3.1.1 Radiolabeled H_3 agonists

Due to the availability of various compounds with a reasonably high affinity, currently, several radioligands for the H_3 receptor are available. With the initial description of (R)-α-methylhistamine (Fig. 2) as a selective ligand for the H_3 receptor [16], the tritiated compound has been used as a radioligand for the H_3 receptor [16, 90]. Saturable binding of $[^3H]$(R)-α-methylhistamine to membranes of rat cerebral cortex can be found, yielding a K_D-value of 0.3–0.4 nM and (depending on the laboratory) a receptor density of 30–130 fmol/mg of protein [16, 90, 91]. The $[^3H]$(R)-α-methylhistamine binding site was pharmacologically characterized as an H_3 receptor by e.g. the stereoselective displacement by the enantiomers of α-methylhistamine [90]. Yet, some observations argue against the simple labeling of the pharmacologically defined H_3 receptor. Both monophasic and biphasic inhibition (Hill coefficient of 0.48) of the binding was observed for the H_3 antagonist burimamide [90, 91]. Moreover, whereas the affinity of the antagonists corresponded rather well with their potency in the histamine release assay, agonists showed a 5- to 10-fold higher activity in the $[^3H]$(R)-α-methylhistamine binding assay. This last finding might be explained by the selective labeling of the high affinty state of the G-protein-coupled receptor [90]. The $[^3H]$(R)-α-methylhistamine binding sites were furthermore strangly affected by calcium and guanine nucleotides [90]. In the presence of calcium a high and low $[^3H]$(R)-α-methylhistamine affinity was observed; only the low affinity component was sensitive to guanine nucleotides, whereas normally the high affinity component of agonist binding is affected. Finally, in kinetic experiments evidence for the presence of two separate sites was reported [91, 92]. Yet, the two sites are indistinguishable at equilibrium as the Hill coefficients of several displacers are close to unity [91]. At this point it is not clear how this apparent heterogeneity should be explained.

Also N^{α}-methylhistamine (Fig. 2) has been used to label the H_3 receptor. This compound has been labeled to a higher specific activity and thus provides a higher sensitivity than $[^3H]$(R)-α-methylhistamine. This ligand binds with high affinity (K_D = 0.4 nM) to a simple class of H_3-receptors in guinea-pig brain (41 fmol/mg protein) which were characterized as H_3-receptors by means of displacement studies [51]. Detailed analysis of the binding data (kinetics, Hill-coefficients) was not provided, which excludes the possibility of revealing heterogeneity. Recently West et al. [93] used the same probe to identify H_3 receptors in rat brain. Whereas under equilibrium conditions $[^3H]N^{\alpha}$-methylhistamine labels a single site (K_D = 0.4

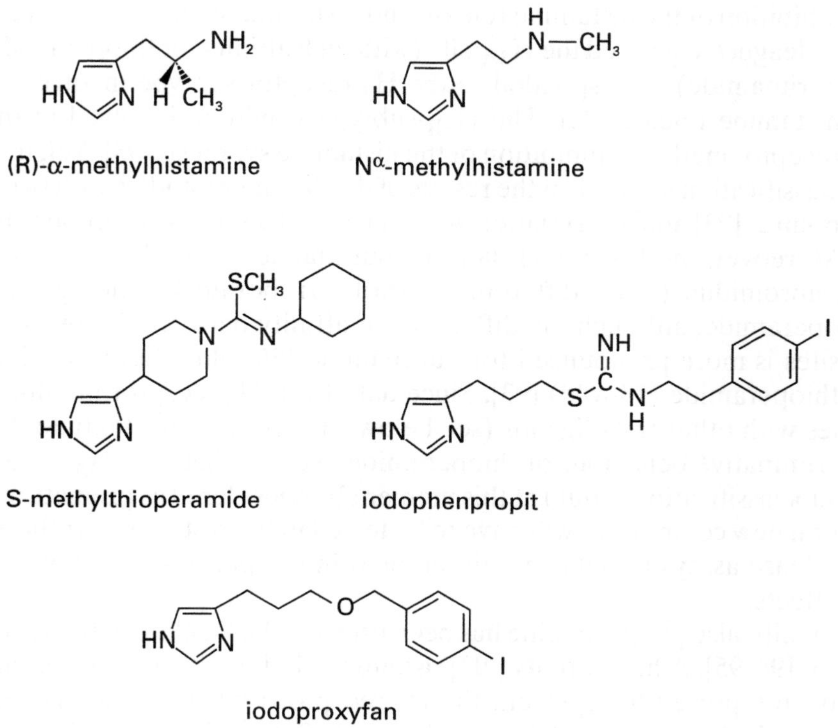

Fig. 2
Structures of the H_3 receptor ligands that have been described as potential radioligands for the histamine H_3 receptor.

nM, 73 fmol/mg protein), displacement studies with thioperamide and burimamide revealed biphasic displacement curves, indicating a heterogeneity of the binding site [93]. The binding of [^{3}H]N$^\alpha$-methylhistamine was inhibited for 50% by guanine nucleotides. In the presence of the GTP analogue GTPγS, thioperamide and burimamide only bound to the high affinity-sites, leading West et al. [93] to suggest that [^{3}H]N$^\alpha$-methylhistamine labels two different receptor proteins with different sensitivity to GTPγS. Although [^{3}H]N$^\alpha$-methylhistamine does not discriminate between these sites, burimamide and thioperamide show different affinities towards these two sites [93]. In the presence of GTPγS [^{3}H]N$^\alpha$-methylhistamine binding to only one site is inhibited, resulting in monophasic displacement curves for thioperamide and burimamide [93]. Based on the observed difference (8-fold) in potency of thioperamide in the H_3 receptor mediated inhibition of the histamine release and histamine synthesis [16], West and colleagues suggested the H_{3A}-site (with high affinity for thioperamide and burimamide) corresponded to the H_3 receptor subtype involved in the histamine release [93]. The H_{3B}-subtype would be involved in the H_3 receptor mediated inhibition of the histamine synthesis [93]. Yet, the subclassification is based on the results of displacement studies with two compounds [93] and a correlation with functional data on only thioperamide. Moreover, the functional data for burimamide (5-fold difference) and impromidine (4-fold difference) do not corroborate the findings with thioperamide, although the difference in affinity between the two binding sites is more pronounced for burimamide (36-fold difference) than for thioperamide (13-fold) [93]. Since data from H_3 receptor binding studies with other radioligands (see below) do also not substantiate the discriminative behaviour of thioperamide, we feel that the H_{3A}- and H_{3B}-subclassification should at this moment be considered as premature. Several new compounds will have to be tested in the histamine synthesis and release assays to delineate differences in the pharmacology of the two effects.

Finally, also [^{3}H]histamine has been used for the labeling of the H_3 receptor [94, 95]. A high affinity [^{3}H]histamine binding site in rat forebrain has been reported to represent the H_3-receptor [95]. This binding site was already described in 1980 by Barbin et al. [96]. [^{3}H]histamine binding can be inhibited by guanine nucleotides [94, 95]. In view of the reported labeling of other less well-defined proteins by [^{3}H]histamine [97] we consider the use of this ligand as inappropriate, although under some well-defined conditions it might label the H_3 receptor.

From these data it is apparent that the binding characteristics of the labeled agonists are complex and yet poorly understood. In contrast to many other receptor systems the low affinity binding of [^{3}H](R)-α-methylhistamine is inhibited by guanine nucleotides instead of the high affinity agonist binding [90]. Moreover, [^{3}H]N$^\alpha$-methylhistamine binding is only partially inhibited by guanine nucleotides, and displacement studies with thioperamide and burimamide suggested that the observed GTPγS effects are due to labeling of different receptor proteins and not to labeling of high and low affinities sites of the same receptor proteins [93].

Despite these problems, the use of the radiolabeled agonists has provided important information on the presence of H_3 receptors in guinea pig brain [51, 91] and some peripheral tissues [51, 90]. [^{3}H](R)-α-methylhistamine and [^{3}H]N$^\alpha$-methylhistamine have, furthermore, been used for autoradiographic studies in guinea pig lung and the brain of various species [73, 98, 99]. The use of these ligands even allowed the observations of a dynamic regulation of the H_3 receptor expression after unilateral enucleation [100] and reserpine [101] treatment.

3.1.2 Radiolabeled H_3 antagonists

To resolve some of the described problems that are related to the use of radiolabeled agonists (see section 3.1.1), a search for a radiolabeled antagonist was initiated by various laboratories. Yanai et al. [102] recently reported on the use of S-[^{3}H]-methylthioperamide (Fig. 2) to radiolabel the H_3 receptor. At 4°C this radioligand labels a saturable site in the rat forebrain, resulting in a K_D value of 2 nM and a receptor density of 551 fmol/mg protein [102]. For [^{3}H](R)-α-methylhistamine the density of binding sites on the same membranes amounted 189 fmol/mg protein [102]. Unfortunately, the binding of S-[^{3}H]-methylthioperamide has not been characterized in detail. Displacement of the binding was only investigated for thioperamide and the two isomers of α-methylhistamine [102]. Yet, the expected stereospecificity of the binding was observed [102]. Moreover, the displacement of the S-[^{3}H]-methylthioperamide binding was biphasically displaced by the agonist (R)-α-methylhistamine ([102], an observation that finally corroborates previous reports on the complex agonist binding characteristics for other receptor systems. This compound has also been used to obtain autoradiographic images from rat brain [102]. The autoradiographic images are essentially the same as those obtained with [^{3}H]-(R)-α-methylhistamine, although the resolution with the radiolabeled agonist was slightly better [102]. Yet, the tissue distribution of the S-[^{3}H]-methylthioperamide binding does not parallel the [^{3}H]-(R)α-methylhistamine binding [102]. As already mentioned before, a 3-fold difference in maximum binding capacity was observed for the rat forebrain; even greater differences were observed in some peripheral tissues [102]. Whereas almost no specific [^{3}H]-(R)α-methylhistamine binding was found in rat liver, adrenal and stomach, high levels of S-[^{3}H]-methylthioperamide binding were observed [102]. These last observations question the appropriate labeling of the H_3 receptor by S-[^{3}H]-methylthioperamide; the authors state themselves that "thioperamide and its related derivatives may have considerable levels of non-H_3 receptor binding sites in central and peripheral tissues" [102]. Further studies are therefore needed to clarify the characteristics of this H_3 antagonist radioligand.

Recently in our laboratory, a new series of H_3 receptor antagonists was developed from the highly selective and potent H_3 receptor agonist imetit (see Table 16, [57, 60]). The highly active compound, clobenpropit, is at this moment the most potent H_3 receptor antagonist *in vitro* and is a valuable tool in pharmacological studies [18, 25, 70, 81, 103]. Following these developments an iodonated analogue of clobenpropit was prepared [68]. Iodophenpropit (Fig. 2) is also a very potent H_3 receptor antagonist [68, 69] and shows only a moderate affinity for the H_1 and H_2 receptor [68]. Therefore it has been radiolabeled with [^{125}I]iodine [68] and the resulting [^{125}I]iodophenpropit appears to be a suitable radiolabel for the H_3 receptor [69, 70]. It shows saturable, high affinity binding to rat brain cortex membranes resulting in a pK_D value of 9.2 and a receptor density of 268 fmol/mg protein [70]. For [^{125}I]iodophenpropit ca. 60% specific binding was found around the K_D value for the binding to the rat brain cortex membranes. With this percentage of specific binding dissociation constants for various H_3 receptor ligands can be determined accurately [70]. The specific [^{125}I]iodophenpropit binding is inhibited by several H_3 antagonists (e.g thioperamide, clobenpropit) in a monophasic way and an H_3 receptor pharmacology [69, 70]. Yet, displacement of the [^{125}I]iodophenpropit binding by the two H_3 antagonists burimamide and dimaprit resulted in biphasic displacement curves, which were insensitive to guanine nucleotide treatment [70].

The data of the biphasic displacement by antagonists do not substantiate the previous suggestion of West et al. [93] of receptor heterogeneity on the basis of thioperamide and burimamide. The [^{125}I]iodophenpropit binding data also stress that the pharmacology of the [^{125}I]iodophenpropit binding site is different from the [^{3}H]Nα-methylhistamine binding sites. Future studies should clarify these differences and the apparent heterogeneity of the different binding sites.

Displacement of the specific [^{125}I]iodophenpropit binding by several H_3 receptor agonists showed a clear stereoselectivity for the enantiomers of α-methylhistamine and a displacement to the same level as is found with the tested antagonists [70]. Agonist displacement resulted in shallow, biphasic displacement curves for all tested agonists. The biphasic displacement curves were shifted rightwards by guanine nucleotides, indicating the coupling to G-proteins [70]. These features are in good agreement with known characteristics of agonist displacement of antagonists radioligands. [^{125}I]iodophenpropit has been used for the autoradiographic localization of the H_3 receptor in the rat brain, which showed essentially a similar localization as obtained with the radiolabeled agonists [70].

Besides [^{125}I]iodophenpropit also another iodonated antagonist has been introduced for radiolabeling of the H_3 receptor. Ligneau et al. [84] recently selected from a series of ethers (see Table 24) the compound iodoproxyfan (Fig. 2). This compound was reported to be an H_3 antagonist at the guinea pig ileum (pA_2 = 8.3 [86], pA_2 = 9.0 [84]), and in the [^{3}H]histamine release from rat brain cortex slices (pA_2 = 8.5 [84]). Saturation analysis of [^{125}I]iodoproxyfan binding to rat striatal membranes resulted in a pK_D value of 10.2 and a receptor density of 78 fmol/mg protein [84]. The specific binding of [^{125}I]iodoproxyfan to rat striatal membranes amounted to ca. 50% at the K_D, a percentage that is comparable to the previously described specific [^{125}I]iodophenpropit binding [70]. The autoradiographic localization of the [^{125}I]iodoproxyfan binding in rat brain is in general agreement with the results obtained with radiolabeled agonists [84]. Moreover, the [^{125}I]iodoproxyfan binding is displaced by many H_3 receptor active ligands and also stereospecifically by the enantiomers of α-methylhistamine [84]. Yet the displacement of the [^{125}I]iodoproxyfan binding by several H_3 agonists and antagonist results in a rather complicated picture. Firstly, H_3 antagonists displaced the total [^{125}I]iodoproxyfan (30 pM) binding almost completely, whereas all the agonists only displaced 65% of the total binding [84]. The specific binding was therefore defined by the agonist displacement curves. For the tested antagonists no clear distinction between the defined specific and non-specific binding sites is observed, which might give problems for the estimation of pseudo-Hill coefficients and K_i values [84]. Secondly, displacement of the [^{125}I]iodoproxyfan binding by thioperamide and burimamide resulted in very steep displacement curves with pseudo-Hill coeficients of 1.7 and 1.9, respectively [84]. The reason for these observations is currently unknown [84]. Future studies should clarify the observed complexities of the [^{125}I]iodoproxyfan binding and thereby show the usefulness of [^{125}I]iodoproxyfan as a radiolabel for the H_3 receptor.

3.1.3 Conclusions

In conclusion, the recent introduction of the radiolabeled antagonists might allow a more detailed analysis of the H_3 receptor binding sites. Due to the high specific activity of [^{125}I]-iodoproxyfan and [^{125}I]-iodophenpropit the presence of H_3 receptors in peripheral tissues can perhaps be studied. Due to the antagonistic nature of the radioligand the interpretation of the binding studies might be more straightforward and hopefully it will soon be clear if the reported complexity of [^{3}H]agonist binding is simply inherent in the use of agonists as radioligands or is e.g. due to H_3 receptor subtypes. Yet, as described above in detail, also the characteristics of the antagonist radioligand binding are not always well understood. Future studies have to delineate which radioligand should be used for H_3 receptor labeling. Finally, [^{125}I]-iodoproxyfan and [^{125}I]-iodophenpropit might be the lead structures for the development of a highly potent and sensitive photoaffinity label. As has previously been shown for both the H_1- and H_2 receptor, the introduction of an azido-moiety in the aromatic ring might give rise to a useful photoaffinity probe [104, 105], which would give valuable information on the receptor protein.

3.2 The H_3 receptor protein

For a rational drug design detailed knowledge of the protein target is indispensable. Unfortunately, so far no detailed information is available for the H_3 receptor. Yet, with the development of selective radioligands (see section 3.1) some information has been obtained and will be presented in this section.

In recent years, some information on the biochemical properties of the other histamine receptor proteins has been obtained. For both the H_1 and H_2 receptor, photoaffinity labels were developed and used to identify the binding peptides of the receptor proteins [104, 105]. Due to the low abundance of histamine H_3 receptors in various tissues and since only recently highly sensitive radioligands were available, the biochemical investigations of the H_3 receptor have been limited. Using $[^3H]$histamine as radioligand the solubilization of the bovine H_3 receptor from brain tissue was reported [94]. In membranes of bovine whole brain, $[^3H]$histamine labels a binding site with a K_D-value of 4.6 ± 1.3 nM and a B_{max} of 78 ± 20 fmol/mg protein [94]. This site showed a pharmacology of a typical H_3 receptor and these properties were retained after solubilization with the detergent digitonin [94]. Size-exclusion chromatography revealed an apparent molecular weight of 220.000 kDa for the solubilized histamine H_3 receptor [94]. This value is probably overestimated due to protein-associated digitonin, but more interestingly also because of the possible co-solubilization of a G-protein [94]. It appeared that the $[^3H]$histamine binding to bovine membranes could be inhibited by guanine-nucleotides [94], indicative of the coupling of the H_3 receptor to a G-protein. The guanine nucleotide sensitivity was retained after solubilization [94], indicating a relatively tight coupling of the H_3 receptor with a G-protein.

Despite the lack of tissues with high levels of H_3 receptor expression, Cherifi et al. [106] recently reported the purification of the H_3 receptor protein from the human gastric tumoral cell line HGT-1. Using $[^3H]N^{\alpha}$-methylhistamine high affinity binding sites were demonstrated (K_D = 0.6 nM, B_{max} = 54 fmol/mg protein). The $[^3H]N^{\alpha}$-methylhistamine binding could be inhibited by GTPγS and was effectively solubilized with Triton X-100 [106]. After gel filtration and Sepharose-thioperamide affinity chromatography the $[^3H]N^{\alpha}$-methylhistamine binding site was 90,225-fold purified [106]. The purified protein showed still a high affinity for $[^3H]N^{\alpha}$-

methylhistamine (K_D = 5.8 nM) and the [^{3}H]N$^\alpha$-methylhistamine binding could be potently inhibited by thioperamide or R-α-methylhistamine [106]. The purified sites had a molecular mass of approximately 70 kDa in SDS-polyacrylamide gel electrophoresis [106].
Besides the reported purification [106], the recent developments in the field of molecular biology of histamine receptors might also soon give rise to detailed information on the molecular properties of the H_3 receptor. First of all, the cloning of the genes encoding for the H_1 and H_2 receptors [107–113] might facilitate the cloning of the gene encoding for the H_3 receptor by homology screening. In view of the apparent lack of a reasonable homology between the H_1 receptor and the H_2 receptor [107] it is, however, not certain that such an approach will be successful. The iodinated radioligands [^{125}I]iodophenpropit [69, 70] and [^{125}I]iodoproxyfan [84] might be useful for the cloning of the gene encoding for the H_3 receptor by expression cloning, whereas the reported purification of the H_3 receptor protein [106]. could also be an important step for the cloning of its encoding gene.

3.3 Receptor subtypes

At this moment no clear evidence for H_3 receptor heterogeneity has been presented. Yet, some reports indicated the potential need for a subdivision of the H_3 receptor. As already discussed (see sections 3.1.1 and 3.1.2) the results, obtained in radioligand binding studies, are not always straightforward and some suggestions for H_3 receptor subtypes have been made on the basis of especially such studies. Since radioligand binding studies on their own can never prove the existence of receptor subtypes, the suggestion for H_3 heterogeneity should be handled with great caution. Nevertheless, also in functional studies some preliminary indications for H_3 receptor heterogeneity have been presented. For both betahistine (**288**) and phenylbutanoylhistamine (**224**) Arrang and co-workers described H_3 receptor antagonism, measured in the [^{3}H]-histamine release assay in the rat cortex [45, 89]. Yet, both compounds are almost inactive when measured at the guinea pig intestine (NANC-induced contractions) [40] or the rat entorhinal cortex ([^{3}H]-acetylcholine release) [24]. Moreover, a pharmacological characterization of the H_3 receptor that is involved in the inhibition of serotonin from porcine enterochromaffin cells, showed that betahistine and phenylbutanoylhistamine were again unable to block the effects of (R)-α-methylhistamine [114]. Impromidine or burimamide were also unable to antagonize the effects of (R)-α-methylhistamine, whereas

thioperamide could inhibit the H_3 receptor responses with a pA_2 value of 8.4 [114].
Altogether, these data present some preliminary evidence for H_3 receptor heterogeneity. Yet one should stress that no extensive studies within one laboratory have been performed. Moreover, in view of the wide array of H_3 selective drugs that are currently known, an extensive screening of several compounds in the aforementioned assay systems might yield the final proof for the existence of receptor subtypes. This information is indispensable for valid structure-activity relationships and thus future drug development.

4 Clinical application of H_3 receptor ligands

In the past, successful drugs have been developed on the basis of their interaction with the histamine receptors. With the acknowledgement of the (patho)physiological role(s) of histamine [115], intensive research started for "antihistamines" (now known as H_1 antagonists) which were thought to be useful as anti-allergic agents [116]. Many compounds, the classical antihistamines and the modern non-sedative H_1 blockers have been developed and introduced since then, especially for treating allergic conditions [4]. During the sixties the classification of H_1- and H_2 receptors [8] led to the development of H_2 antagonists as anti-ulcer agents [9]. Later on some attention has been given to the potential application of H_2 agonists as cardiostimulants [117]. After the definition of the H_3 receptor as a presynaptic receptor, affecting many different neuronal systems, the last decade research has been directed towards the use of H_3 agonists and antagonists as therapeutical agents [118].
So far no H_3-ligands have been introduced into therapy, but intensive research has suggested several putative applications. H_3 receptors regulate important processes in the airways, suggesting that the application of H_3 agonists might be benificial in asthmatic conditions. It has been reported that H_3 agonists reduce NANC- and cholinergic neurotransmission in airways and reduce microvascular leakage [3, 32, 39]. Moreover, H_3 receptor stimulation causes relaxation in the airways [119], has been sugggested to reduce the antigen-induced histamine release of from airway mast cells from ovalbumine-sensitized guinea pigs [120] and recently has been shown to reduce [^{3}H]-histamine synthesis in rat lung mast cells via a C-fiber-mast cell feedback loop [38]. So far (R)-α-methylhistamine has been tested once in provoked-asthma; yet the success was limited [96], but this might have been due to the H_1 agonistic activity of this agonist

[7, 121]. Future tests with other agonists like imetit and immepip might give relevant information on the potential use of these ligands for airway disorders.

In view of the reported inhibition of both the NANC-, cholinergic-, and serotonergic transmission in the GI tract [31, 33, 37, 40–42, 122] H_3 receptor agonists could perhaps be used as anti-diarrhoeals. Furthermore, various H_3 receptor agonist have also been reported to be able to reduce the acid secretion in a variety of experimental models [30, 123]. In several *in vivo* studies in cat [124] and dog [125, 126], H_3 receptor stimulation was shown to inhibit gastric acid secretion after activation of cholinergic pathways or pentagastrin administration. These data suggest that H_3 receptors are located on enterochrommaffin-like (ECL) cells, which after stimulation, release histamine to stimulate the parietal cell. These findings seem to be supported by recent *in vitro* experiments with a relatively pure, rabbit ECL cell preparation [127]. In this cell preparation H_3 receptor stimulation was reported to reduce the histamine synthesis [127]. Although these findings suggest a potential therapeutic application of H_3 agonists, one should mention that species differences appear to be important. For instance, in the rat H_3 receptor modulation of gastric acid secretion is absent [128]. Moreover, in view of already existing therapies a potential use of the agonists in gastric acid secretion disorders is unlikely.

As is the case with the H_3 agonists, so far no definite therapeutical use has been identified for the H_3 antagonists. Following the observations that the H_3 receptors can influence the release of several important neurotransmitters in the brain, various applications may be predicted. It has e.g. been known for several years that histamine is involved in the regulation of sleep and wakefulness [1, 2]. The circadian rhythm of histamine levels in the brain is thought to be associated with this process [129]. Many lines of evidence indicate that an interaction of histamine with the postsynaptic H_1 receptor is probably involved in the regulation of wakefulness. This hypothesis explains the sedative properties of brain-penetrating H_1 receptor antagonists [130] and also provides a rational basis for the observed CNS-effects with H_3 receptor ligands in rat and cats [19, 131]. It is known that direct injection of histamine in the posterior hypothalamus leads to an increase in wakefulness; this effect could be inhibited by the H_1 receptor antagonist mepyramine [132]. In line with these findings is the observation that increasing the brain histamine levels in W/Wv mice with the H_3 antagonist thioperamide leads to an increase of the locomotor activity [19]. This effect on locomotion after H_3 receptor blockade could be reversed by concomitant application of the H_3 agonist (R)-α-methylhistamine and fully blocked with mepyramine, indicating an interaction of released histamine with the H_1 receptor [19]. Moreover, in freely moving cats oral administration of (R)-α-methylhistamine caused a significant decrease in deep slow wave sleep, while administration of thioperamide enhanced the wakefulness [131]. Again the arousal effect of thioperamide was inhibited by mepyramine [131]. These data indicate that histaminergic neurons are critically involved in arousal mechanisms and that H_3 receptor antagonists could be valuable in narcolepsy and certain attention deficit disorders.

Brain histamine levels and the postsynaptic H_1 receptor are also important in epilepsy [2]. Histamine and the H_1 receptor agonist 2-thiazolylethylamine both reduce seizure susceptibility on electrically- and pentylenetetrazole-induced convulsions in mice [133], whereas there have been some reports that H_1 antagonist treatment increases epileptic discharges in mice and humans [2]. Moreover, in epileptic patients higher H_1 receptor densities in the electrical focal in the temporal neocortex were found in a recent [^{11}C]doxepin PET-study [134], indicating a functional upregulation of H_1 receptors to counteract the epileptical discharges in this brain area. As expected, elevation of brain histamine levels via administration of the H_3 receptor antagonists thioperamide [135] or clobenpropit [18] in mice resulted in an inhibition of an electrically-induced epileptic attacks. This antiepileptic effect could be inhibited by an H_1 receptor antagonist [18, 135]. Although these findings suggest a potential therapeutical application of antagonists in epilepsy, the overall inhibitory effects of the H_3 antagonists were somewhat limited and question therefore the potential usefulness in therapy.

Application of H_3 receptor antagonists could also be envisaged in eating disorders. There are clear indications that histaminergic neurotransmission via H_1 receptors is involved in the regulation of food intake [1, 2, 136]. This observation forms the rational basis for the reported side-effects of weight gain after H_1 antagonist treatments. In rats the application of thioperamide results in a decrease in food intake [137, 138], suggesting a putative application of H_3 receptor antagonists in obesity.

Application of H_3 antagonists has also been suggested for the treatment of motion sickness and vertigo. There are strong indications that the histaminergic system is involved in the pathophysiology of motion sickness [1, 2]. Several H_1 antagonists are known to be of use in prophylaxis and treatment of motion sickness [2]. Recently, thioperamide was reported to be effective in a animal model for motion sickness [139]. These data are interesting, since betahistine has been described as a H_3 antagonist [89] and is known for its therapeutic usefulness in vertigo [140].

Finally, a very important therapeutic application of H_3 receptor ligands could be in the field of dementia. The role of histamine in memory processes has been neglected in the last decades, but is gaining interest in view of some recent findings. It has been known for some time that intracerebroventricular application of histamine can facilitate memory [141, 142]. Histamine has been found to increase the NMDA-currents in hippocampal neurons via an interaction with the polyamine regulatory binding site on the NMDA channel [143, 144]. Moreover, preliminary findings indicate that via this mechanism histamine can facilitate the induction of long-term potentiation in rat hippocampal slices [145]. In view of the findings that in Alzheimer patients in some brain areas histamine levels are reduced [146], the regulatory H_3 receptor system might be a target for normalization of histaminergic transmission and thus brain function. Since a loss of cholinergic transmission is often regarded as one of the underlying mechanisms of reduced memory (see e.g. [147] and references therein), the reported findings that H_3 receptor blockade can increase acetylcholine release [23, 148] might also be of importance in this respect. If H_3 antagonists might indeed be useful in this field, the concommitant increase in wakefulness can be regarded as a potential advantage over muscarinic agonists. Unfortunately, no detailed studies have been published so far. Only two, contradictory studies appeared. In one preliminary study thioperamide was reported to improve learning in rats [148]; yet, in another study, (R)-α-methylhistamine was reported to exert the same effect [149]. In the near future more studies will certainly be performed to elucidate the potential role of the H_3 receptor in memory processes.

5 Concluding remarks

During the last decade impressive progress has been made in the field of the H_3 receptor. Many selective agonists (R)-α-methylhistamine, imetit, immepip) and antagonists (thioperamide, clobenpropit) have been developed and made available for pharmacologists. The availability of selective ligands has resulted in the recognition of the role of the H_3 receptors in a wide variety of physiological responses. Moreover, with the development of radiolabeled ligands new techniques for the characterization of the H_3 receptor protein became available and have e.g. resulted in the identification of two isolated cell lines that endogenously express H_3 receptors. Moreover, the recently described iodonated radioligands [^{125}I]iodophenpropit and (probably) [^{125}I]iodoproxyfan are new important tools for a future characterization of the H_3 receptors in various tissues, which express the H_3 receptor in low amounts. These highly sensitive probes might also be very useful for an expression cloning approach to obtain the gene encoding the H_3 receptor. The availability of the H_3 receptor gene will be an important step towards the rational design of new H_3 receptor drugs. Moreover, the expression of such an H_3 receptor gene in various cell systems might also be an important improvement for the elucidation of the signal transduction of the H_3 receptor subtype. Finally, in the following years it will become clear if the H_3 receptor can actually be regarded as a therapeutical target. Especially for the H_3 antagonists interesting therapeutical potentials can be expected.

Acknowledgement

The work of Dr. Leurs was made possible by a fellowship of the Royal Netherlands Academy of Arts and Sciences.

References

1 J.C. Schwartz, J.M. Arrang, M. Garbarg, H. Pollard, and M. Ruat: Physiol. Rev. *71*, 1 (1991).
2 K. Onodera, A. Yamatodani, T. Watanabe, and H. Wada: Prog Neurobiol. *42*, 685 (1994).
3 P.J. Barnes, in: J.C.Schwartz.and H.L. Haas (Eds.), The histamine receptors, Wiley-Liss, New York (1992), p. 253.
4 J. Ring, F. Sedlmeier, H. Van der Helm, T. Mayr, U. Walz, H. Ibel, H. Riepel, B. Przybilla, H.J. Reimann, and W. Dorsch, in: J. Ring (Ed.), New Trends in Allergy, Springer-Verlag: Berlin (1985), p. 44.
5 P.K. Rangachari: Am. J. Physiol. *262*, G1 (1992).
6 S.J. Hill: Pharmacol. Rev. *42*, 45 (1990).
7 R. Leurs, H. Van der Goot, and H. Timmerman, in: B. Testa (Ed.), Advances in Drug Research, Vol. 20. Academic Press: London (1990), p. 217.
8 A.S.F. Ash and H.O. Schild: Br. J. Pharmac. *27*, 427 (1966).
9 J.W. Black, W.A.M. Duncan, G.J. Durant, C.R. Ganellin, and M.E. Parsons: Nature *236*, 385 (1972).
10 J.M. Arrang, M. Garbarg, and J.C. Schwartz: Nature *302*, 832 (1983).
11 J.M. Arrang, M. Garbarg, and J.C. Schwartz: Neurosci. *23*, 149 (1987).
12 K.E. Barke and L.B. Hough: J. Neurochem. *63*, 238 (1994).
13 T. Mochizuki, A. Yamatodani, K. Okakura, M. Takemura, N. Inagaki, and H. Wada: Arch. Pharmacol. *343*, 190 (1991).
14 Y. Itoh, R. Oishi, M. Nishibori, and K. Saeki: J. Neurochem. *56*, 769 (1991).
15 H. Prast, M. Prast, and A. Philippu: Agents Actions *41*, C64 (1994).

16 J.M. Arrang, M. Garbarg, J.C. Lancelot, J.M. Lecomte, H. Pollard, M. Robba, W. Schunack, and J.C. Schwartz: Nature *327*, 117 (1987).
17 M. Garbarg, J.M. Arrang, A. Rouleau, X. Ligneau, M.D.T. Tuong, J.C. Schwartz, and C.R. Ganellin: J. Pharmacol. Exp. Ther. *263*, 304 (1992).
18 H. Yokoyama, K. Onodera, K. Maeyama, E. Sakurai, K. Iinuma, R. Leurs, H. Timmerman, and T. Watanabe: Eur. J. Pharmacol. *260*, 23 (1994).
19 N. Sakai, K. Onodera, K. Maeyama, K. Yanai, and T. Watanabe: Life Sci. *48*, 2397 (1991).
20 R. Oishi, Y. Itoh, M. Nishibori, and K. Saeki: J. Neurochem. *52*, 1388 (1989).
21 M. Garbarg, M.D. Trung Tuong, C. Gros, and J.C. Schwartz: Eur. J. Pharmacol. *164*, 1 (1989).
22 N. Sakai, A. Sakurai, E. Sakurai, K. Yanai, K. Maeyama, and T. Watanabe: Biochem. Biophys. Res. Commun. *185*, 121 (1992).
23 T. Mochizuki, K. Okakuramochizuki, A. Horii, Y. Yamamoto, and A. Yamatodani: J. Neurochem. *62*, 2275 (1994).
24 J. Clapham and G.J. Kilpatrick: Br. J. Pharmacol. *107*, 919 (1992).
25 E. Schlicker, B. Malinowska, M. Kathmann, and M. Gothert: Fundam. Clin. Pharmacol. *8*, 128 (1994).
26 E. Schlicker, K. Fink, M. Detzner, and M. Gothert: J. Neural. Transm. *93*, 1 (1993).
27 E. Schlicker, K. Fink, M. Hinterthaner, and M. Göthert: Arch. Pharmacol. *340*, 633 (1989).
28 E. Schlicker, A. Behling, G. Lümmen, and M. Göthert: Arch. Pharmacol. *345*, 489 (1992).
29 E. Schlicker, R. Betz, and M. Göthert: Arch. Pharmacol. *337*, 588 (1988).
30 G. Bertaccini, G. Coruzzi, and E. Poli: Aliment. Pharmacol. Therap. *5*, 585 (1991).
31 R.C. Vollinga, O.P. Zuiderveld, H. Scheerens, A. Bast, and H. Timmerman: Meth. Find. Exp. Clin. Pharmacol. *14*, 747 (1992).
32 M. Ichinose, C.D. Stretton, J.C. Schwartz, and P.J. Barnes: Br. J. Pharmacol. *97*, 13 (1989).
33 G. Coruzzi, E. Poli, and G. Bertaccini: J. Pharmacol. Exp. Ther. *258*, 325 (1991).
34 E. Poli, G. Coruzzi, and G. Bertaccini: Life Sci. *48*, PL63 (1991).
35 E. Schlicker, W. Schunack, and M. Göthert: Arch. Pharmacol. *342*, 497 (1990).
36 G.J. Molderings, G. Weissenborn, E. Schlicker, J. Likungu, and M. Gothert: Arch. Pharmacol. *346*, 46 (1992).
37 H. Schworer, S. Katsoulis, and K. Racke: Gastroenterology *102*, 1906 (1992).
38 V. Dimitriadou, A. Rouleau, M.D.T. Tuong, G.J.F. Newlands, H.R.P. Miller, G. Luffau, J.C. Schwartz, and M. Garbarg: Clin. Sci. *87*, 151 (1994).
39 M. Ichinose and P.J. Barnes: Eur. J. Pharmacol. *174*, 49 (1989).
40 S.J. Taylor and G.J. Kilpatrick: Br. J. Pharmacol. *105*, 667 (1992).
41 R. Leurs, M.M. Brozius, M.J. Smit, A. Bast, and H. Timmerman: Br. J. Pharmacol., *102*, 179 (1991).
42 G.J. Menkveld and H. Timmerman: Eur. J. Pharmacol. *186*, 343 (1990).
43 J.G. Van der Werf, G.J. Bijloo, A. Van der Vliet, A. Bast, and H. Timmerman: Agents Actions *20*, 239 (1987).
44 J.C. Eriks, H. Van der Goot, G.J. Sterk, and H. Timmerman: J. Med. Chem. *35*, 3239 (1992).
45 R. Lipp, H. Stark, and W. Schunack, in: J.C. Schwartz and H.L. Haas (Eds.), Receptor Biochemistry and Methodology, Wiley-Liss, New York (1992), p. 57.

46 R. Lipp, J.M. Arrang, M. Garbarg, P. Luger, J.C. Schwartz, and W. Schunack: J. Med. Chem. *35*, 4434 (1992).
47 R. Lipp, J.M. Arrang, J. Buschmann, M. Garbarg, P. Luger, W. Schunack, and J.C. Schwartz, in: H. Timmerman and H. Van der Goot (Eds.), New perspectives in Histamine Research, Birkhauser Verlag: Basel (1991), p. 277.
48 J.M. Arrang, M. Garbarg, J.C. Schwartz, R. Lipp, H. Stark, W. Schunack, and J.M. Lecomte, in: H. Timmerman and H. Van der Goot (Eds.), New Perspectives in Histamine Research, Birkhauser Verlag: Basel (1991), p.55.
49 J.M. Arrang, M. Garbarg, W. Schunack, J.C. Schwartz, and R. Lipp, (1987), Eur. Patent Appl. pO214058.
50 N.-Y. Shih, R. Aslanian, A.T. Lupo Jr., L. Duguma, S. Orlando, J.J. Piwinski, M.J. Green, A.K. Ganguly, M. Clark, S. Tozzi, W. Kreutner, and J.A. Hey. Poster presented at New Perspectives in Histamine Research 1994. Riding Mountain National Park, Manitoba, Canada.
51 A. Korte, J. Myers, N.Y. Shih, R.W. Egan, and M.A. Clark: Biochem. Biophys. Res. Comm. *168*, 979 (1990).
52 A. Burger, M. Bernabe, and P.W. Collins: J. Med. Chem. *13*, 33 (1970).
53 J.C. Schwartz, J.M. Arrang, M. Garbarg, and W. Schunack, in: A.F. Harms (Ed.), Innovative Approaches in Drug Research, Elsevier Science Publishers BV: Amsterdam (1986), p.73.
54 J.M. Arrang, J.C. Schwartz, and W. Schunack: Eur. J. Pharmacol. *117*, 109 (1985).
55 J.F. Van der Werf, A. Bast, G.J. Bijloo, A. Van der Vliet, and H. Timmerman: Eur. J. Pharmacol. *138*, 199 (1987).
56 N.Y. Shih, Int. Patent Appl. (PCT) (1993) p. WO 93.
57 H. Van der Goot, M.J.P. Schepers, G.J. Sterk, and H. Timmerman: Eur. J. Med. Chem. *27*, 511 (1992).
58 W. Howson, M.E. Parsons, P. Raval, and G.T.G. Swayne: Bioorg. Med. Chem. Lett. *2*, 77 (1992).
59 C.R. Ganellin, B. Bangandersen, Y.S. Khalaf, W. Tertiuk, J.M. Arrang, M. Garbarg, X. Ligneau, A. Rouleau, and J.C. Schwartz: Bioorg. Med. Chem. Lett. *2*, 1231 (1992).
60 R. Leurs and H. Timmerman: Prog. Drug Res. *39*, 127 (1992).
61 R.C. Vollinga, J.P. De Koning, F.P. Jansen, R. Leurs, W.M.P.B. Menge, and H. Timmerman: J. Med. Chem. *37*, 332 (1994).
62 N.Y. Shih, Int. Patent Appl. (PCT) (1993), p. WO 93.
63 N.Y. Shih, Int. Patent Appl. (PCT) (1993). p. WO 93.
64 R. Lipp, W. Schunack, and J.M. Arrang: Poster presented at Xth Int. Symp. Med. Chem. Budapest, 239 (1988).
65 R.C. Vollinga, W.M.P.B. Menge, R. Leurs, and H. Timmerman: J. Med. Chem. *38*, 266 (1995).
66 R.C. Vollinga: (unpublished results).
67 J.M. Arrang, M. Garbarg, J.C.M. Lancelot, J.M. Lecomte, M.F. Robba, and J.C. Schwartz, Eur. Pat. Appl. (1986) p. EP 0.
68 W.M.P.B. Menge, H. Van der Goot, H. Timmerman, J.L.H. Eersels, and J.D.M. Herscheid: J. Lab. Comp. Radiopharm. *31*, 781 (1992).
69 F.P. Jansen, B. Rademaker, A. Bast, and H. Timmerman: Eur. J. Pharmacol. *217*, 203 (1992).
70 F.P. Jansen, W. T.S., H.P. Voss, H.W.M. Steinbusch, R.C. Vollinga, B. Rademaker, A. Bast, and H. Timmerman: Br. J. Pharmacol. *113*, 355 (1994).

71 J.C. Schwartz, J.M. Arrang, M. Garbarg, J.M. Lecomte, C.R. Ganellin, A. Fkyerat, W. Tertiuk, W. Schunack, R. Lipp, H. Stark, and K. Puran, Int. Patent Appl. (PCT) (1993) p. WO 93.
72 E. Schlicker, M. Kathmann, S. Reidemeister, H. Stark, and W. Schunack: Br. J. Pharmacol. *112*, 1043 (1994).
73 J.C. Schwartz, J.M. Arrang, M. Garbarg, and H. Pollard: Agents Actions *30*, 13 (1990).
74 R.C. Vollinga, W.M.P.B. Menge, R. Leurs, and H. Timmerman: J. Med. Chem. *38*, 2244 (1995).
75 E. Barocelli, V. Ballabeni, A. Caretta, F. Bordi, C. Silva, G. Morini, and M. Impicciatore: Agents Actions *38*, 158 (1993).
76 Y.S. Khalaf, C.R. Ganellin, S.K. Hosseini, W. Tertiuk, J.M. Arrang, and N. Defontaine. Presented at European Histamine Research Society XIXth Annual Meeting. 1990, Kuopio, Finland.
77 F. Bordi, M. Mor, P.V. Plazzi, C. Silva, G. Morini, A. Caretta, E. Barocelli, and M. Impicciatore: Farmaco *47*, 1343 (1992).
78 M. Amin Khan, G.J. Durant, S. Ghodsi-Hovseplan, A.A. El-Assadi, W. Hoss, W.S. Messer jr., and R.C.A. Frederickson: Med. Chem. Res. *3*, 428 (1993).
79 H. Stark, R. Lipp, W. Schunack, J.M. Arrang, N. Defontaine, and J.C. Schwartz: Poster presented at New Perspectives in Histamine Research 1990. Noordwijkerhout, The Netherlands.
80 R. Mierzwa, A. King, M.A. Conover, S. Tozzi, M.S. Puar, M. Patel, S.J. Coval, and S.A. Pomponi: J. Nat. Prod-Lloydia *57*, 175 (1994).
81 M. Kathmann, E. Schlicker, M. Detzner, and H. Timmerman: Arch. Pharmacol. *348*, 498 (1993).
82 S.A. Pomponi, V.P. Gullo, A.C. Horan, M.G. Patel, and S. Coval, US Patent (1993), Fla. p.5.
83 K. Purand, H. Stark, X. Ligneau, M. Garbarg, J.C. Schwartz, and W. Schunack: Poster presented at European Histamine Research Society XXIIIrd Annual Meeting 1994. Budapest, Hungary.
84 X. Ligneau, M. Garbarg, M.L. Vizuette, J. Diaz, K. Purand, H. Stark, W. Schunack, and J.C. Schwartz: J. Pharmacol. Exp. Ther. *271*, 452 (1994).
85 A. Hüls, K. Purand, H. Stark, X. Ligneau, M. Garbarg, J.C. Schwartz, and W. Schunack: Poster presented at European Histamine Research Society XXIIIrd Annual Meeting 1994. Budapest, Hungary.
86 W. Schunack, K. Purand, A. Hüls, H. Stark, X. Ligneau, M. Garbarg, and J.C. Schwartz: Poster presented at XIIth Int. Congress of Pharmacology (IUPHAR) 1994. Montreal, Quebec, Canada.
87 M. Kathmann, E. Schlicker, and M. Gothert: Psychopharmacology *116*, 464 (1994).
88 A. Alves Rodrigues, F.P. Jansen, R. Leurs, H. Timmerman, and G.D. Prell: Br. J. Pharmacol. *114*, 1523 (1995).
89 J.M. Arrang, M. Garbarg, T.T. Quach, M. Dam Trung Tuong, E. Yeramian, and J.C. Schwartz: Eur. J. Pharmacol. *111*, 73 (1985).
90 J.M. Arrang, J. Roy, J.L. Morgat, W. Schunack, and J.C. Schwartz: Eur. J. Pharmacol. *188*, 219 (1990).
91 G.J. Kilpatrick and A.D. Michel, in: H.Timmerman and H.van der Goot (Eds.), New Perspectives in Histamine Research, Birkhäuser Verlag, Basel (1991), p. 69.
92 R.E. West, A. Zweig, R.T. Granzow, M.I. Siegel, and R.W. Egan: J. Neurochem. *55*, 1612 (1990).

93 R.E. West, A. Zweig, N.-Y. Shih, M.I. Siegel, R.W. Egan, and M.A. Clark: Mol. Pharmacol. *38*, 610 (1990).
94 A. Zweig, M.I. Siegel, R.W. Egan, M.A. Clark, R.G.L. Shorr, and R.E. West: J. Neurochem. *59*, 1661 (1992).
95 P. Cumming, C. Shaw, and S.R. Vincent: Synapse *8*, 144 (1991).
96 G. Barbin, J.M. Palacois, E. Rodergas, J.C. Schwartz, and M. Garbarg: Mol. Pharmacol. *18*, 1 (1980).
97 W.G. Sinkins, M. Kandel, S.I. Kandel, W. Schunack, and J.W. Wells: Mol. Pharmacol. *43*, 569 (1993).
98 M.I. Martinez-Mir, H. Pollard, J. Moreau, J.M. Arrang, M. Ruat, E. Traiffort, J.C. Schwartz, and J.M. Palacois: Brain Res. *526*, 322 (1990).
99 H. Pollard, J. Moreau, J.M. Arrang, and J.C. Schwartz: Neuroscience *52*, 169 (1993).
100 Y. Nakagawa, K. Yanai, J.H. Ryu, M. Kiyosawa, M. Tamai, and T. Watanabe: Brain Res. *643*,74 (1994).
101 P. Cumming and S.R. Vincent: Brain Res. *602*, 53 (1993).
102 K. Yanai, J.H. Ryu, N. Sakai, T. Takahashi, R. Iwata, T. Ido, K. Murakami, and T. Watanabe: Jpn. J. Pharmacol. *65*, 107 (1994).
103 J.C. Barnes, J.D. Brown, N.P. Clarke, J. Clapham, D.J. Evans, and C.T. Oshaughnessy: Eur. J. Pharmacol. *250*, 147 (1993).
104 M. Ruat, M. Korner, M. Garbarg, C. Gros, J.C. Schwartz, W. Tertiuk, and C.R. Ganellin: Proc. Natl. Acad. Sci. *85*, 2743 (1988).
105 M. Ruat, E. Traiffort, M.L. Bouthenet, J.C. Schwartz, J. Hirschfeld, A. Buschauer, and W. Schunack: Proc. Natl. Acad. Sci. *87*, 1658 (1990).
106 Y. Cherifi, C. Pigeon, M. Leromancer, A. Bado, F. Reyldesmars, and M.J.M. Lewin: J. Biol. Chem. *267*, 25315 (1992).
107 M. Yamashita, H. Fukui, K. Sugama, Y. Horio, S. Ito, H. Mizuguchi, and H. Wada: Proc. Natl. Acad. Sci. USA *88*, 11515 (1991).
108 M. Ruat, E. Traiffort, J.M. Arrang, R. Leurs, and J.C. Schwartz: Biochem. Biophys. Res. Commun. *179*, 1470 (1991).
109 I. Gantz, M. Schaffer, J. DelValle, G. Logdson, V. Campbell, M. Uhler, and T. Yamada: Proc. Natl. Acad. Sci. USA *88*, 429 (1991).
110 I. Gantz, G. Munzert, T. Tashiro, M. Schaffer, L. Wang, J. DelValle, and T. Yamada: Biochem. Biophys. Res. Commun. *178*, 1386 (1991).
111 H. Fukui, K. Fujimoto, H. Mizuguchi, K. Sakamoto, Y. Horio, S. Takai, K. Yamada, and S. Ito: Biochem. Biophys. Res. Commun. *201*, 894 (1994).
112 K. Fujimoto, Y. Horio, K. Sugama, S. Ito, Y.Q. Liu, and H. Fukui: Biochem. Biophy.s Re.s Commun. *190*, 294 (1993).
113 M.D. Debacker, W. Gommeren, H. Moereels, G. Nobels, P. Vangompel, J.E. Leysen, and W.H.M.L. Luyten: Biochem. Biophys. Res. Commun. *197*, 1601 (1993).
114 H. Schworer, A. Reimann, G. Ramadori, and K. Racke: Arch. Pharmacol. *350*, 375 (1994).
115 H.H. Dale and P.P. Laidlaw: J. Physiol. *41*, 318 (1910).
116 D. Bovet and A.M. Staub: C.R. Soc. Biol. *124*, 547 (1937).
117 S.B. Felix, A. Buschauer, and G. Baumann, in: H.Timmerman.and H. Van der Goot (Eds.), New perspectives in histamine research, Birkhäuser Verlag: Basel (1991), p. 257.
118 H. Timmerman: J. Med. Chem. *33*, 4 (1990).
119 J.L. Burgaud and N. Oudart: Brit. J. Pharmacol. *109*, 960 (1993).
120 M. Ichinose and P.J. Barnes: J. Allerg. Clin. Immunol. *86*, 491 (1990).

121 J.A. Hey, M. Del Prado, R.W. Egan, W. Kreutner, and R.W. Chapman: Eur. J. Pharmacol. *211*, 421 (1992).
122 J.P. Trzeciakowski: J. Pharm. Exp. Therap. *243*, 874 (1987).
123 M.J.M. Lewin, A. Bado, Y. Cherifi, and F. Reyldesmars: J. Biol. Med. *65*, 607 (1992).
124 A. Bado, F. Hervatin, and M.J.M. Lewin: Am. J. Physiol. *260*, G631 (1991).
125 G. Soldani, G. Mengozzi, L. Intorre, G. De Giorgi, G. Coruzzi, and G. Bertaccini: Arch. Pharmacol. *347*, 61 (1993).
126 G. Soldani, L. Intorre, S. Bertini, E. Luchetti, G. Coruzzi, and G. Bertaccini: Arch. Pharmacol. *350*, 218 (1994).
127 F. Hollande, J.P. Ball, and R. Magous: Am. J. Physiol. *265*, G1039 (1993).
128 G. Coruzzi, M. Adami, and G. Bertaccini: Pharmacol. *44*, 190 (1992).
129 T. Mochizuki, A. Yamatodani, K. Okakura, A. Horii, N. Inagaki, and H. Wada: Physiol. Behav. *51*, 391 (1992).
130 A.N. Nicholson, P.A. Pascoe, C. Turner, C.R. Ganellin, P.M. Greengrass, A.F. Casy, and A.D. Mercer: Br. J. Pharmacol. *104*, 270 (1991).
131 J.S. Lin, K. Sakai, G. Vannimercier, J.M. Arrang, M. Garbarg, J.C. Schwartz, and M. Jouvet: Brain Res. *523*, 325 (1990).
132 J.C. Lin, K. Sakai, and M. Louvet: C. R. Acad. Sci. *303*, 469 (1986).
133 H. Yokoyama, K. Onodera, K. Iinuma, and T. Watanabe: Pharmacol. Biochem. Behav. *47*, 503 (1994).
134 K. Iinuma, H. Yokoyama, T. Otsuki, K. Yanai, T. Watanabe, T. Ido, and M. Itoh: Lancet *341*, 238 (1993).
135 H. Yokoyama, K. Onodera, K. Iinuma, and T. Watanabe: Eur. J. Pharmacol. *234*, 129 (1993).
136 T. Sakata, K. Ookuma, K. Fujimoto, K. Fukagawa, and H. Yoshimatsu: Brain Res. Bull. *27*, 371 (1991).
137 T. Doi, T. Sakata, H. Yoshimatsu, H. Machidori, M. Kurokawa, L.A.L.W. Jayasekara, and N. Niki: Brain Res. *641*, 311 (1994).
138 A. Oohara, H. Yoshimatsu, M. Kurokawa, R. Oishi, K. Saeki, and T. Sakata: J. Neurochem. *63*, 677 (1994).
139 T. Yabe, C. De Waele, M. Serafin, N. Vibert, J.M. Arrang, M. Muhlethaler, and P.P. Vidal: Exp. Brain. Res. *93*, 249 (1993).
140 A.J.E.M. Fischer: Acta Otolaryngol. *479*, 24 (1991).
141 M.A.M.R. De Almeida and I. Izquierdo: Arch. Int. Pharmacodyn. *283*, 193 (1986).
142 M.A.M.R. De Almeida and I. Izquierdo: Arch. Int. Pharmacodyb. *291*, 202 (1988).
143 J.M. Bekkers: Science *261*, 104 (1993).
144 V.S. Vorobjev, I.N. Sharonova, I.B. Walsh, and H.L. Haas: Neuron *11*, 837 (1993).
145 R.E. Brown, H.L. Haas, and K.G. Reymann: Soc. Neurosci. Abstr. *20*, 1515 (1994).
146 I.M. Mazurkiewicz-Kwilecki and S. Nsonwah: Can. J. Physiol. Pharmacol. *67*, 75 (1989).
147 L.M. Bierer, V. Haroutunian, S. Gabriel, P.J. Knott, L.S. Carlin, D.P. Purohit, D.P. Perl, J. Schmeidler, P. Kanof, and K.L. Davis: J. Neurochem. *64*, 749 (1995).
148 J.C. Barnes, J. Clapham, R.P. Dennes, G.L. Kilpatrick, F.H. Marshall, C.T. O'Shaughnessy, and E. Cavicchini: Soc. Neurosci. Abstr. *19*, P1813 (1993).
149 C.P.S. Smith, A.J. Hunter, and G.W. Bennett: Psychopharmacology *114*, 651 (1994).

Progress in Drug Research, Vol. 45 (E. Jucker, Ed.)

Serotonin uptake inhibitors: Uses in clinical therapy and in laboratory research

By Ray W. Fuller

Lilly Research Laboratories, Eli Lilly and Company, Lilly Corporate Center, Indianapolis, IN 46285, USA

1 Introduction

Shortly after serotonin was discovered to be present in the brain in 1953, it was suspected to be a neurotransmitter there. Just over 40 years later, much has been learned about brain serotonin neurons and their physiological roles. One contributor to this advance in knowledge has been a group of compounds that selectively inhibit serotonin uptake. The study of these compounds in laboratory animals has not only given insight into the operation of serotonin neurons themselves and how the synthesis and release of serotonin is controlled, but also has helped in the understanding of physiological roles of serotonin neurons. Moreover, these serotonin uptake inhibitors have been therapeutically useful in treating mental depression, bulimia and obsessive-compulsive disorder in humans, and there is some indication they may have therapeutic effects in a variety of other diseases. The continued study of these compounds will further increase our knowledge about the role of serotonin in disease and may lead to ways of enhancing their therapeutic effects.

2 Selectivity of serotonin uptake inhibitors

The target for serotonin uptake inhibitors is the transporter present on the outer neuronal membrane of serotonin neurons. For years, it has been possible to study *in vitro* the transport of radioactive serotonin and other monoamines by pinched-off nerve endings or synaptosomes prepared from brain homogenates. The tricyclic antidepressant drugs were found to be inhibitors of this monoamine transport, and it was postulated that blockade of serotonin uptake and blockade of norepinephrine uptake were mechanisms of their antidepressant efficacy. Numerous selective inhibitors of serotonin uptake were later identified, which do not inhibit norepinephrine or dopamine uptake except at much higher concentrations *in vitro* and which inhibit only serotonin uptake at doses ordinarily used *in vivo*.

Fig. 1 shows the chemical structures of seven selective inhibitors of serotonin uptake. Additional selective inhibitors of serotonin uptake have been described and characterized, but have been studied to a lesser extent than those shown. These seven compounds represent a chemically diverse group; they are highly selective in their pharmacologic actions and they share no other known activity in common apart from inhibition of serotonin uptake. The references given in the figure describe various experimental methods that have been used to document selective inhibition of serotonin uptake by these compounds in laboratory animals. Commonly used methods include *ex vivo* measurement of serotonin uptake by brain synaptosomes from animals treated with the uptake inhibitors at various times previously; antagonism of serotonin depletion by agents that deplete serotonin by a transporter-dependent mechanism, such as p-chloroamphetamine, H75/12 (4-methyl-α-ethyl-m-tyramine), or fenfluramine; potentiation of 5-hydroxytryptophan (5HTP)-induced head twitches or other effects; or reduction in brain concentrations of 5-hydroxyindoleacetic acid (5HIAA) or in some other measure of serotonin turnover.

All of the selective uptake inhibitors listed in Fig. 1 have been shown in double-blind clinical studies to be effective in the treatment of mental depression [1–3]. Two other antidepressant drugs – trazodone and nefazodone – are sometimes referred to as serotonin uptake inhibitors. These compounds are relatively weak inhibitors of serotonin uptake by brain synaptosomes *in vitro*, but *in vivo* they are not effective as serotonin uptake inhibitors at doses that antagonize $5HT_2$ receptors (their predominant pharmacologic action). Serotonin uptake inhibition does not occur at doses of trazodone and nefazodone that are ordinarily used in laboratory animals [4, 5], and it is unlikely that significant inhibition of serotonin uptake occurs at doses of trazodone and nefazodone that are used in treating mental depression. Those two compounds are not further considered in this review. Also not included is clomipramine, which is a selective inhibitor of serotonin uptake in the test tube but becomes nonselective *in vivo* due to prominent actions of its desmethyl metabolite to inhibit norepinephrine uptake.

In laboratory animals, all of the compounds listed in Fig. 1 are selective inhibitors of serotonin uptake and have generally similar pharmacologic effects. There may be significant differences among them clinically, but as a class they represent an improvement over the tricyclic antidepressant drugs in avoiding the prevalent anticholinergic actions of the earlier drugs, in not having direct cardiac effects, and in being safer in overdose. All of these characteristics presumably result from their greater specificity of pharmacologic action.

The rat [6, 7], mouse [8] and human [9, 10] serotonin transporters have been cloned. They can be expressed in suitable host cells in which they are functionally active in transporting serotonin. This has not been a particularly important advantage technically over the use of synaptosomes or blood platelets as a serotonin-transporting unit for *in vitro* studies. However, the cloning of the transporter and the ability to measure messenger RNA encoding for it have facilitated further studies of its distribution, structural specificity, ionic mechanisms and regulation [11–17]. The serot-

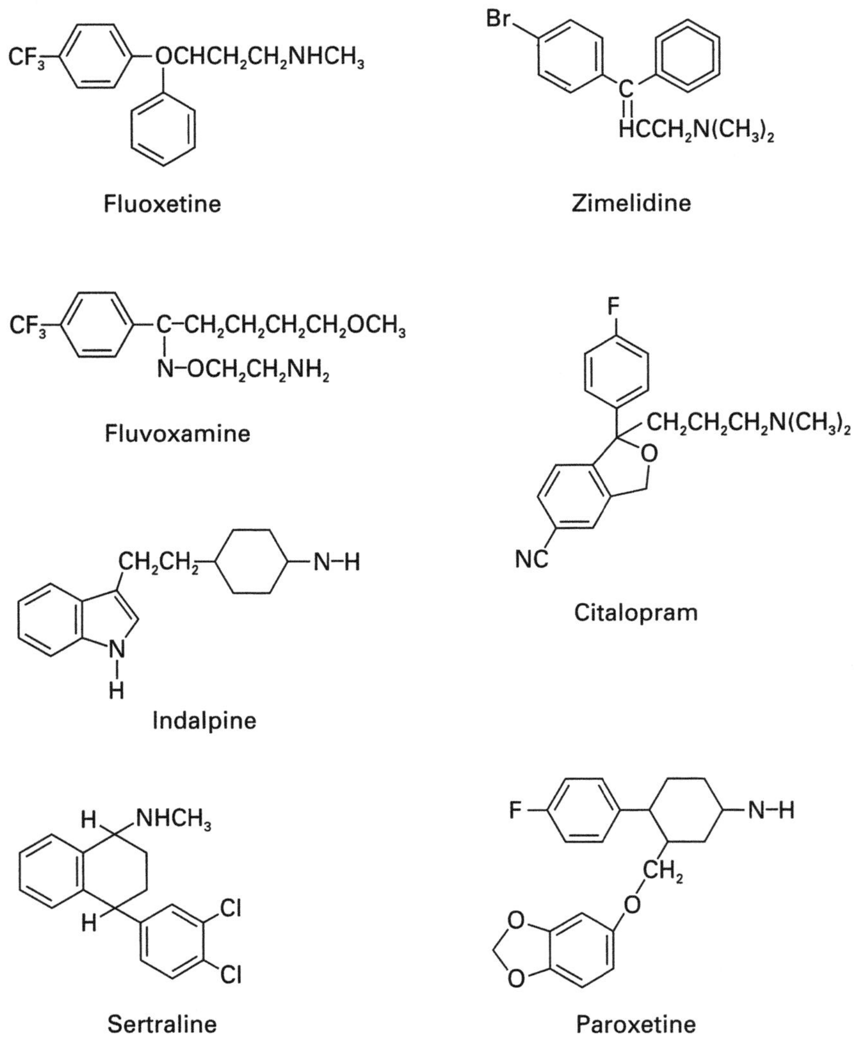

Fig. 1.
Chemical structures of some selective inhibitors of serotonin uptake: fluoxetine [275], paroxetine [276], fluvoxamine [277], citalopram [278], zimelidine [279], indalpine [280] and sertraline [248]. At the time this figure was prepared, the number of references retrieved from PaperChase was fluoxetine, 1720; fluvoxamine, 766; zimelidine (zimeldine), 438, paroxetine, 343; citalopram, 239; sertraline, 116; and indalpine, 30, giving some indication of the extent to which these compounds have been characterized and used as experimental probes.

onin transporter in humans appears to be encoded by a single gene located on chromosome 17 [10]. The transporter protein has twelve membrane-spanning segments, a feature common to other sodium-dependent transporters [7, 13].

3 Enhanced input to diverse postsynaptic receptors on widespread target neurons

Serotonin neurons in the central nervous system have their cell bodies in clusters of cells in raphe nuclei along the midline in the brain stem, and they send ascending and descending projections to many parts of the brain and to the spinal cord [18]. Indeed, Jacobs and Azmitia [18] consider that among currently known neuronal systems, serotonin neurons represent the most expansive circuitry in the central nervous system. Serotonin nerve terminals are found in nearly all parts of the brain, regions that are involved in the control of many bodily functions regulated by the brain, including behavior, movement, appetite, sexual activity, pain, blood pressure, body temperature, and endocrine secretion.

One of the major developments in serotonin pharmacology in recent years has been the recognition that all serotonin receptors are not alike and the elucidation of multiple subtypes of serotonin receptors. Presently there are at least 14 distinct serotonin receptor subtypes that have been cloned: $5HT_{1A}$, $5HT_{1B}$ (or $5HT_{1D\beta}$), $5HT_{1D}$ (also called $5HT_{1D\alpha}$), $5HT_{1E}$, $5HT_{1F}$, $5HT_{2A}$, $5HT_{2B}$, $5HT_{2C}$, $5HT_3$, $5HT_4$, $5HT_{5A}$, $5HT_{5B}$, $5HT_6$ and $5HT_7$ [19]. Serotonin activates all of these receptors, albeit with different sensitivities, but some of their pharmacologic properties are different; selective agonists and antagonists acting directly at each of the receptor subtypes are being sought and found. When serotonin uptake inhibitors increase extracellular concentrations of serotonin, that serotonin can activate all of these receptors that are present at a given serotonergic synapse. Thus various effects of serotonin uptake inhibitors in laboratory animals and in humans (discussed below) are presumably mediated by increased activation of one or more of these receptors by serotonin.

Tork [20], Descarries et al. [21] and others have pointed out that some serotonin nerve terminals in some parts of the brain do not form tight synaptic junctions with specific target neurons but instead terminate in a field of neurons. Tork has referred to this as a "drip-irrigation" system in which serotonin released into the extracellular fluid can diffuse to affect multiple neurons in the region provided they have serotonin receptors. In this type of arrangement, one might anticipate the serotonin receptors would need to be sensitive to low concentrations of serotonin, whereas within a synaptic junction the local concentrations of serotonin might be much higher so that junctional receptors could require higher concentrations of serotonin for activation.

4 Brain microdialysis studies with serotonin uptake inhibitors; insight into dynamics of serotonin neurons

The administration of serotonin uptake inhibitors causes an increase in extracellular serotonin that has been measured in various brain regions by microdialysis followed by liquid chromatography with electrochemical detection [22]. This increased amount of extracellular serotonin results in greater activation of postsynaptic serotonin receptors on target neurons and of presynaptic autoreceptors on serotonin nerve terminals and serotonin cell bodies [23]. The increased activation of postsynaptic receptors represents an increase in serotonergic neurotransmission and causes numerous physiological consequences, to be discussed below. The increased activation of the autoreceptors causes a decrease in the rate of firing of serotonin neurons and a decrease in the rate of serotonin synthesis and release by those neurons. These compensatory changes result in the increase in extracellular serotonin being less than it would have been after uptake inhibition if serotonin had continued to be made and released at the same rate. Although the excessive (very intense) activation of postsynaptic serotonin receptors causes effects in rats that can be observed – components of the "serotonin behavioral syndrome" such as head weaving, reciprocal forepaw treading, hindlimb abduction which leads to flat body posture, Straub tail, and lower lip retraction [24] – such effects are not observed after the administration of uptake inhibitors alone. But they can be observed when uptake inhibitors are administered along with a serotonin precursor or a monoamine oxidase inhibitor [24]. The explanation seems to be that the increase in extracellular serotonin concentration following uptake inhibition alone is not sufficient to activate the postsynaptic serotonin receptors to the extent necessary to cause these serotonin behavioral syndrome symptoms, because the compensatory adjustments in the serotonin neurons limit the increase in extracellular serotonin. When those compensatory changes are avoided or bypassed by the administration of a monoamine oxidase inhibitor or a serotonin precursor with the uptake inhibitor, then extracellular serotonin concentrations become higher and the components of the serotonin behavioral syndrome are observed [25].

Although we have measured higher concentrations of extracellular serotonin when a $5HT_{1A}$ receptor antagonist is coadministered with an uptake inhibitor and have seen functional consequences in excess of those produced by uptake inhibition alone [26], we have not noticed components of the serotonin behavioral syndrome in those rats. It may be that this combination of drugs produces increases in extracellular serotonin that are not quite as large as those produced by an uptake inhibitor combined with a serotonin precursor or with a monoamine oxidase inhibitor. More quantitative comparisons of extracellular serotonin increases in various brain regions after these treatments may clarify the relationships between extracellular serotonin and the behavioral syndrome.

It is important to recognize that the decrease in serotonin neuron firing and the decrease in serotonin synthesis following serotonin uptake inhibition are due at least in part to the increased extracellular concentrations of serotonin acting on autoreceptors. Serotonin transmission – how well serotonin neurons are signalling their target neurons – is increased for that same reason, the increase in serotonin concentrations extracellularly. The decrease in 5HIAA concentrations in cerebrospinal fluid found in untreated depressed patients, particularly with aggressive/impulsive/suicidal symptoms [27], is properly interpreted as indicative of reduced serotonin formation and release, hence reduced serotonergic transmission. A decrease in 5HIAA caused by serotonin uptake inhibitors should not be interpreted in that same way. 5HIAA is not thought to have a physiological function, so the concentrations of 5HIAA are not in themselves important functionally. 5HIAA levels may provide some index of serotonin function, but the interpretation of 5HIAA changes must be done with caution. A change in 5HIAA in the endogenous state without drug intervention, may indicate the direction in which serotonin function is changed. A decrease in 5HIAA may indicate serotonin function is decreased. On the other hand, a decrease in 5HIAA following an uptake inhibitor or a monoamine oxidase inhibitor does not indicate serotonin transmission is decreased. In both cases, serotonin transmission is increased because both pre- and postsynaptic receptors are seeing increased concentrations of serotonin. When serotonin uptake inhibitors are given and cause an increase in extracellular serotonin, that serotonin acts on autoreceptors to cause a decrease in firing of serotonin neurons and in serotonin synthesis and release (hence in the *activity* of serotonin neurons) and acts on postsynaptic target receptors so that serotonergic *neurotransmission* is increased. The activity of serotonin neurons – how rapidly they are firing and releasing serotonin – is not the same as how well they are transmitting signals in this case.

5 Functional consequences of increased serotonergic neurotransmission

Animals treated with serotonin uptake inhibitors look normal in gross appearance, but numerous effects that seem to be consequences of increased serotonergic transmission have been measured. Some of those are described below.

5.1 Neurochemical effects

Probably the best known and most studied neurochemical change after administration of a serotonin uptake inhibitor is a decrease in serotonin turnover [28, 29]. Tissue concentrations of serotonin are not changed, or at most are only slightly increased, but tissue concentrations of 5HIAA are significantly decreased. The dose-dependence and duration of 5HIAA lowering parallel the inhibition of serotonin uptake. The decrease in 5HIAA concentration is a consequence of decreased serotonin synthesis and turnover. Serotonin synthesis measured by the rate of 5HTP accumulation after decarboxylase inhibition is also decreased (Table 1), as is the rate of decrease in serotonin concentration after treatment with p-chlorophenylalanine to inhibit tryptophan hydroxylation and the rate of increase in 5HIAA after inhibition of its efflux by probenecid, two other measures of serotonin turnover [28]. The decrease in serotonin turnover coincides with a decrease in serotonin neuron firing measured electrophysiologically [30], which is a consequence of increased extracellular concentrations of serotonin [31, 32].

Changes in turnover of neurotransmitters would certainly be expected in postsynaptic target neurons, but relatively little is known about what these neuronal targets for serotonergic input are in various brain regions. An increase in MHPG sulfate (3-methoxy-4-hydroxy-phenylethyleneglycol sulfate), the metabolite of norepinephrine, has been observed in rat hypothalamus following fluoxetine administration, indicating an increase in norepinephrine turnover [33]. Those results are consistent with the findings of Smythe et al. [34] that the combination of fluoxetine with L-5HTP increased hypothalamic concentrations of another norepinephrine metabolite, 3,4-dihydroxyphenylethyleneglycol (DHPG). Microdialysis studies have shown that fluoxetine increases extracellular concentrations of norepinephrine in hypothalamus and in frontal cortex (but not hippocampus) in rats [K. W. Perry and R. W. Fuller, unpublished data]. These changes are attributed to increased norepinephrine release and turnover when serotonergic input to norepinephrine neurons is magnified by flu-

Table 1.
Decreased 5HTP accumulation after decarboxylase inhibition as an index of decreased serotonin synthesis in rat brain regions following fluoxetine administration.

	5HTP, nmoles/g	
Brain region	Control	Fluoxetine-treated
Midbrain	1.48 ± 0.11	0.96 ± 0.11* (–35%)
Hypothalamus	1.25 ± 0.08	0.64 ± 0.06* (–49%)
Brain stem	0.89 ± 0.08	0.67 ± 0.05* (–25%)
Striatum	0.68 ± 0.08	0.31 ± 0.04* (–54%)
Hippocampus	0.64 ± 0.03	0.31 ± 0.04* (–52%)
Cortex	0.54 ± 0.02	0.22 ± 0.02* (–59%)

* Significant difference from control group ($p < .05$)

m-Hydroxybenzylhydrazine (NSD 1015) (100 mg/kg i.p.) was injected 30 minutes before measurements were made and 1 hr after fluoxetine hydrochloride (10 mg/kg i.p.). Mean values ± standard errors for 5 rats per group are shown. The experiment was performed by Kenneth W. Perry.

oxetine; similar changes are produced by direct-acting serotonin agonists and by serotonin-releasing drugs.

In the dorsal hippocampus in rats, serotonergic input appears to facilitate acetylcholine release. The serotonin uptake inhibitor citalopram increased extracellular concentrations of acetylcholine measured by microdialysis, as did the serotonin-releasing drugs d-fenfluramine and d-norfenfluramine [35]. In the prefrontal cortex but not in the nucleus accumbens in rats, extracellular concentrations of dopamine were increased by fluoxetine and by other antidepressant drugs [36]. More neurochemical effects of these sorts, representing consequences of increased serotonergic input to target neurons, are likely to be found after the administration of serotonin uptake inhibitors.

5.2 Behavioral effects

In rats treated with a single dose of fluoxetine or some other selective inhibitor of serotonin uptake, no increased or decreased locomotion or other visible change in behavior is observed. But when certain specific behaviors are looked for, characteristic behavioral changes can be measured. A well-studied example is a decrease in aggression, a behavioral

Table 2.
Inhibition of aggressive behavior in several species by serotonin uptake inhibitors

Species	Uptake inhibitor	Type of aggression	Reference
Rat	Fluoxetine	Spontaneous muricide	Gibbons et al.[37]; Stark et al. [40]
Rat	Fluoxetine	Muricide induced by p-chlorophenylalanine	Berzsenyi et al. [38]
Rat	Fluoxetine	Spontaneous and p-chlorophenylalanine-induced muricide	Kostowski et al. [39]
Rat	Fluoxetine, indalpine	Muricide induced by raphe lesion or by p-chlorophenylalanine	Molina et al. [41]
Rat	Fluoxetine, citalopram	Muricide induced by raphe lesion or by p-chlorophenylalanine	Molina et al. [42]
Rat	Paroxetine	Muricide induced by raphe lesion or by olfactory bulbectomy	Yamamoto et al. [43]
Rat	Fluoxetine	Intraspecies aggression induced by footshck	Datla et al. [45]
Vervet monkey	Fluoxetine	Intraspecies aggression spontaneously occurring in natural setting	Raleigh et al. [48]
Mouse	Zimelidine Fluoxetine	Isolation-induced aggression	Ogren et al. [44]; R. J. Katz [personal communication]
Mouse	Fluoxetine	Resident-intruder aggression	Wagner et al. [46]
Mouse	Zimelidine	Heightened resident-intruder aggression in transgenic mice overexpressing human growth factor alpha	Hilakivi-Clark and Goldberg [274]
Golden hamster	Fluoxetine	Resident-intruder aggression, spontaneous or induced by vasopressin	Ferris and Delville [47]; Ferris [personal communication]

change that is only observed in a setting where aggression is manifest. Table 2 lists multiple studies in which some type of aggressive behavior in animals has been reduced by one or more inhibitors of serotonin uptake. Muricidal (mouse-killing) aggression in rats is decreased by fluoxetine and by other inhibitors of serotonin uptake, whether that aggression is occurring spontaneously in a certain strain of rats or has been induced by chemical or electrolytic lesions or by inhibition of serotonin synthesis [37–43]. Other types of aggressive behavior in rats and in mice are also inhibited by serotonin uptake inhibitors [44–46]. Territorial aggression in golden hamsters, induced by central injection of vasopressin [47] or occurring spontaneously [C. F. Ferris, personal communication], is inhibited by fluoxetine.

A particularly interesting decrease in aggressive behavior by fluoxetine was observed in monkeys by Raleigh et al. [48]. They studied social behavior in troops of monkeys living in natural conditions. Each troop consisted of three male monkeys, three or more female monkeys, and their offspring. In such troops, one male monkey was always dominant, the leader of the troop. The experimental protocol involved removing the dominant male and observing which of the two remaining male monkeys became dominant during the ensuing weeks. One of the two remaining males was treated with placebo, and the other received a treatment to increase or to decrease serotonin function. Tryptophan, the amino acid precursor to serotonin, or fluoxetine was given to increase serotonin function. Cyproheptadine, a serotonin receptor antagonist, or fenfluramine, a serotonin depletor, was given to decrease serotonin function. In all cases, the male monkey given a treatment to increase serotonin function became dominant over the male monkey given placebo, and the male monkey given placebo became dominant over the male monkey given a drug to decrease serotonin function. The acquisition of dominance did not mean the monkeys were more aggressive. Indeed, measurement of specific behaviors revealed that fluoxetine-treated monkeys showed *less* aggression and more positive social interactions (e.g., approaching other monkeys and staying near or grooming them), as did tryptophan-treated monkeys. Drugs that decrease serotonin function *increased* aggression and reduced the positive social interactions.

The decrease in aggressive behavior after fluoxetine treatment has been observed in various animal species, with different types of aggressive behavior occurring spontaneously or induced by various means. Several studies in humans (to be discussed below) are consistent in suggesting that fluoxetine can reduce aggressive behavior. The animal data also are consistent with a larger body of data showing decreased aggressive behavior after administration of direct-acting serotonin receptor agonists, serotonin precursors and serotonin-releasing drugs [42, 48–50].

Another behavioral effect of fluoxetine is an increase in acquisition rate for a passive avoidance task in olfactory bulbectomized rats in whom that rate had been decreased [51]. The effect produced by direct injection of fluoxetine into the amygdala was attenuated by metergoline, supporting a serotonergic mechanism [52]. Zimelidine mimicked fluoxetine in increasing passive avoidance behavior in olfactory bulbectomized rats in a step-down task, and metergoline blocked the effect of fluoxetine [53]. Fluoxetine enhanced memory processing in mice and blocked amnesia induced by a protein synthesis inhibitor or by an anticholinergic drug [54].

5.3 Inhibition of food intake

One important function of brain serotonin neurons appears to be the regulation of food intake. Studies with serotonin uptake inhibitors have provided much data supporting and elucidating this idea. Fluoxetine was shown to decrease food intake in meal-fed rats after single doses and to act synergistically with 5HTP [55]. Chronic administration of fluoxetine to rats [56, 57] or to mice [58] decreased food intake and decreased body weight, as did chronic administration of other serotonin uptake inhibitors and other drugs that increase serotonin function in other ways [59–61]. Fluoxetine and other serotonin uptake inhibitors have also been shown to decrease carbohydrate intake preferentially in rats with a choice of foods [62–68], to decrease stress-induced eating in nonfasted rats [69], and to decrease hyperphagia induced by insulin or 2-deoxyglucose injection in rats [70, 71], whereas appetite suppressant drugs acting through other mechanisms (e.g., dopamine release) do not have these characteristics. In addition, fluoxetine (and the serotonin-releasing drug fenfluramine) had a different effect on the microstructure of ingestive behavior in rats than did amphetamine and phenylpropanolamine, drugs acting via a catecholaminergic mechanism [72].

Although fluoxetine decreases food intake in numerous experimental settings in rats, in one interesting example it increased food intake. Altemus et al. [73] described what may be an animal model of obsessive-compulsive disorder. Rats with 90-minute daily access to food normally thrive, but when they have access to a running wheel, these rats run excessively, decrease their food intake, and may die of malnutrition. In these rats, fluoxetine significantly attenuated wheel running, anorexia and weight loss. The efficacy of serotonin uptake inhibitors in treating obsessive-compulsive disorder in humans (discussed below) supports the predictive value of this model.

5.4 Decreased alcohol drinking

In rats with a choice of drinking water or an ethanol solution, fluoxetine caused a decrease in total ethanol intake and a decrease in ethanol intake as a percentage of total fluid intake during the period of days that it was administered [74]. Similar effects have been reported with other serotonin uptake inhibitors such as zimelidine [74, 75] and sertraline [76]. Fluoxetine also reduced ethanol intake in rats genetically predisposed to prefer ethanol to water [77].

5.5 Neuroendocrine effects

Secretion of glucocorticoids from the adrenal cortex is regulated by ACTH (adrenocorticotropin) released from the anterior pituitary gland, and ACTH release in turn is controlled by CRF (corticotropin-releasing factor). Serotonin neurons make synaptic contact with CRF neurons in the paraventricular nucleus of the hypothalamus in rats [78], and serotonin or serotonin agonists increase CRF release from rat hypothalamus *in vitro* [79]. Fluoxetine administration to rats increases corticosterone [80] and ACTH [81] concentrations in systemic blood and increases CRF concentration in the hypophyseal portal blood from the hypothalamus [81]. The ability of fluoxetine to increase serum corticosterone concentration is potentiated by L-5HTP and is mimicked by other serotonin uptake inhibitors, by direct-acting serotonin agonists, and by serotonin-releasing drugs [82]. Bianchi et al. [83] have reported that fluoxetine reduces inflammatory edema, following injection of brewer's yeast into the rat hind paw, by activating pituitary-adrenocortical secretion. Fluoxetine combined with L-5HTP, but not fluoxetine alone, increased serum prolactin concentration in rats [30, 84].

5.6 Anticonvulsant effects

Serotonin uptake inhibitors have anticonvulsant effects in some animal models. Siegel and Murphy [85] reported that fluoxetine inhibited amygdala-kindled seizures in cats, as did stimulation of the nucleus raphe centralis, which contains serotonin neuronal cell bodies. Dailey et al. [86] showed that fluoxetine decreased sound-induced convulsions in genetically epilepsy-prone rats of both moderate and severe seizure liability, at doses that increased extracellular concentrations of serotonin in the thalamus. Support for a serotonergic mechanism in these effects was provided by Yan et al. [87], who showed that coadministration of L-5HTP potentiated the effect of fluoxetine in these rats.

Pasini et al. [88] observed that bilateral focal injection of fluoxetine into the substantia nigra of rats protected against convulsive seizures evoked by focal injection of bicuculline methiodide into the area tempestas, an epileptogenic site within the deep prepiriform cortex. Prendiville and Gale [89] also found that systemic injection of fluoxetine had anticonvulsant effects in this model. Fluoxetine is also reported to enhance the anticonvulsant effects of phenytoin, carbamazepine and ameltolide in the maximal electroshock seizure test in mice [90].

5.7 Analgesia

In some experimental paradigms, fluoxetine has been shown to have analgesic effects [91–93]. Fluoxetine also is reported to potentiate analgesic effects of morphine [94,95]. Citalopram, fluvoxamine, zimelidine, paroxetine, sertraline and fluoxetine are reported to inhibit acetic acid-induced writhing in a standard analgesic test in mice [96, 97]. These findings are consistent with a large body of evidence that serotonin neurons in the central nervous system modulate pain perception and responsiveness [98, 99].

5.8 Other physiological effects

Fluoxetine administration to rats and cats has been shown to decrease rapid-eye-movement sleep without significant effects on other stages of sleep [100]. The effect in cats was potentiated by coadministration of L-5HTP. A chemical analog of fluoxetine that did not block serotonin uptake failed to mimic the ability of fluoxetine to suppress rapid-eye-movement sleep in rats [101]. Fluoxetine also reduced rapid-eye-movement sleep in hamsters [102]. Zimelidine has also been reported to reduce rapid-eye-movement sleep in rats and in cats [103], with similar effects in rats reported for paroxetine and indalpine [104, 105].

The combination of fluoxetine with L-5HTP, but not fluoxetine alone, significantly reduced blood pressure in genetically hypertensive rats and in rats made hypertensive by treatment with deoxycorticosterone and saline [106], perhaps a consequence of altering central serotonergic pathways that modulate blood pressure.

5.9 Functional effects: uptake inhibitors vs. releasers

Serotonin uptake inhibitors and serotonin-releasing drugs such as p-chloroamphetamine and fenfluramine increase extracellular concentrations of serotonin and produce some of the same functional consequences acutely, such as reduction in food intake and elevation of serum corticosterone concentration [60, 107]. The serotonin-releasing drugs can lead to depletion of serotonin stores at later times and produce opposite kinds of effects to serotonin uptake inhibitors or to their acute effects, e.g., increases in aggressive behavior [37, 48, 108].

Recent microdialysis studies have shown that the acute increase in extracellular serotonin concentration produced by serotonin-releasing drugs (fenfluramine and p-chloroamphetamine) can be much larger than the increase produced by serotonin uptake inhibitors, because the increase by serotonin-releasing drugs is not dependent upon neuronal firing and is not limited by compensatory reductions in firing of serotonin neurons [109–110]. The large increase in extracellular serotonin elicited by fenfluramine acutely is antagonized by fluoxetine or sertraline [109, 111], because the release of serotonin by fenfluramine occurs through a transporter-dependent mechanism. Marsden et al. [112] have shown by *in vivo* voltammetry that the large increase in extracellular serotonin elicited by p-chloroamphetamine is antagonized by fluoxetine pretreatment.

These data on extracellular serotonin agree well with previous literature on functional effects. For example, serotonin-releasing drugs (fenfluramine and p-chloroamphetamine) produce certain functional changes that uptake inhibitors do not produce; examples are increases in serum prolactin concentration [113–115] and some signs of the serotonin behavioral syndrome [116, 117]. Uptake inhibitors antagonize the increase in serum prolactin and the serotonin behavioral syndrome symptoms elicited by these serotonin-releasing drugs [114, 115, 117], just as they antagonize the large increase in extracellular serotonin measured by microdialysis or voltammetry. Apparently the elevation of serum prolactin and the emergence of the serotonin behavioral syndrome require large concentrations of extracellular serotonin beyond those produced by uptake inhibition alone.

6 Means of further enhancement of serotonergic function

As mentioned above, compensatory decreases in serotonin synthesis and release limit the extent to which extracellular serotonin concentrations are increased after uptake inhibitors are given. That limitation presumably keeps serotonergic transmission within physiological bounds so that signs of excessive serotonergic receptor activation, such as the serotonin behavioral syndrome in rats, are not seen when uptake inhibitors are given. A major advantage of uptake inhibitors used in clinical medicine is that they have comparatively few side effects (see below). Thus, the ability of the serotonin neurons to control the degree of increased neurotransmission resulting from uptake inhibition makes uptake inhibition perhaps one of the least intrusive ways of intervening in serotonin function. It is possible that for certain therapeutic applications, the needed degree of increase in serotonergic neurotransmission is greater than can be achieved by uptake inhibition alone. For that reason, there has been interest in boosting the functional effects of uptake inhibitors by coadministration of a second agent that can enhance their effects on extracellular serotonin.

The coadministration of a serotonin precursor to increase serotonin formation and release is one means of enhancing the effect of serotonin uptake inhibitors. L-Tryptophan and L-5HTP are the amino acid precursors to serotonin. One advantage of L-tryptophan is that it is converted to serotonin only in cells that normally form serotonin, that is in cells including serotonin neurons that contain the enzyme tryptophan-5-hydroxylase. L-5HTP can be converted to serotonin anywhere the aromatic L-amino acid decarboxylase is present, leading to the possibility of nonspecific effects. But there are other important considerations. Conversion to serotonin is not the major metabolic pathway for L-tryptophan. L-Tryptophan is extensively used for protein synthesis, and its main pathway of catabolism is via tryptophan oxygenase or tryptophan pyrrolase. The immediate product of that catabolism is N-formyl-kynurenine, and numerous other breakdown products are subsequently formed, some of which have biological activity. For instance, quinolinic acid is one metabolic product from L-tryptophan, and quinolinic acid is an agonist at excitatory amino acid receptors. During et al. [118] have measured extracellular concentrations of quinolinic acid and of serotonin in rat brain after the systemic administration of L-tryptophan. At a 100 mg/kg dose of L-tryptophan needed to produce a modest increase in extracellular serotonin (less than two-fold), a large increase in extracellular quinolinic acid (over 80-fold) was found. L-Tryptophan is neither an efficient nor a specific means of increasing serotonin formation.

The coadministration of L-5HTP with a serotonin uptake inhibitor magnifies many pharmacological consequences of uptake inhibition (such as reduced food intake [55], anticonvulsant effects [87], and sleep effects [100]), and the combination produces some serotonergic effects that uptake inhibitors alone do not cause (such as increases in serum prolactin concentration [30, 76], lowering of blood pressure in spontaneously hypertensive rats [106], and suppression of milk drinking in nonfasted rats [119]). These functional consequences no doubt occur because the extracellular concentrations of serotonin in brain regions are higher when an uptake inhibitor (fluoxetine) and L-5HTP are coadministered than when either agent is administered alone, shown in microdialysis studies [120].

The synergism between fluoxetine and L-5HTP has also been demonstrated in limited clinical studies. Postanoxic intention myoclonus is a condition that has been treated with L-5HTP [121]. Van Woert et al. [122] found that fluoxetine alone had minimum benefit in this disorder, but in two patients receiving fluoxetine, the coadministration of L-5HTP, at doses several-fold lower than those ordinarily needed, produced better therapeutic responses than had been observed earlier with high doses of L-5HTP alone, and the combination had fewer side effects. Further therapeutic trials of the combination in other diseases would be of interest.

As mentioned above, the reduction in firing of serotonin neurons after administration of uptake inhibitors is apparently mediated by increased action of extracellular serotonin on the somatodendritic autoreceptors, which are $5HT_{1A}$ receptors, on serotonin neurons. The decrease in serotonin synthesis and release after uptake inhibition also result presumably from increased activation of terminal autoreceptors which are probably $5HT_{1B}$ and $5HT_{1D}$ receptors on serotonin neurons. Another means of boosting the increases in extracellular serotonin following uptake inhibition should be to block these autoreceptors. Hjorth [123] has shown that penbutolol, a $5HT_{1A}$ receptor antagonist (and a β adrenergic receptor blocker), enhances the increase in extracellular serotonin in ventral hippocampus caused by systemic injection of citalopram, a serotonin uptake inhibitor, in rats. Subsequently, Hjorth and Auerbach [124] have shown that local application of serotonin uptake inhibitors via the microdialysis probe into the rat hippocampus markedly increases extracellular serotonin there and that subsequent systemic injection of the uptake inhibitor reduces that elevated extracellular concentration, presumably as a consequence of increasing serotonin action on $5HT_{1A}$ autoreceptors in cell body regions so that firing of serotonin neurons (and release of serotonin at their terminals) is reduced. Antagonists of $5HT_{1A}$ receptors prevent that action of systemically injected uptake inhibitors. Thus the coadministration of a $5HT_{1A}$ receptor antagonist can remove one controlling mechanism that normally limits the extent to which uptake inhibition increases extracellular serotonin.

Artigas et al. [125] have reported preliminary observations from non-blinded clinical studies that coadministration of pindolol, another β adrenergic blocker that also antagonizes $5HT_{1A}$ receptors, with serotonin uptake inhibitors results in faster onset of antidepressant activity and efficacy in patients refractory to treatment with uptake inhibitors alone. If these results can be confirmed in double blind controlled studies, the most likely interpretation will be that block of $5HT_{1A}$ autoreceptors magnified the increase in extracellular serotonin produced by uptake inhibition, and that the greater increase in activation of serotonin receptors on postsynaptic target neurons gave better antidepressant benefit than could be achieved after uptake inhibition alone. Such a combination of drugs might be useful in other conditions besides depression (see following section). Ideally the $5HT_{1A}$ receptor antagonist would not have other pharmacologic effects such as β adrenergic receptor blockade. Appropriate antagonists of the terminal autoreceptors on serotonin neurons ($5HT_{1B}$ or $5HT_{1D}$ receptors?) might have similar benefit in combination with uptake inhibitors.

7 Therapeutic effects of serotonin uptake inhibitors

As mentioned above, the widespread distribution of serotonin neurons has led to the consideration that their dysfunction might be involved in the etiology of a variety of psychiatric and neurologic diseases, and that drugs which modify serotonin function might be useful in treating those diseases. Table 3 lists many of the diseases in which serotonin uptake inhibitors have been evaluated clinically. Although there is no reason to think that serotonin uptake inhibitors will be useful in managing all of those diseases or even efficacious in all of them, the possibility that they may be active in some of those diseases and the fact they have even been tried in a variety of diseases partly reflect the recognition that serotonin neurons can influence a lot of different physiologic functions under the control of the central nervous system. As the efficacy of serotonin uptake inhibitors becomes more precisely defined in these various conditions [126], our understanding of the physiological roles of serotonin and its relevance to these diseases will have grown.

7.1 Mental depression

The most widespread therapeutic use of selective inhibitors of serotonin uptake has been in the treatment of mental depression. Zimelidine was the first selective inhibitor of serotonin uptake to be marketed worldwide, and fluoxetine was the first such agent to be marketed in the United States. Zimelidine later had to be removed from the market because of side effects that were apparently unrelated to its inhibition of serotonin uptake. Subsequently, several other selective inhibitors of serotonin uptake have been introduced into therapeutic use in treating depression. Nierenberg [127] reviewed all available literature and concluded that serotonin uptake

Table 3.
Diseases in which selective inhibitors of serotonin uptake have demonstrated or potential therapeutic use

Approved in some countries	
Mental depression	Obsessive-compulsive disorder
Bulimia	
Investigational	
Obesity	Panic disorder
Post-traumatic stress disorder	Borderline personality disorder
Type 2 diabetes	Alcoholism
Aggression/violence	Late luteal phase dysphoric disorder
Trichotillomania	Cataplexy
Chronic pain	Headache or migraine
Obsessional jealousy	Whole body dysmorphic disorder
Attention-deficient disorder with hyperactivity	

inhibitors are as effective as tricyclic antidepressant drugs in treating severe depression.

The efficacy of as many as a dozen different serotonin uptake inhibitors in the treatment of mental depression [128], compounds of diverse chemical structure (refer to Fig. 1) whose only known shared pharmacologic action is the selective inhibition of serotonin uptake, is compelling evidence that inhibition of the serotonin transporter is the initial molecular event that leads to their antidepressant efficacy. Further support for that interpretation has come from ongoing studies at Yale University School of Medicine, in which a tryptophan-free mixture of amino acids has been given to interrupt serotonin biosynthesis in the brain [129, 130]. When this amino acid mixture was given to depressed patients whose symptoms had been alleviated effectively by treatment with a compound that inhibits serotonin uptake selectively (e.g., fluoxetine), depressive symptoms transiently recurred, presumably during the period when serotonin synthesis was expected to be reduced. In contrast, patients who had responded to desipramine, a norepinephrine uptake inhibitor, did not show recurrence of symptoms when given the amino acid mixture. The interpretation is that serotonin is indeed essential to the antidepressant efficacy of fluoxetine (and other serotonin uptake inhibitors) but not of desipramine. Consistent with that interpretation is the report by Feder [131] that cyproheptadine, a serotonin receptor antagonist, reverses the antidepressant response to fluoxetine.

Table 4.
Major advantages of selective inhibitors of serotonin uptake compared to tricyclic drugs in the treatment of mental depression.

Pharmacologic characteristic	Clinical consequence
Low affinity for muscarinic receptors	Low incidence of anticholinergic side effects, e.g., dry mouth, blurred vision, constipation, etc.
Low affinity for α_1 adrenergic receptors	Low incidence of orthostatic hypotension (caused by block of peripheral α_1 receptors) and low incidence of sedation (caused by block of central α_1 receptors).
Low affinity for histamine H_1 receptors	Low incidence of drowsiness
Lack of direct effects on the heart	Low incidence of electrocardiogram changes, low toxicity in overdose

Because fluoxetine and other selective inhibitors of serotonin uptake do not block muscarinic receptors, histamine H_1 receptors and α_1 adrenergic receptors as the tricyclic antidepressant drugs do, it was expected that these newer agents would lack some of the prominent side effects of the older drugs (Table 4). Clinical experience has borne out that anticholinergic side effects such as dry mouth, blurred vision and others, antihistaminic side effects such as drowsiness, and effects like postural hypotension and sedation which may result from α_1 adrenergic receptor blockade, are not commonly seen with the serotonin uptake inhibitors [132–134]. Because the latter drugs do not have direct effects on the heart, they also are less likely to alter the electrocardiogram than are the tricyclic antidepressant drugs [135–138]. The specificity of pharmacologic action and relative infrequency of side effects probably account for the conclusion from an open clinical trial that fluoxetine may be more suitable than tricyclic drugs for treating depressive comorbidity in medically ill patients [139] and for the attractiveness of serotonin uptake inhibitors in the long-term maintenance therapy of depression [140] as well as in the treatment of depression in the elderly [141].

An important advantage of the selective inhibitors of serotonin uptake that has become clear with their increased use is their greater safety in overdose, also likely to be a result of their more specific pharmacologic action. Overdose with tricyclic antidepressant drugs has sometimes been used as a means of suicide in depressed patients, and this is much less likely with the selective inhibitors of serotonin uptake [132, 142–146]. Excessive weight gain, which has sometimes been a limitation of tricyclic antidepressant drugs, is also less likely with fluoxetine and other serotonin uptake inhibitors [147, 148].

7.2 Other psychiatric disorders

Extensive data, particularly for fluoxetine, fluvoxamine and sertraline, indicate that serotonin uptake inhibitors are effective in obsessive-compulsive disorder [149–154]. There are several reports that serotonin uptake inhibitors are effective in treating panic disorder. In particular, case reports, open trials and small double-blind studies have been positive for fluvoxamine [155–157] and for fluoxetine [158–160]. Fluvoxamine, fluoxetine and sertraline have been reported to be beneficial in social phobia based on limited clinical studies [161–165], but further controlled clinical studies may be necessary to establish the efficacy of these drugs [166]. Open-label and double-blind clinical trials have found selective inhibitors of serotonin uptake to be beneficial in patients with post-traumatic stress disorder [167–169]. Small, non-blinded clinical trials of fluoxetine in patients with borderline personality have suggested that it has beneficial effects [170–172], though double-blind studies would be required to demonstrate more definitively if serotonin uptake inhibitors are therapeutically useful in this disorder. A rationale for trying serotonin uptake inhibitors in impulsive aggression has been advanced [173], and small studies have suggested they can have beneficial effects [174–177]. Fava et al. [178] have defined anger attacks (intense spells of anger with symptoms of autonomic arousal) in some depressed patients and reported that fluoxetine was beneficial in reducing anger and hostility in these patients.

Studies in small numbers of patients have suggested that serotonin uptake inhibitors may be beneficial in patients with trichotillomania, compulsive hair pulling. Stanley et al. [179] treated five female patients with fluoxetine and found significant improvements in four of the patients. Koran et al. [180] reported that in 13 adult patients with long-standing trichotillomania who completed an 8- to 12-week open trial with fluoxetine, mean Yale-Brown obsessive-compulsive scale scores decreased markedly. Winchel et al. [181] studied 12 adult patients given fluoxetine in a 16-week trial and found significant improvement in severity scores. However, a small double-blind crossover study in 15 patients with trichotillomania failed to demonstrate the efficacy of fluoxetine [182].

Zubieta and Alessi [183] reviewed evidence that serotonin neurons can modulate motor activity, impulsive aggression, and learning and memory and advocated the need for more research with serotonergic drugs in disruptive behavior disorders such as attention-deficit disorder with hyperactivity (ADHD). In an open label study of 19 children and adolescents with ADHD, nearly 60% were judged to be at least moderately improved after treatment with fluoxetine for 6 weeks [184]. In another open study, fluoxetine was combined with methylphenidate in an 8-week trial in 32 patients, all of whom showed positive therapeutic responses [185].

Consistent with findings in rats, serotonin uptake inhibitors have been reported to decrease alcohol intake in humans. Naranjo et al. [186–188] have reported that zimelidine, citalopram and fluoxetine reduce alcohol intake in controlled studies. Gorelick and Paredes [189] found only a transient and small reduction by fluoxetine of voluntary alcohol intake in a group of alcohol-dependent subjects. There is limited evidence that serotonin uptake inhibitors are clinically useful in treating alcoholism in non-depressed patients.

In 30 patients with whole body dysmorphic disorder, more than half of those treated with fluoxetine and clomipramine showed a complete or partial response [190]. Some patients with pathological jealousy have a predominant obsessional component to their jealous thoughts, so the efficacy of serotonin uptake inhibitors in obsessive-compulsive disorder led to their trial in this condition. Open-label studies have shown serotonin uptake inhibitors to be useful in some patients with pathological jealousy [191].

7.3 Obesity, eating disorders, metabolic disorders

Consistent with its appetite suppressant activity in laboratory animals, fluoxetine studied in depressed patients was observed not to cause the weight gain commonly found with tricyclic antidepressant drugs and to cause loss of body weight in patients who were obese. Clinical trials in non-depressed obese subjects confirmed the efficacy of fluoxetine in promoting weight loss, presumably mainly if not entirely by reducing food intake [192, 193]. However, treatment of obesity is not an approved indication for fluoxetine or other selective inhibitors of serotonin uptake. Although suppression of food intake is generally considered to be the major basis for the anti-obesity effects of serotonin uptake inhibitors, there have been some suggestions that the involvement of serotonin in the hypothalamic control of energy balance may include actions on caloric utilization as well as intake [194–197], effects possibly mediated through different serotonin receptor subtypes [198]. Weight loss apparently can sometimes occur without a decrease in food intake [199].

Large, double-blind placebo-controlled studies have shown that fluoxetine is effective in treating bulimia [200], and limited data suggest that other serotonin uptake inhibitors may also be effective [201–203]. The Fluoxetine Bulimia Nervosa Collaborative Study Group [204] reported results from a multicenter study of 387 bulimic women treated on an outpatient basis. Fluoxetine at 60 mg daily was superior to placebo in decreasing the frequency of weekly binge-eating and vomiting episodes, and fluoxetine at 20 mg daily was less effective. Serotonin may be more of a regulator of food intake than simply a suppressor of food intake [205, 206]. For that reason, fluoxetine has been given to patients with anorexia nervosa in preliminary studies, with some reports of beneficial results [207–210].

Gray et al. [211] studied fluoxetine given for 24 weeks in a double-blind study in 48 obese, type 2 non-insulin dependent diabetic patients. There was significantly more weight loss with fluoxetine than with placebo, and subjects in the fluoxetine group also were maintained on a lower insulin dose compared to the placebo group. The authors felt that fluoxetine may be of benefit in such patients. O'Kane et al. [212] also suggested that fluoxetine might prove to be a useful adjunct therapy in 19 obese type 2 diabetic patients where short-term weight loss and a decrease in carbohydrate intake are indicated, based on a 12-month double-blind trial of fluoxetine 60 mg daily. Significant weight reduction was observed throughout the study, although fasting blood glucose and glycosylated hemoglobin levels were decreased only at 3 and 6 months but not at 9 or 12 months. An involvement of serotonin in the hypothalamic control of caloric intake and possibly other aspects of energy balance may be the basis for these effects.

7.4 Neurologic disorders

Some studies of serotonin uptake inhibitors in migraine have been based on the rationale that serotonin from blood platelets may initiate vasoconstrictive events which trigger migraine. Chronic treatment with uptake inhibitors depletes platelet serotonin, so the likelihood of a migraine attack being triggered should be reduced. Some evidence has been presented that migraine attack frequency is reduced by serotonin uptake inhibitors during the time platelet serotonin content is decreased [213–216]. However, not all trials have shown efficacy of serotonin uptake inhibitors in the prophylaxis of migraine [217].

Another rationale why serotonin uptake inhibitors might be effective in migraine can be based on sumatriptan, a recently introduced drug which aborts migraine attacks [218, 219]. Sumatriptan is a serotonin analog whose antimigraine effect has been attributed to $5HT_{1D}$ receptor activation but might be mediated by a different serotonin receptor subtype [220]. If that receptor is innervated by serotonergic nerve terminals, then a serotonin uptake inhibitor might be expected to mimic the action of sumatriptan, although serotonin uptake inhibitors have not been shown to abort a migraine attack.

A third reason why serotonin uptake inhibitors might be useful in migraine could relate to their enhancement of central serotonergic pathways than modulate pain (discussed above). That mechanism might make uptake inhibitors effective in other pain syndromes as well as migraine. Numerous clinical reports support the idea that antidepressant drugs including serotonin uptake inhibitors can be useful in treating some types of chronic pain. Eisendrath and Kodama [221] described a patient with chronic abdominal pain who responded well to fluoxetine. Fluoxetine [217] and paroxetine [222] are reportedly effective in the treatment of chronic daily headache.

Paroxetine was effective against diabetic neuropathy symptoms in preliminary studies [223–225], but the results with fluoxetine have been conflicting [226, 227]. Overall, the possible utility of serotonin uptake inhibitors in managing various types of pain needs to be defined in more large, well-controlled clinical trials.

Another neurologic syndrome in which serotonin uptake inhibitors may be effective is postanoxic intention myoclonus. As discussed above, the combination of fluoxetine with the serotonin precursor, L-5HTP, has been reported to have therapeutic benefit in two such patients [122].

The potential usefulness of serotonin uptake inhibitors in treating some symptoms of Alzheimer's disease has been investigated. Serotonin concentration, along with other parameters of serotonin neurons, is decreased in some regions of brains from patients with Alzheimer's disease [228], and the possibility that dysfunction of serotonergic transmission contributes to some of the behavioral abnormalities in Alzheimer's diseases such as agitation and aggression has been suggested [229]. Available data suggest that serotonin uptake inhibitors may not improve cognitive function in Alzheimer's disease patients [230, 231] but may reduce aggressive and agitated behavior [231, 232]. The lack of anticholinergic actions of serotonin uptake inhibitors contributes to their suitability for treatment of depressive symptoms in Alzheimer's disease patients [233], because anticholinergic actions can exacerbate memory impairment [234–235].

7.5 Other disorders

In a double-blind study of late luteal phase dysphoric disorder (premenstrual syndrome), Menkes et al. [236] found marked improvement in 15 of 16 women treated with fluoxetine 20 mg daily. Elks [237] reported beneficial responses to fluoxetine 20 mg daily in an open trial of 14 women with severe symptoms of premenstrual syndrome. Pearlstein and Stone [238] reported that all patients showed remission or partial remission after treatment with 20–40 mg daily of fluoxetine. Symptoms recurred in most women after treatment discontinuation and remitted again with reinstitution of treatment. Mortola [239] suggested that three classes of agents are efficacious and widely used to treat premenstrual syndrome – benzodiazepines, serotonin uptake inhibitors, and gonadotropin-releasing hormone agonists – although there currently are no approved medications for this indication in the United States.
Frey and Darbonne [240] reported a pilot study in which fluoxetine reduced the number of cataplectic episodes by 92% in six patients with cataplexy treated with 20 mg daily for 20 weeks. Such data seem consistent with anticataplectic effects of fluoxetine that had been described earlier in dogs (mentioned above).
Serotonin generally suppresses sexual activity. Serotonin uptake inhibitors can cause unwanted effects on sexual function, e.g., loss of libido or delayed orgasm, but may have beneficial effects in some conditions such as erectile failure and premature ejaculation [241].

8 Why are serotonin uptake inhibitors potentially useful in many different diseases?

As discussed above, serotonin neurons in brain are very widespread in their projections [18, 20, 21]. Serotonin nerve terminals are found in many different parts of the brain that are involved in regulating many different physiological functions. For that reason, serotonin neurons may influence many different things, including behavior, pain, appetite, sleep, movement, blood pressure, hormone secretion, and so on. Serotonin neurons might play some part in the pathophysiology of a variety of psychiatric, neurologic and other disorders. Importantly, drugs that modify serotonin function have potential therapeutic application in many different disorders. The widespread distribution of serotonin neurons in brain is the neuroanatomic basis for why selective inhibitors of serotonin uptake have been tried in many different disorders and seem to have therapeutic utility in diseases in addition to mental depression, including bulimia, obsessive-compulsive disorder, trichotillomania, premenstrual syndrome, and perhaps others.

As pointed out by Jacobs and Azmitia [18], serotonin can modulate a large number of different behavioral and physiological processes but seems not to be essential for those processes to occur. Animals in whom serotonin neurons have been lesioned surgically or chemically (by drugs such as 5,6- or 5,7-dihydroxytryptamine or p-chloroamphetamine) are relatively normal in appearance, although numerous subtle alterations can be detected [242, 243]. The role of serotonin neurons may typically be in the "fine-tuning" of processes regulated by the brain, a characteristic that may make serotonin neurons an attractive site for drug intervention in the treatment of human diseases.

9 Serotonin transporters outside the brain

Although the focus in this review has been on serotonin neurons within the brain, serotonin neurons also occur outside the brain, particularly in the gastrointestinal tract [244, 245]. These neurons also have serotonin transporters and are expected to be influenced by uptake inhibitors, although much less is known about the physiological consequences of blocking uptake by those gastrointestinal neurons.

Blood platelets contain a serotonin transporter that appears to be identical to the brain serotonin transporter [246]. Fluoxetine inhibits the uptake of serotonin by blood platelets with about the same potency as it inhibits the uptake of serotonin by brain synaptosomes *in vitro* [247], as is true for other serotonin uptake inhibitors as well. Blood platelets do not synthesize serotonin, but instead the serotonin which they store has been obtained entirely by uptake from blood plasma. Inhibition of that uptake over a prolonged period decreases platelet content of serotonin [247, 248]. The study of serotonin uptake inhibitors in humans is facilitated by the existence of the platelet transporter. Currently there are no direct means of measuring inhibition of serotonin uptake in brain in patients treated with uptake inhibitors. Eventually, imaging techniques may permit the measurement of occupancy of transporter sites [249–251] or the increased extracellular serotonin concentration resulting from uptake inhibition. It is now possible, however, to take blood platelets from humans treated with uptake inhibitors and show that the uptake of serotonin by those platelets *in vitro* is inhibited and to show that the content of serotonin in those platelets is reduced as a consequence of prolonged inhibition of the transporter [230, 252, 253]. These measurements have helped in choosing doses of serotonin uptake inhibitors to be tested for efficacy in depression or in other diseases.

10 Adaptive changes after repeated administration of uptake inhibitors

A puzzling feature of antidepressant drugs has always been their delayed onset of therapeutic efficacy. Since 1974, there has been investigation of the ability of tricyclic antidepressant drugs given chronically to rats to cause adaptive decreases in β adrenergic receptors in brain [254, 255]. Most likely the chronic inhibition of norepinephrine transport maintained increased synaptic concentrations of norepinephrine, and the β adrenergic receptors downregulated as a consequence of continued overexposure to the neurotransmitter, norepinephrine. It was suspected that this gradual downregulation was responsible for the onset of antidepressant efficacy in humans. Such a causal relationship has yet to be proven, however, in part because true antidepressant efficacy cannot be demonstrated in laboratory animals where the β adrenergic receptor has been measured, and as yet means are not available for showing downregulation of β adrenergic receptors in humans in whom depressive symptoms are being measured. When fluoxetine was found not to cause downregulation of β adrenergic receptors in rat brain [256–257], some predicted that selective inhibitors of serotonin uptake would not be effective as antidepressant drugs, but that prediction has proven to be untrue. Apparently downregulation of β adrenergic receptors is not a characteristic common to all classes of antidepressant drugs but may instead be a marker for drugs which cause prolonged increases in extracellular norepinephrine concentration.

There has been interest in studying possible adaptive changes in serotonin receptors associated with chronic treatment with serotonin uptake inhibitors, in part because such changes might be causally linked to the onset of antidepressant activity in humans. Early reports that $5HT_2$ receptors in rat brain were not decreased after chronic treatment with serotonin uptake inhibitors [258, 259] have been confirmed [260], whereas $5HT_1$ receptors labeled with tritiated serotonin were found to be decreased [259, 261, 262]. Later, it was recognized that the tritiated serotonin was not labeling a single receptor site, and the elucidation of serotonin receptor heterogeneity revealed the number of specific receptors that might be undergoing adaptive changes. Unfortunately, specific radioligands are not yet available for labeling each of the serotonin receptor subtypes currently known, so further, more detailed investigations of receptor changes after chronic treatment with serotonin uptake inhibitors have not yet been completed.

de Montigny and colleagues [263, 264] have presented electrophysiologic evidence that autoreceptors on serotonin neurons can desensitize after chronic treatment with selective inhibitors of serotonin uptake. They have postulated that the immediate increase in serotonergic neurotransmission after uptake inhibitors is inadequate to produce antidepressant efficacy due to the adaptive decrease in serotonin neuron firing and in serotonin release; when the autoreceptors that modulate those adaptive decreases desensitize, then serotonin is released at its pre-drug rate, and because serotonin uptake is still inhibited there now results a larger increase in serotonergic neurotransmission sufficient to alleviate depressive symptoms. This attractive idea is supported by some microdialysis data in rats showing that uptake inhibitors cause larger increases in extracellular serotonin after chronic treatment than after single doses [265, 266], but conclusive evidence that these mechanisms are involved in the delayed onset of antidepressant efficacy in humans is still lacking.

There have been conflicting reports about whether $5HT_{1A}$ autoreceptors downregulate following treatment of rats with serotonin uptake inhibitors. Welner et al. [267] reported a decrease in $5HT_{1A}$ sites labeled with tritiated 8-OH-DPAT in the dorsal raphe nucleus after chronic treatment with fluoxetine, whereas Hensler et al. [268] found no change in $5HT_{1A}$ sites labeled with tritiated 8-OH-DPAT in the dorsal raphe nucleus or in other brain regions after chronic treatment with citalopram or sertraline. Functional studies have also not been entirely consistent. de Montigny et al. [269] found that i.v. LSD suppressed firing of serotonin neurons to a lesser extent after chronic treatment with citalopram, suggesting reduced sensitivity of the somatodendritic autoreceptor known to be a $5HT_{1A}$ receptor. Invernizzi et al. [270] found that chronic administration of citalopram to rats led to diminished reduction by 8-OH-DPAT of extracellular serotonin concentrations in the cortex, interpreted as desensitization of somatodendritic $5HT_{1A}$ receptors. Rutter et al. [266] reported similar findings, that 8-OH-DPAT reduced extracellular serotonin concentrations less in the diencephalon, after chronic treatment with fluoxetine. However, Hjorth and Auerbach [271] found no alteration in the ability of 8-OH-DPAT to reduce extracellular serotonin in the frontal cortex and hippocampus after chronic treatment with citalopram and suggested that cell body $5HT_{1A}$ autoreceptors do not desensitize.

Terminal autoreceptors which modulate serotonin release, probably $5HT_{1B}$ and $5HT_{1D}$ receptors, have been reported to desensitize after chronic treatment with serotonin uptake inhibitors based on electrophysiologic studies. de Montigny and colleagues [263, 264, 269] reported enhanced efficacy of electrical stimulation of afferent serotonergic pathway in suppressing the firing of postsynaptic CA3 hippocampal neurons after the chronic treatment of rats with fluoxetine, paroxetine or citalopram, and interpreted the findings as due to desensitization of terminal autoreceptors that normally limit the effect of the electrical stimulation.

More experimental evidence is needed on the extent to which presynaptic and postsynaptic serotonin receptors or perhaps the transporter itself [272] change in number or in function after chronic treatment with serotonin uptake inhibitors. If changes are unequivocally shown to occur, the question of whether they are related to clinical therapeutic effects such as the treatment of mental depression will have to be addressed. Until methods are available for assessing receptor changes in humans, in whom antidepressant efficacy can be monitored, establishing a causal relationship between receptor adaptation and onset of antidepressant efficacy will be difficult.

11 Serotonin uptake inhibitors as research tools

Apart from their therapeutic applications in humans, selective inhibitors of serotonin uptake have been useful research tools for experiments in laboratory animals. The reference citations in Fig. 1 give some indication of the relative utilization of the compounds in that regard. Although reference citations include papers that characterize the serotonin uptake inhibitors and that investigate their therapeutic actions, a portion of the citations are of papers in which the compounds are used as research tools. The compounds vary in their potency and degree of selectivity *in vitro*, but in all cases they can be given at appropriate doses *in vivo* to inhibit serotonin uptake selectively. Citalopram is probably the most highly selective of the compounds *in vitro* in respect to inhibiting serotonin uptake not norepinephrine or dopamine uptake; according to Hyttel [273], it is nearly 5000-fold selective for serotonin vs. norepinephrine and over 20,000-fold selective for serotonin vs. dopamine in blocking synaptosomal uptake. Some investigators simply think of the compounds as selective inhibitors of serotonin uptake and add concentrations as high as 10^{-5} M expecting selectivity. Selectivity is relative, of course. Generally these compounds block serotonin uptake selectively in the range of 10^{-9} to 10^{-7} M concentrations *in vitro*, but at concentrations as high as 10^{-5} M, they all interact with other transporters or with receptors, i.e. are not selective in their actions. It is important to use appropriate concentrations *in vitro* and to use appropriate doses *in vivo*. At properly chosen doses of each of the compounds in Fig. 1, it is possible to block serotonin uptake *in vivo* without blocking norepinephrine or dopamine uptake and, in most cases, without known interactions with any neurotransmitter receptors. At those doses, the compounds can be valuable research tools for investigating the role of serotonin neurons in some physiological or behavioral phenomenon, for preventing platelet uptake of serotonin, for preventing unspecific effects of 6-hydroxydopamine (a catecholamine neurotoxin) on serotonin neurons, and for other applications of that sort.

12 Summary and conclusions

Fluoxetine, zimelidine, sertraline, paroxetine, fluvoxamine, indalpine and citalopram are the selective inhibitors of serotonin uptake that have been most widely studied. Some of these compounds are or have been used clinically in the treatment of mental depression, obsessive-compulsive disorder and bulimia, and therapeutic benefit has been claimed in additional diseases as well. By blocking the membrane uptake carrier which transports serotonin from the extracellular space to inside the serotonin nerve terminals, these compounds increase extracellular concentrations of serotonin and amplify signals sent by serotonin neurons. Because serotonin neurons are widespread in the central nervous system, the functional consequences of blocking serotonin uptake are diverse, but are generally subtle. Animals treated with serotonin uptake inhibitors look normal in gross appearance, but effects such as reduced aggressive behavior, decreased food intake and altered food selection, analgesia, anticonvulsant activity, endocrine changes and neurochemical changes have been demonstrated and characterized. Serotonin uptake inhibitors have helped in revealing some dynamics of serotonin neurons; for example, when uptake is inhibited and extracellular serotonin concentration increases, presynaptic as well as postsynaptic receptors for serotonin are activated to a greater degree. A consequence of increased activation of autoreceptors on serotonin cell bodies and nerve terminals is a reduction in firing of serotonin neurons and a decrease in serotonin synthesis and release. The result is a limit on the degree to which extracellular serotonin and serotonergic neurotransmission are increased. The study of selective inhibitors of serotonin uptake, which began over two decades ago, is giving added insight into the role of serotonin in brain function and in disease, and will define better the scope of therapeutic uses of these agents.

References

1 M. Asberg, B. Eriksson, B. Martensson, L. Traskman-Bendz and A. Wagner: J. Clin. Psychiat. *47* Suppl. 23 (1986).
2 P. Bech and P. Cialdella: Int. Clin. Psychopharmacol. *6* Suppl 5, 45 (1992).
3 P.R. Finley: Ann. Pharmacother. *28*, 1359 (1994).
4 R.W. Fuller, H.D. Snoddy and M. L. Cohen: Neuropharmacology *23*, 539 (1984).
5 S.K. Hemrick-Luecke, H.D. Snoddy and R.W. Fuller: Life Sci. *55*, 479 (1994).
6 R.D. Blakely, H.E. Berson, R.T. Fremeau, Jr., M.G. Caron, M.M. Peek, H.K. Prince and C.C. Bradley: Nature *354*, 66 (1991).
7 B.J. Hoffman, E. Mezey and M.J. Brownstein: Science *254*, 579 (1991).
8 P. Gregor, A. Patel, S. Shimada, C.L. Lin, J.M. Rochelle, S. Kitayama, M.F. Seldin and G.R. Uhl: Mamm. Genome *4*, 283 (1993).
9 K.P. Lesch, C.S. Aulakh, B.L. Wolozin, T.J. Tolliver, J.L. Hill and D.L. Murphy: Brain Res. Mol. Brain Res. *17*, 31 (1993).
10 S. Ramamoorthy, A.L. Bauman, K.R. Moore, H. Han, T. Yang-Feng, A.S. Chang, V. Ganapathy and R.D. Blakely: Proc. Natl. Acad. Sci. USA *90*, 2542 (1993).
11 M.C. Austin, C.C. Bradley, J.J. Mann and R.D. Blakely: J. Neurochem. *62*, 2362 (1994).
12 H. Gu, S.C. Wall and G. Rudnick: J. Biol. Chem. *269*, 7124 (1994).
13 K.P. Lesch, B.L. Wolozin, H.C. Estler, D.L. Murphy and P. Riederer: J. Neural Transm. *91*, 67 (1993).
14 R.D. Blakely, K.R. Moore and Y. Qian: Soc. Gen. Physiol. Ser. *48*, 283 (1993).
15 B.J. Hoffman: Pharmacopsychiatry *27*, 16 (1994).
16 J.F. Lopez, D.T. Chalmers, D.M. Vazquez, S.J. Watson and H. Akil: Biol. Psychiatry *35*, 287 (1994).
17 S. Mager, C. Min, D. J. Henry, C. Chavkin, B. J. Hoffman, N. Davidson and H. A. Lester: Neuron *12*, 845 (1994).
18 B. L. Jacobs and E. C. Azmitia: Physiol. Rev. *72*, 165 (1992).
19 D. Hoyer, D. E. Clarke, J. R. Fozard, P. R. Hartig, G. R. Martin, E. J. Mylecharane, P. R. Saxena and P. P. A. Humphrey: Pharmacol. Rev. *46*, 157 (1994).
20 I. Tork: Ann. N. Y. Acad. Sci. *600*, 9 (1990).
21 L. Descarries, M. A. Audet, G. Doucet, S. Garcia, S. Oleskevich, P. Seguela, J.-J. Soghomonian and K.C. Watkins: Ann. N. Y. Acad. Sci. *600*, 81 (1990).
22 R.W. Fuller: Life Sci. *55*, 163 (1994).
23 R.W. Fuller: J. Clin. Psychiat. *53* Suppl. 10, 36 (1992).
24 A.R. Green and D.J. Heal: In: Neuropharmacology of Serotonin, pp. 326–365, A. R. Green, Ed., 1985.
25 R. Ortmann: Drug Develop. Res. *4*, 593 (1984).
26 R.W. Fuller: Submitted for publication (1995).
27 G.L. Brown and M I. Linnoila: J. Clin. Psychiat. *51* Suppl. 4, 31 (1990).
28 R.W. Fuller, K.W. Perry and B B. Molloy: Life Sci. *15*, 1161 (1974).
29 R.W. Fuller and D.T. Wong: Fed. Proc. *36*, 2154 (1977).
30 J.A. Clemens, B.D. Sawyer and B.Cerimele: Endocrinology *100*, 692 (1977).
31 N. Limberger, K. Starke and E.A. Singer: Naunyn-Schmiedeberg's Arch. Pharmacol. *342*, 363 (1990).
32 G.C. Rigdon and C.M. Wang: Drug Develop. Res. *22*, 135 (1991).
33 K. W. Perry and R. W. Fuller: Soc. Neurosci. Abstr. *17*, 1178 (1991).
34 G.A. Smythe, R.M. Gleeson and B.M. Stead: Neuroendocrinology *47*, 389 (1988).

35 S. Consolo, R. Bertorelli, G. Russi, M. Zambelli and H. Ladinsky: J. Neurochem. *62*, 2254 (1994).
36 G. Tanda, E. Carboni, R. Frau and G. Di Chiara: Psychopharmacology *115*, 285 (1994).
37 J.L. Gibbons, M. Glusman, G.A. Barr, W.H. Bridger and S F. Leibowitz: Soc. Neurosci. Abstr. *4* (1978).
38 P. Berzsenyi, E. Galateo and L. Valzelli: Aggress. Behav. *9*, 333 (1983).
39 W. Kostowski, L. Valzelli, W. Kozak and S. Bernasconi: Pharmacol. Res. Commun. *16*, 265 (1984).
40 P. Stark, R.W. Fuller and D.T. Wong: J. Clin. Psychiatry *46*, 7 (1985).
41 V. Molina, S. Gobaille and P. Mandel: Aggress. Behav. *12*, 201 (1986).
42 V. Molina, L. Ciesielski, S. Gobaille, F. Isel and P. Mandel: Pharmacol. Biochem. Behav. *27*, 123 (1987).
43 T. Yamamoto, S. Shibata, T. Shimazoe, K. Iwasaki, M. Ohno, Y. Minamoto, Y. Furuya, K. Miyamoto, S. Watanabe, and S. Ueki: Nippon Yakurigaku Zasshi *94*, 189 (1989).
44 S.O. Ogren, A.C. Holm, A.L. Renyi and S.B. Ross: Acta Pharmacol. Toxicol. *47*, 71 (1980).
45 K.P. Datla, S.K. Mitra and S.K. Bhattacharya: Indian J. Exp. Biol. *29*, 631 (1991).
46 G. C. Wagner, H. Fisher, N. Pole, T. Borve and S. K. Johnson: J. Stud. Alcohol. Suppl. *11*, 185 (1993).
47 C. F. Ferris and Y. Delville: Psychoneuroendocrinology *19*, 593 (1994).
48 M.J. Raleigh, M.T. McGuire, G.L. Brammer, D.B. Pollack and A. Yuwiler: Brain Res. *559*, 181 (1991).
49 B.S. Eichelman: Ann. Rev. Med. *41*, 149 (1990).
50 B. Olivier, J. Mos, J. van der Heyden, J. Schipper, M. Tulp, B. Berkelmans and P. Bevan: In: Ethopharmacology of Agonistic Behavior in Animals and Humans, pp. 162–186, B. Olivier, J. Mos and P.F. Brain, Eds., 1987.
51 C.L. Broekkamp, D. Garrigou and K.G. Lloyd: Pharmacol. Biochem. Behav. *13*, 643 (1980).
52 D. Garrigou, C.L. Broekkamp and K.G. Lloyd: Psychopharmacology *74*, 66 (1981).
53 D. Joly and D.J. Sanger: Pharmacol. Biochem. Behav. *24*, 199 (1986).
54 J.F. Flood and A. Cherkin: Psychopharmacology *93*, 36 (1987).
55 A.J. Goudie, E.W. Thornton and T.J. Wheeler: J. Pharm. Pharmacol. *28*, 318 (1976).
56 N. Rowland, S.M. Antelman and D. Kocan: Eur. J. Pharmacol. *81*, 57 (1982).
57 D.T. Wong, L.R. Reid, F.P. Bymaster and P.G. Threlkeld: J. Neural Trans. *64*, 251 (1985).
58 T.T. Yen, D.T. Wong and K.G. Bemis: Drug Develop. Res. *10*, 37 (1987).
59 J.E. Blundell: Neuropharmacology *23*, 1537 (1984).
60 R.W. Fuller and D.T. Wong: Drug Develop. Res. *17*, 1 (1989).
61 J.A. Nielsen, D.S. Chapin, J.L. Johnson, Jr., and L.K. Torgersen: Am. J. Clin. Nutr. *55* Suppl. 1, 185S (1992).
62 S.H. Kim and R.J. Wurtman: Physiol. Behav. *42*, 319 (1988).
63 S.F. Leibowitz, J.T. Alexander, W.K. Cheung and G.F. Weiss: Pharmacol. Biochem. Behav. *45*, 185 (1993).
64 S.Q. Luo and E.T. Li: Brain Res. Bull. *24*, 729 (1990).
65 S.Q. Luo, T. Ransom and E.T. Li: Life Sci. *46*, 1643 (1990).
66 G.F. Weiss, N. Rogacki, A. Fueg, D. Buchen, J.S. Suh, D.T. Wong and S.F. Leibowitz: Psychopharmacology *105*, 467 (1991).

67 J J. Wurtman and R.J. Wurtman: Science *198*, 1178 (1977).
68 J.J. Wurtman and R.J. Wurtman: Curr. Med. Res. Opin. *6* (Suppl. 1), 28 (1979).
69 S.M. Antelman, N. Rowland and C. Kocan: In: Anorectic Agents: Mechanisms of Action and Tolerance, pp. 45–62, S. Garattini and R. Samanin, Eds., 1981.
70 M.O. Carruba, S. Ricciardi, P. Spano and P. Mantegazza: Life Sci. *36*, 1739 (1985).
71 D.T. Wong, L.R. Reid and P.G. Threlkeld: Pharmacol. Biochem. Behav. *31*, 475 (1988).
72 K.E. Asin, J.D. Davis and L. Bednarz: Psychopharmacology *109*, 415 (1992).
73 M. Altemus, J.R. Glowa and D. L. Murphy: Psychopharmacol. Bull. *29*, 397 (1993).
74 G.E. Rockman, Z. Amit, Z.W. Brown, C. Bourque and S.-O. Ogren: Neuropharmacology *21*, 341 (1982).
75 Z. Amit, E.A. Sutherland, K. Gill and S.O. Ogren: Neurosci. Biobehav. Rev. *8*, 35 (1984).
76 K. Gill, Z. Amit and B.K. Koe: Alcohol *5*, 349 (1988).
77 J.M. Murphy, M.B. Waller, G.J. Gatto, W.J. McBride, L. Lumeng and T.-K. Li: Alcohol *2*, 349 (1985).
78 Z.S. Liposits, C. Phelix and W.K. Paull: Histochemistry *86*, 541 (1987).
79 A.E. Calogero, R. Bernardini, A.N. Margioris, G. Bagdy, W.T. Gallucci, P J. Munson, L. Tamarkin, T.P. Tomai, L. Brady, P.W. Gold and G.P. Chrousos: Peptides *10*, 189 (1989).
80 R.W. Fuller, H.D. Snoddy and B.B. Molloy: Life Sci. *19*, 337 (1976).
81 D.M. Gibbs and W. Vale: Brain Res. *280*, 176 (1983).
82 R.W. Fuller: Frontiers in Neuroendocrinology *13*, 250 (1992b).
83 M. Bianchi, P. Sacerdote and A.E. Panerai: Eur. J. Pharmacol. *263*, 81 (1994).
84 L. Krulich: Life Sci. *17*, 1141 (1975).
85 J. Siegel and G.J. Murphy: Brain Res. *174*, 337 (1979).
86 J.W. Dailey, Q.S. Yan, P.K. Mishra, R.L. Burger and P.C. Jobe: J. Pharmacol. Exp. Ther. *260*, 533 (1992).
87 Q.S. Yan, P.C. Jobe and J.W. Dailey: Eur. J. Pharmacol. *252*, 105 (1994).
88 A. Pasini, A. Tortorella and K. Gale: Brain Res. *593*, 287 (1992).
89 S. Prendiville and K. Gale: Epilepsia *34*, 381 (1993).
90 J.D. Leander: Epilepsia *33*, 573 (1992).
91 J.A. Harvey and K.J. Simansky: In: Serotonin: Current Aspects of Neurochemistry and Function, pp. 125–151, B. Haber, S. Gabay, M.R. Issidorides and S.G.A. Alivisatos, Eds., 1981.
92 R.B. Messing, L. Phebus, L.A. Fisher and L.D. Lytle: Psychopharmacol. Commun. *1*, 511 (1975).
93 R.B. Messing, L.A. Fisher, L. Phebus and L.D. Lytle: Life Sci. *18*, 707 (1976).
94 A.A. Larson and A.E. Takemori: Life Sci. *21*, 1807 (1977).
95 M.D. Hynes and R.W. Fuller: Drug Develop. Res. *2*, 33 (1982).
96 D.W. Robertson, J.H. Krushinski, R.W. Fuller and J.D. Leander: J. Med. Chem. *31*, 1412 (1988).
97 M. Rafieian-kopaei and R.D.E. Sewell: J. Pharm. Pharmacol. *46* Suppl. 2, 1088 (1994).
98 B.P. Richardson: Adv. Biosci. *85*, 335 (1992)
99 P.K. Eide and K. Hole: Cephalalgia *13*, 75 (1993).
100 I.H. Slater, G.T. Jones and R.A. Moore: Neuropharmacology *17*, 383 (1978).
101 R.H. Pastel and J.D. Fernstrom: Brain Res. *436*, 92 (1987).
102 B. Gao, W.C. Duncan, Jr., and T.A. Wehr: Psychopharmacology *106*, 321 (1992).
103 L. Sommerfelt, E.R. Hauge and R. Ursin: J. Neural Trans. *68*, 127 (1987).

104 H. Kleinlogel and H.R. Burki: Neuropsychobiology *17*, 206 (1987).
105 S. Kafi-De St Hilaire, H. Merica and J.M. Gaillard: Eur. J. Pharmacol. *98*, 413 (1984).
106 R.W. Fuller, D.R. Holland, T.T. Yen, K.G. Bemis and N.B. Stamm: Life Sci. *25*, 1237 (1979).
107 R.W. Fuller: Neuroendocrinology *32*, 118 (1981).
108 M.H. Sheard and M. Davis: Eur. J. Pharmacol. *40*, 295 (1976).
109 K.E. Sabol, J.B. Richards and L.S. Seiden: Brain Res. *585*, 421 (1992).
110 P. Kalen, R.E. Strecker, E. Rosengren and A. Bjorklund: J. Neurochem. *51*, 1422 (1988).
111 J.J. Rutter and S.B. Auerbach: J. Pharmacol. Exp. Ther. *265*, 1319 (1993).
112 C.A. Marsden, J. Conti, E. Strope, G. Curzon and R.N. Adams: Brain Res. *171*, 85 (1979).
113 R.W. Fuller, H.D. Snoddy and J.A. Clemens: Endocr. Res. Commun. *7*, 77 (1980).
114 A. Quattrone, G. Schettini, G.F. Di Renzo, S. Amoroso and L. Annunziato: Adv. Biochem. Psychopharmacol. *31*, 229 (1982).
115 L.D. Van de Kar, J.H. Urban, K.D. Richardson and C.L. Bethea: Neuroendocrinology *41*, 283 (1985).
116 M.E. Trulson and B.L. Jacobs: Eur. J. Pharmacol. *36*, 149 (1976).
117 J.H. Growdon: Neurology *27*, 1074 (1977).
118 M.J. During, A. Freese, M.P. Heyes, K.J. Swartz, S.P. Markey, R.H. Roth and J.B. Martin: FEBS Letters *247*, 438 (1989).
119 R.W. Fuller and J.E. Owen: Res. Commun. Chem. Pathol. Pharmacol. *34*, 137 (1981).
120 K.W. Perry and R.W. Fuller: Life Sci. *50*, 1683 (1992).
121 M.H. Van Woert and D. Rosenbaum: Adv. Neurol. *26*, 107 (1979).
122 M.H. Van Woert, I. Magnussen, D. Rosenbaum and E. Chung: Clin. Neuropharmacol. *6*, 49 (1983).
123 S. Hjorth: J. Neurochem. *60*, 776 (1993).
124 S. Hjorth and S.B. Auerbach: Eur. J. Pharmacol. *260*, 251 (1994).
125 F. Artigas, V. Perez and E. Alvarez: Arch. Gen. Psychiatry *51*, 248 (1994).
126 W. F. Boyer: Int. Clin. Psychopharmacol. *6* Suppl 5, 5 (1992).
127 A.A. Nierenberg: J. Clin. Psychiatry *55*, 55 (1994).
128 L. Lemberger, R.W. Fuller and R.L. Zerbe: Clin. Neuropharmacol. *8*, 299 (1985).
129 P.L. Delgado, L.H. Price, H.L. Miller, R.M. Salomon, J. Licinio, J.H. Krystal, G.R. Heninger and D.S. Charney: Psychopharmacol. Bull. *27*, 321 (1991).
130 R.M. Salomon, H.L. Miller, P.L. Delgado and D.Charney: Int. Clin. Psychopharmacol. *8* Suppl. 2, 41 (1993).
131 R. Feder: J. Clin. Psychiat. *52*, 163 (1991).
132 P. E. Stokes: Clin. Ther. *15*, 216 (1993).
133 S. Kasper, G. Hoflich, H.P. Scholl and H.J. Moller: Human Psychopharmacol. Clin. Exper. *9*, 1 (1994).
134 M.V. Rudorfer, H.K. Manji and W.Z. Potter: Drug Safety *10*, 18 (1994).
135 D.S. Chutka: Geriatrics *45*, 55 (1990).
136 C. Fisch and S.B. Knoebel: Drug Investigation *4*, 305 (1992).
137 H. Kuhs and G.A.E. Rudolf: Psychopharmacology *102*, 379 (1990).
138 J.W. Upward, J.G. Edwards, A. Goldie and D.G. Waller: Brit. J. Clin. Pharmacol. *26*, 399 (1988).
139 F.J. Huyse, W.A. Zwaan and R. Kupka: J. Psychosom. Res. *38*, 695 (1994).
140 R.M.A. Hirschfeld and A.F. Schatzberg: Am. J. Med. *97*, S33–S38 (1994).
141 M.G. Harris and P. Benfield: Drugs & Aging *6*, 64 (1995).

142 D.J. Borys, S.C. Setzer, L.J. Ling, J.J. Reisdorf, L.C. Day and E.P. Krenzelok: Clin. Toxicol. *28*, 331 (1990).
143 D.J. Borys, S.C. Setzer, L.J. Ling, J.J. Reisdorf, L.C. Day and E.P. Krenzelok: Am. J. Emerg. Med. *10*, 115 (1992).
144 N. Freemantle, A. House, F. Song, J.M. Mason and T.A. Sheldon: BMJ *309*, 249 (1994).
145 S. Kapur, T. Mieczkowski and J.J. Mann: J. Am. Med. Assoc. *268*, 3441 (1992).
146 R.D.T. Farmer: Hum. Psychopharmacol. Clin. *S13* (1994).
147 M.H. Fernstrom and D.J. Kupfer: Psychiat. Res. *26*, 265 (1988).
148 E. Frank, D.J. Kupfer, C.M. Bulik and J.A. Levenson: J. Affect. Dis. *20*, 165 (1990).
149 G. Chouinard: Int. Clin. Psychopharmacol. *7*, 37 (1992).
150 W.K. Goodman, L.H. Price, P.L. Delgado, J. Palumbo, J.H. Krystal, L.M. Nagy, S.A. Rasmussen, G.R. Heninger and D.S. Charney: Arch. Gen. Psychiat. *47*, 577 (1990).
151 J.H. Greist, J.W. Jefferson, K.A. Kobak, D.J. Katzelnick and R.C. Serlin: Arch. Gen. Psychiat. *52*, 53 (1995).
152 C.W. Jackson, W.A. Morton and R.B. Lydiard: South. Med. J. *87*, 310, 1994.
153 G.D. Tollefson, A.H. Rampey, Jr., J.H. Potvin, M.A. Jenike, A J. Rush, R.A. Dominguez, L.M. Koran, M.K. Shear, W. Goodman and L.A. Genduso: Arch. Gen. Psychiat. *51*, 559 (1994).
154 A. Wood, G.D. Tollefson and M. Birkett: Int. Clin. Psychopharmacol. *8*, 301 (1993).
155 D.W. Black, R. Wesner, W. Bowers and J. Gabel: Arch. Gen. Psychiat. *50*, 44 (1993).
156 J.A. Den Boer and H.G. Westenberg: Int. Clin. Psychopharmacol. *3*, 59 (1988).
157 R. Hoehn-Saric, D.R. McLeod and P.A. Hipsley: J. Clin. Psychopharmacol. *13*, 321 (1993).
158 A.K. Louie, T.B. Lewis and R.A. Lannon: J. Clin. Psychiat. *54*, 435 (1993).
159 F.R. Schneier, M.R. Liebowitz, S.O. Davies, J. Fairbanks, E. Hollander, R. Campeas and D.F. Klein: J. Clin. Psychopharmacol. *10*, 119 (1990).
160 L. Solyom, C. Solyom and B. Ledwidge: Canad. J. Psychiat. *36*, 378 (1991).
161 B. Birmaher, G.S. Waterman, N. Ryan, M. Cully, L. Balach, J. Ingram and M. Brodsky: J. Am. Acad. Child Adolescent Psychiatry *33*, 993 (1994).
162 B. Black, T.W. Uhde and M.E. Tancer: J. Clin. Psychopharmacol. *12*, 293 (1992).
163 J.A. Den Boer, I.M. Van Vliet and H.G. Westenberg: Prog. Neuropsychopharmacol. Biol. Psychiat. *18*, 625 (1994).
164 M. Van Ameringen, C. Mancini and D.L. Streinger: J. Clin. Psychiatry *54*, 27 (1993).
165 M. Van Ameringen, C. Mancini and D.L. Streinger: J. Affect. Disord. *31*, 141 (1994).
166 R.D. Marshall, F.R. Schneier, B.A. Fallon, J. Feerick and M.R. Liebowitz: J. Clin. Psychiat. *55* Suppl, 33 (1994).
167 L.M. Nagy, C.A. Morgan III, S.M. Southwick and D.S. Charney: J. Clin. Psychopharmacol. *13*, 107 (1993).
168 C.G. Fichtner, R.C. Arora and J.W. Crayton: Life Sci. *54*, PL39 (1994).
169 B.A. Vanderkolk, D. Dreyfuss, M. Michaels, D. Shera, R. Berkowitz, R. Fisler and G. Saxe: J. Clin. Psychiatry *55*, 517 (1994).
170 J.R. Cornelius, P.H. Soloff, J.M. Perel and R.F. Urich: J. Clin. Psychopharmacol. *11*, 116 (1991).
171 P.J. Markovitz, J.R. Calabrese, S.C. Schulz and H.Y. Meltzer: Am. J. Psychiat. *148*, 1064 (1991).
172 M.J. Norden: Prog. Neuropsychopharmacol. Biol. Psychiatry *13*, 885 (1989).
173 H.M. Van Praag, R. Kahn, G.M. Asnis, C.Z. Lemus and S.L. Brown: Biol. Psychiat. *22*, 205 (1987).

174 E.F. Coccaro: Int. Clin. Psychopharmacol. *7*, 3 (1992).
175 E.F. Coccaro, J.L. Astil, J.L. Herbert and A.G. Schut: J. Clin. Psychopharmacol. *10*, 373 (1990).
176 R.J. Kavoussi, J. Liu and E.F. Coccaro: J. Clin. Psychiat. *55*, 137 (1994).
177 P.I. Markowitz: J. Clin. Psychopharmacol. *12*, 27 (1992).
178 M. Fava, J.H. Rosenbaum, J. Pava, M.K. McCarthy, R.J. Steingard and E. Bouffides: Am. J. Psychiatry *150*, 1158 (1993).
179 M.A. Stanley, T.C. Bowers, A.C. Swann and D.J. Taylor: J. Clin. Psychiat. *52*, 282 (1991).
180 L.M. Koran, A. Ringold and W. Hewlett: Psychopharmacol. Bull. *28*, 145 (1992).
181 R.M. Winchel, J.S. Jones, B. Stanley, A. Molcho and M. Stanley: J. Clin. Psychiat. *53*, 304 (1992).
182 G.A. Christenson, T.B. Mackenzie, J.E. Mitchell and A.L. Callies: Am. J. Psychiat. *148*, 1566 (1991).
183 J.K. Zubieta and N.E. Alessi: J. Child. Adoles. Psychopharmacol. *3*, 11 (1993).
184 L. Barrickman, R. Noyes, S. Kuperman, E. Schumacher and M. Verda: J. Am. Acad. Child. Adolesc. Psychiat. *30*, 762 (1991).
185 G.D. Gammon and T.E. Brown: J. Child Adoles. Psychopharmacol. *3*, 1 (1993).
186 C.A. Naranjo, C.X. Poulos, K.E. Bremner and K.L. Lanctot: Intl. Clin. Psychopharmacol. *9*, 163 (1994).
187 C.A. Naranjo, E.M. Sellers, C.A. Roach, D.V. Woodley, M. Sanchez-Craig and K. Sykora: Clin. Pharmacol. Ther. *35*, 374 (1984).
188 C.A. Naranjo, E.M. Sellers, J.T. Sullivan, D.V. Woodley, K. Kadlec and K. Sykora: Clin. Pharmacol. Ther. *41*, 266 (1987).
189 D.A. Gorelick and A. Paredes: Alcohol Clin. Exp. Res. *16*, 261 (1992).
190 K.A. Phillips, S.L. McElroy, P.E. Keck, Jr., H.G. Pope, Jr. and J.I. Hudson: Am. J. Psychiatry *150*, 302 (1993).
191 D.J. Stein, E. Hollander and S.C. Josephson: J. Clin. Psychiatry *55*, 30 (1994).
192 D.J. Goldstein, A.H. Rampey, Jr., G.G. Enas, J.H. Potvin, L.A. Fludzinski and L.R. Levine: Int. J. Obes. Relat. Metab. Disord. *18*, 129 (1994).
193 M. McGuirk and T. Silverstone: Int. J. Obesity *14*, 361 (1990).
194 K. Arase, T. Sakaguchi and G.A. Bray: Pharmacol. Biochem. Behav. *29*, 675 (1988).
195 P. Even and S. Nicolaidis: Appetite *7*, 141 (1986).
196 N.J. Fuller, M. Ashwell and D.M. Stirling: Proc. Nutr. Soc. Engl. Scot. *47*, 79A (1988).
197 N.J. Rothwell and M.J. Stock: Int. J. Obes. *11*, 319 (1987).
198 S. Bovetto and D. Richard: Am. J. Physiol. *37*, R14–R20 (1995).
199 C.G. Fichtner and B.G. Braun: Ann. Pharmacother. *28*, 1350 (1994).
200 A. Wood: Int. Clin. Psychopharmacol. *8*, 295 (1993).
201 J.L. Ayuso-Gutierrez, M. Palazon and J.L. Ayuso-Mateos: Int. J. Eat. Disord. *15*, 245 (1994).
202 H.M. Gardiner, C.P. Freeman, D.K. Jesinger and S.A. Collins: Int. J. Obes. Relat. Metab. Disord. *17*, 301 (1993).
203 J.M. Robert and R.B. Lydiard: Am. J. Psychiat. *150*, 1753 (1993).
204 Fluoxetine Bulimia Nervosa Collaborative Study Group: Arch. Gen. Psychiat. *49*, 139 (1992).
205 D.C. Jimerson, M.D. Lesem, W.H. Kaye, A.P. Hegg and T.D. Brewerton: Biol. Psychiat. *28*, 443 (1990).
206 S.F. Leibowitz: Drugs *39* Suppl 3, 33 (1990).
207 J.M. Ferguson: Am. J. Psychiat. *144*, 1239 (1987).

208 H.E. Gwirtsman, B.H. Guze, J. Yager and B. Gainsley: J. Clin. Psychiat. *51*, 378 (1990).
209 W.H. Kaye, T.E. Weltzin, L.K. Hsu and C.M. Bulik: J. Clin. Psychiat. *52*, 464 (1991).
210 S. Lee: J. Clin. Psychiat. *52*, 240 (1991).
211 D.S. Gray, K. Fujioka, W. Devine and G.A. Bray: Int. J. Obesity *16* Suppl 4, S67–S72 (1992).
212 M. O'Kane, P.G. Wiles and J.K. Wales: Diabet. Med. *11*, 105 (1994).
213 C. Adly, J. Straumanis and A. Chesson: Headache *32*, 101 (1992).
214 J. Bank: Headache *34*, 476 (1994).
215 E. Syvalahti, P. Kangasniemi and S.B. Ross: Curr. Ther. Res. *25*, 299 (1979).
216 I. Zeeberg, M. Orholm, J. Dalsgaard-Nielsen, P. Le Fevre Honore and J.J. Larsen: Acta Neurol. Scand. *674*, 452 (1981).
217 J.R. Saper, S.D. Silberstein, A.E. Lake III and M.E. Winters: Headache *34*, 497 (1994).
218 M.A. Moskowitz and F.M. Cutrer: Ann. Rev. Med. *44*, 145 (1993).
219 G.L. Plosker and D. McTavish: Drugs *47*, 622 (1994).
220 S.D. Silberstein: Headache *34*, 408 (1994).
221 S.J. Eisendrath and K.T. Kodama: Psychosomatics *33*, 227 (1992).
222 C.A. Foster and J. Bafaloukos: Headache *34*, 587 (1994).
223 S.M. Holliday and G.L. Plosker: Drugs Aging *3*, 278 (1993).
224 S.H. Sindrup, L.F. Gram, K. Brosen, O. Eshoj and E.F. Mogensen: Pain *42*, 135 (1990).
225 S.H. Sindrup, E. Grodum, L.F. Gram and H. Beck-Nielsen: Ther. Drug Monit. *13*, 408 (1991).
226 K.A. Theesen and W.R. Marsh: DICP *23*, 572 (1989).
227 M.B. Max, S.A. Lynch, J. Muir, S.E. Shoaf, B. Smoller and R. Dubner: New Engl. J. Med. *326*, 1250 (1992).
228 C.G. Gottfries: J. Neural Trans. *30* Suppl, 33 (1990).
229 A.M. Palmer and S.T. DeKosky: J. Neural Trans. Gen. Sect. *91*, 135 (1993).
230 N.R. Cutler, J. Haxby, A.D. Kay, P.K. Narang, L.J. Lesko, J.L. Costa, M. Ninos, M. Linnoila, W.Z. Potter and J.W. Renfrew: Arch. Neurol. *42*, 744 (1985).
231 C.G. Gottfries and A.L. Nyth: Ann. N. Y. Acad. Sci. *640*, 276 (1991).
232 A.J. Cross: Ann. N. Y. Acad. Sci. *600*, 405 (1990).
233 M.J. Tueth: Geriatrics *50*, 43 (1995).
234 G. Beaumont: Int. Clin. Psychopharmacol. *5* Suppl 3, 61 (1990).
235 P.J. Thompson: Human Psychopharmacol. *6*, 79 (1991).
236 D.B. Menkes, E. Taghavi, P.A. Mason and R.C. Howard: Int. Clin. Psychopharmacol. *8*, 95 (1993).
237 M.L. Elks: Southern Med. J. *86*, 503 (1993).
238 T.B. Pearlstein and A.B. Stone: J. Clin. Psychiatry *55*, 332 (1994).
239 J.F. Mortola: Drug Saf. *10*, 160 (1994).
240 J. Frey and C. Darbonne: Neurology *44*, 707 (1994).
241 P. Power-Smith: Br. J. Psychiatry *164*, 249 (1994).
242 J.H. Jacoby and L.D. Lytle: Ann. N. Y. Acad. Sci. *305*, 1–702 (1978).
243 R.W. Fuller and M.G. Henderson: In: Amphetamine and Its Analogs, pp. 209–242, A.K. Cho and D.S. Segal, Eds., 1994.
244 M.D. Gershon, G.M. Mawe and T.A. Branchek: In: The Peripheral Actions of 5-Hydroxytryptamine, pp. 247–273, J.R. Fozard, Ed., 1989.
245 N.J. Talley: Aliment. Pharmacol. Ther. *6*, 273 (1992).
246 K.P. Lesch, B.L. Wolozin, D.L. Murphy and P. Riederer: J. Neurochem. *60*, 2319 (1993).

247 R.W. Fuller and D.T. Wong: J. Clin. Psychopharmacol. *7* Suppl. 6, 36S (1987).
248 B.K. Koe, A. Weissman, W.M. Welch and R.G. Browne: J. Pharmacol. Exp. Ther. *226*, 686 (1983).
249 T. Brucke, J. Kornhuber, P. Angelberger, S. Asenbaum, H. Frassine and I. Podreka: J. Neural Trans. Gen. Sect. *94*, 137 (1993).
250 U. Scheffel, S. Kim, E.J. Cline and M.J. Kuhar: Synapse *16*, 263 (1994).
251 J.K. Staley, M. Basile, D.D. Flynn and D.C. Mash: J. Neurochem. *62*, 549 (1994).
252 L. Lemberger, H. Rowe, R. Carmichael, R. Crabtree, J.S. Horng, F. Bymaster and D.T. Wong: Clin. Pharmacol. Ther. *23*, 421 (1978).
253 D. Muck-Seler, M. Jakovljevic and Z. Deanovic: J. Affect. Disord. *23*, 157 (1991).
254 J. Vetulani, J.V. Dingell and F. Sulser: The Pharmacologist *16*, 287 (1974).
255 A. Frazer, G. Pandey, J. Mendels, S. Neeley, M. Kane and M.E. Hess: Neuropharmacology *13*, 1131 (1974).
256 R. Mishra, N J. Leith, L. Steranka and F. Sulser: Naunyn-Schmiedeberg's Arch. Pharmacol. *316*, 218 (1981).
257 M.J. Schmidt and J.F. Thornberry: Arch. Int. Pharmacodyn. *229*, 42 (1977).
258 S.J. Peroutka and S.H. Snyder: Science *210*, 88 (1980).
259 A. Dumbrille-Ross and S.W. Tang: Life Sci. *32*, 2677 (1983).
260 D.B. Goodnough and G.B. Baker: J. Neurochem. *62*, 2262 (1994).
261 D.T. Wong and F.P. Bymaster: Res. Commun. Chem. Pathol. Pharmacol. *32*, 41 (1981).
262 K. Fuxe, S.-O. Ogren, L.F. Agnati, P. Eneroth, A.C. Holm and K. Andersson: Neurosci. Lett. *21*, 57 (1981).
263 Y. Chaput, C. de Montigny and P. Blier: Neuropsychopharmacology *5*, 219 (1991).
264 P. Blier, Y. Chaput and C. de Montigny: Naunyn-Schmiedeberg's Arch. Pharmacol. *337*, 246 (1988).
265 N. Bel and F. Artigas: Synapse *15*, 243 (1993).
266 J.J. Rutter, C. Gundlah and S.B. Auerbach: Neurosci. Lett. *171*, 183 (1994).
267 S.A. Welner, C. de Montigny, J. Desroches, P. Desjardins and B.E. Suranyi-Cadotte: Synapse *4*, 347 (1989).
268 J.G. Hensler, G.B. Kovachich and A. Frazer: Neuropsychopharmacology *4*, 131 (1991).
269 C. de Montigny, Y. Chaput and P. Blier: J. Clin. Psychiat. *51* Suppl B, 4 (1990).
270 R. Invernizzi, M. Bramante and R. Samanin: Eur. J. Pharmacol. *260*, 243 (1994).
271 S. Hjorth and S.B. Auerbach: Neuropharmacology *33*, 331 (1994).
272 G. Pineyro, P. Blier, T. Dennis and C. de Montigny: J. Neurosci. *14*, 3036 (1994).
273 J. Hyttel: Prog. Neuro-Psychopharmacol. Biol. Psychiat. *6*, 277 (1982).
274 L.A. Hilakivi-Clarke and R. Goldberg: Eur. J. Pharmarcol. *237*, 101 (1993).
275 R.W. Fuller, D.T. Wong and D.W. Robertson: Med. Res. Rev. *11*, 17 (1991).
276 J. Buus Lassen: Eur. J. Pharmacol. *47*, 351 (1978).
277 V. Claassen, J.E. Davies, G. Hertting and P. Placheta: Br. J. Pharmacol. *60*, 505 (1977).
278 J. Hyttel: Acta Pharmacol. Toxicol. *40*, 439 (1977).
279 S.B. Ross, H. Hall, A.L. Renyi and D. Westerlund: Psychopharmacology *72*, 219 (1981).
280 G. Le Fur, M. Kabouche and A. Uzan: Life Sci. *23*, 1959 (1978).

Progress in Drug Research, Vol. 45 (E. Jucker, Ed.)

Generation of new-lead structures in computer-aided drug design

By Nissim Claude Cohen and Vincenzo Tschinke

Research Department, Pharmaceutical Division, CIBA-GEIGY Limited, CH-4002 Basel, Switzerland

1 Introduction

New and powerful tools are going to alter the perspectives of drug design in the near future. Impressive advances have recently been made in providing automated methods for lead finding in drug design. The spectacular progress made in both computational power and extensive data-storage capacity has made it possible to conceive very ambitious projects directed at lead finding in rational drug design. Computational capacity and memory are no longer limiting factors. Million of operations can be envisaged to process, retrieve, store and verify the structural capabilities of candidate molecules before lead structures conforming to the desired profile are identified and displayed. The aim of this article is to review existing approaches in the design of new lead structures, and to critically discuss some of the trends likely to emerge in the future in this relatively new discipline.

2 Computer-aided drug-design strategies

There are two major strategies currently used in the rational conception of new drugs. In the first, the three-dimensional features of a known protein-receptor site are directly considered (i.e., an X-ray structure or a 3-D model), and in the second the design is based on the comparative analysis of the 3-D structural features of known active and inactive molecules that are interpreted in terms of complementarity with a hypothetical receptor site.

Several years ago, we proposed that these two approaches could best be designated as the "direct" approach and the "indirect" approach [1]. Nowadays the expression "structure-based" is coming into use to qualify the direct approach, but it is ambiguous: 'structure' can refer not only to the receptor, but also to the ligand. To avoid this imprecision, we submit that it would be preferable to differentiate between the "receptor structure-based" and the "pharmacophore-based" approach, and we will use these terms in the present article.

From the experience gained in molecular modelling over the past few years, it is plainly evident that this discipline has widened the horizons of pharmaceutical research and provided useful tools for finding new lead compounds by both approaches. These aspects will be discussed in detail in the following sections.

3 Pharmacophore-based drug design

3.1 Importance of the bioactive conformation

Knowing the bioactive conformation of the ligand as it binds to the receptor or enzyme greatly facilitates the designing of new potent and specific lead molecules. Experience shows that the bioactive conformation of a molecule is not necessarily that found in solution or in the crystal. Rather, it is the specific conformation of lowest energy in the context of the receptor: during the process of complex formation, the protein and the ligand respond to each other's presence. The more flexible the molecule, the more unlikely it is that the bioactive conformation will be the same as that seen in other conditions (in solution, in the crystal, or in the gaseous phase). If an experimental structure for the protein-ligand complex already exits, the information it conveys can be used to design new molecules. In indirect design, this information is not available and the first step in this strategy therefore consists in generating such information.

3.2 The pharmacophore

The indirect drug design approach is based on the recognition of three-dimensional stereochemical and physicochemical features common to sets of active molecules – the pharmacophore. As already mentioned, this recognition results from the comparative analysis of the properties of the different compounds, which are interpreted in terms of complementarity with a hypothetical receptor site.
The pharmacophore consists of a set of molecular fragments in a precise relative location in 3-D; they are supposed to be recognized by the receptor concerned and responsible for the biological activity in question.

3.3 Deriving a pharmacophore model

The visualization in 3-D of molecular properties (steric aspects, electrostatic potentials, hydrophobicity, etc.) is one step towards the determination of similarities and differences between active and inactive compounds. The easiest way to reveal 3-D structural features common to a series of compounds is to use superimposition procedures. This technique has been applied extensively since the early seventies. The superimpositions are obvious when topological analogs are considered; but they are not obvious when chemically unrelated structures are compared. Extensive analyses made in a variety of therapeutic areas have shown how different molecules can elicit similar biological activities when they share common stereochemical features in 3-D. This has led to the development of 3-D pharmacophoric models, which are necessary for the rational design of new lead compounds. Even if the molecular geometries available derive from X-ray crystallography or NMR measurements, a flexible molecule should be represented as a set of low-energy conformers.

The structures are usually aligned on the basis of their atomic positions, but the alignment can be very subjective. The best way to reduce subjectivity is to compare the molecules in 3-D in the actual space of their physicochemical properties (designated sometimes as four-dimensional, 4-D representation). The conformational flexibility of the molecules introduces another level of complication: due to the extreme difficulty of the problem, the modelist often relies on visual judgements to control and modify manually the current conformations.

Superposition and comparison methods, often called "molecular fitting" or "pharmacophore alignment", are the most routinely available for revealing pharmacophores. Table 1 lists some published computer programs based on such concepts.

Computerized superimposition techniques are relatively new and very complex, especially when the multiple-conformation perspective is envisaged. New developments in this field are in progress and should provide a powerful means of obtaining good structural pharmacophore models. The most popular approach to pharmacophore superimposition has been the "active-analog" approach [18], developed by Marshall et al., which uses systematic search to determine the admissible conformation of all molecules in the study, followed by comparison of interatomic distances to select conformers that overlap, based on the proposed pharmacophore. Attempts have been made to take the conformational energies during the fitting process into consideration. Excluded-volume analysis was the classical way to compare geometrically a set of active and inactive molecules in order to reveal essential features, based on the simple idea that regions of inactive molecules that protrude beyond the volume common to the active molecules indicate sterically unfavorable regions of the receptor. Without replacing a complete systematic search, the elegant "ensemble distance geometry" method [19] affords a means of rapidly determining whether any solutions exist and, if so, provides a random sampling of solutions that indicates how uniquely determined the model is. Additional advantages of this approach are that it handles rings naturally, without the ring-closure difficulties encountered in dihedral search methods, and that chirality can be allowed to vary for any specified stereocenters of unknown absolute configuration. The drawback of this approach is that

Table 1.
Computer programs for aligning molecules

	Ref.	Features[a]	Comments
ASP	2	S, Q	Automatic comparison of molecules
MEPCONF	3	Q, F	Search for electrostatic similarity
SPERM	4	S, F	Icosahedron mapping algorithm
OVID and SUPER	5	S	Overlap based on molecular shape
RECEPS	6	S, Q, HB, F, R	Interactive superposition
AUTOFIT	7	S, Q, HB, F, R	Automatic superposition
DISCO	8	S, F	Search for bioactive conformation
CoMFA	9	S, Q	Superposition in the space of properties
BIOCES	10	S, Q, R	Electrostatic complementarity
YING	11	S, Q, R, E	Electrostatic complementarity
LOCKSMITH, LOCK, and KEY	12	L	Search for hydropathic similarity
SEAL	13	S, Q, F	Generation of many superposition modes
CATALYST	14	S, Q, HB, F	Pharmacophore visualization
APEX-3D	15	S, Q, HB, F	Pharmacophore visualization
LIPOT	16	L	Search for lipophilic similarity
YAK	17	R, E	Pseudoreceptor concept

[a] S: shape, steric similarity/complementarity; Q: charge, electrostatic similarity/complementarity; HB: H-bond similarity/complementarity; L: lipophilicity, hydrophobicity similarity; F: molecules treated as flexible; R: receptor complementarity; E: energy refinements.

conformational energies are not considered in the treatment. Most available implementations of this method provide a simple interactive fitting functionality by assuming the molecules to be conformationally rigid, while optionally allowing motion of a few dihedral angles. More recently, flexible-fit computational treatments were developed in which not only the internal rotational degrees of freedom, but also the conformational energies of the individual molecules are taken into account. MAXIMIN [20] is an example in which two alternative methods are possible: a set of flexible molecules can be mapped onto a rigid reference compound, or all the molecules are treated as flexible entities, and the treatment is directed towards the minimization of the conformational variance of the whole set. "Template forcing" [21] is another way to maximize overlaps between molecules, using restrained molecular mechanics and dynamics.
In molecular-fitting treatments, the maximization of the overlaps is generally achieved by geometrical least-squares minimizations, which require a preliminary selection of pairs of atoms expected to be superimposable. The choice of the pairs of atoms is very subjective, being based on a "chem-

ical intuition" of the probable pharmacophore. Less subjective approaches were developed on the basis of maximizing the overlap of a set of molecules by minimizing the exposed area of the entire set while simultaneously ensuring that the energies of the individual molecules remain close to a local minimum [22], combinatorial methods for comparing all possible overlaps of similar atom types [23, 24], and approaches based on three-dimensional electrostatic potential similarity [25, 26], molecular-similarity [27] and molecular-shape analyses [28].

A more physical approach is to force common pharmacophore atoms to interact with a common binding site, defined by hypothetical points of interaction (e.g., dummy atoms or a pseudo-receptor), rather than forcing them to superimpose directly: different (and sometimes identical) chemical moieties can be compared and need not be exactly superimposable [6, 29]. Several approaches make it possible to find similarities between two molecules in terms of preselected electrostatic contours or molecular volumes. In the same perspective, instead of superimposing pairs of atoms in molecular fitting, it would be preferable to superimpose the molecules in the space of their physicochemical properties. Attempts of this type have been made and have proved very promising. The most popular method developed along this line is the CoMFA [9] approach (comparative field analyses) recently developed by Cramer et al. as a new generation of 3D-QSAR method. It is based on the calculation of the interaction of each molecule in a set of superimposed active structures. CoMFA searches and Marshall's method have proved a powerful combination in deriving pharmacophore models [30, 31].

New approaches developed on the multiple conformation definition of a given structure (e.g., a database of minimized conformers) and using three-dimensional substructure and similarity search techniques [32] have shown themselves to be of value in identifying pharmacophore moieties and associated bioactive conformations of molecules [68]. Efforts of this type are current topics in modelling development and are going to extend the range of the tools already available.

3.4 Molecular mimicry and peptidomimetism

Molecular mimicry is a concept of central importance in drug research. Very often the molecules created are conceived as mimics of substances known to interact with the biological system under consideration (i.e., hormones, peptides, transmitters, etc.) For example, peptidomimetic molecules are conceived to mimic the structure of an endogenous peptide. They are converted into a regular organic molecule. The reason is that very

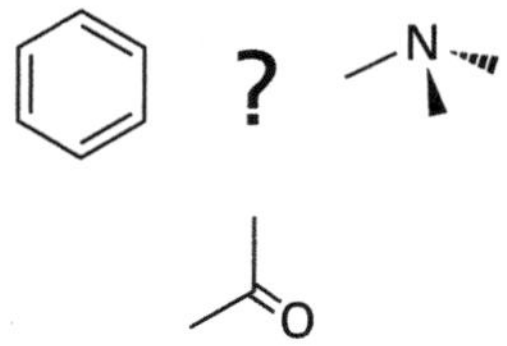

Fig. 1
How to link the recognition fragments of a pharmacophore?

often peptide molecules cannot be developed as drugs. Peptide molecules are in general biologically unstable, poorly absorbed, and rapidly metabolized. A non-peptide molecule should have none of these drawbacks. It is expected that the synthetic molecules may provide the structural diversity necessary to allow the molecule to be optimized for specificity, oral bioavailability, and pharmacokinetic properties. Molecular mimicry can be considered from various points of view and can cover many molecular properties. Actually, this is not really a new approach in drug research; it has been inherent in most attempts aimed at designing drugs in a rational way. New compounds have been, and continue to be conceived on the basis of analogies with the structures of known active reference molecules. Pharmacophore models provide useful means for the design of new lead structures. A central issue in the development of a research project is to find new lead compounds possessing the expected biological activities. Even if series of compounds are already known, medicinal chemists will still often search for a new series chemically unrelated to the known ones. Molecular mimicry and its associated computerized tools constitute the very vector that allows progress to be made in the indirect approaches and, *a fortiori*, in the direct methods.

3.5 How lead structures are obtained

Designing molecules that assemble a set of disconnected functional groups in three dimensions is no trivial task and remains very subjective. A computerized approach may provide a broad-diversity set of solutions that are free from any subjective bias. It is a general feature of computer-aided lead generation that the proposed molecules come from two main sources: they are either extracted from a data-bank of known molecules (the database approach), or generated on the basis of construction algorithms (construction methods) that generate new molecules conforming to desired requirements. One of the advantages of database searching is that it gen-

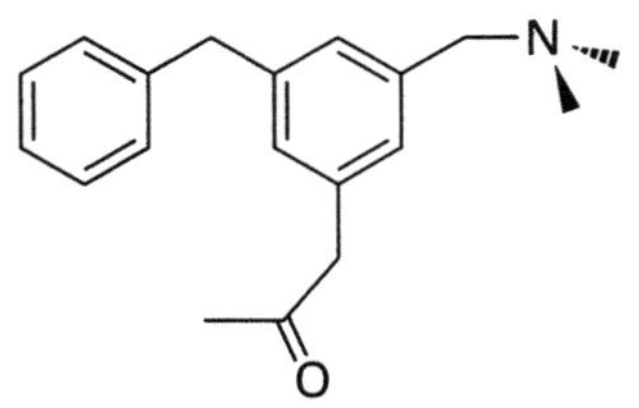

Fig. 2
A possible solution to the query represented in Fig. 1.

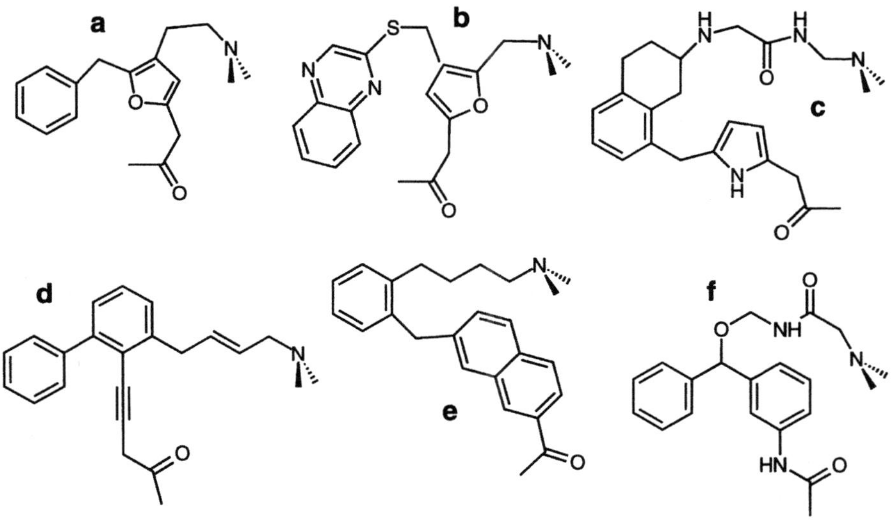

Fig. 3
Other possible solutions to the query represented in Fig. 1 showing the chemical diversity that can be associated with the recognition fragments considered. These results were obtained by the authors, using the NEWLEAD program [61].

erally requires no synthetic effort, which is often not the case in construction methods. On the other hand, the latter have the advantage of not being biased or dependent on a given databank, and they provide the structural diversity necessary to allow a synthetic target to be chosen as a first lead.

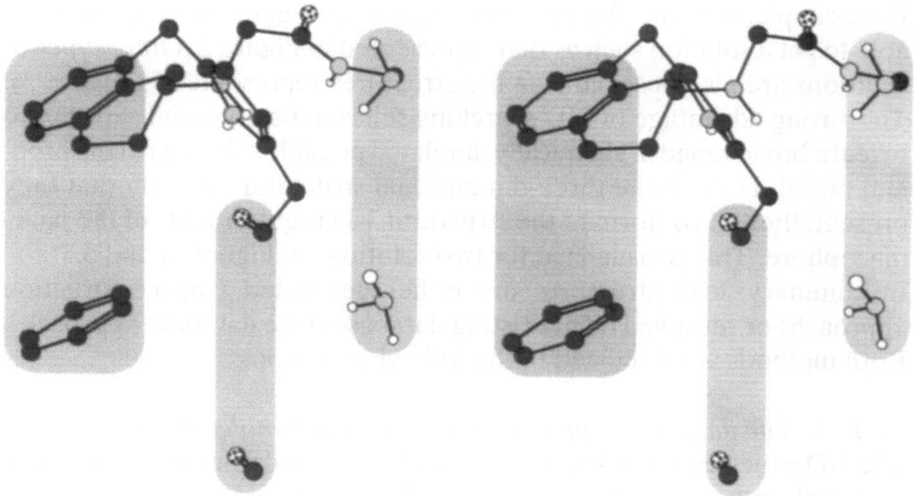

Fig. 4
Stereo view of the structure in Figure 3c superimposed on the pharmacophore example in Fig. 1. Atom patterns: dark grey, Carbon; light grey, Nitrogen; white, Hydrogen; dotted pattern, Oxygen. Hydrogen atoms on carbons are omitted.

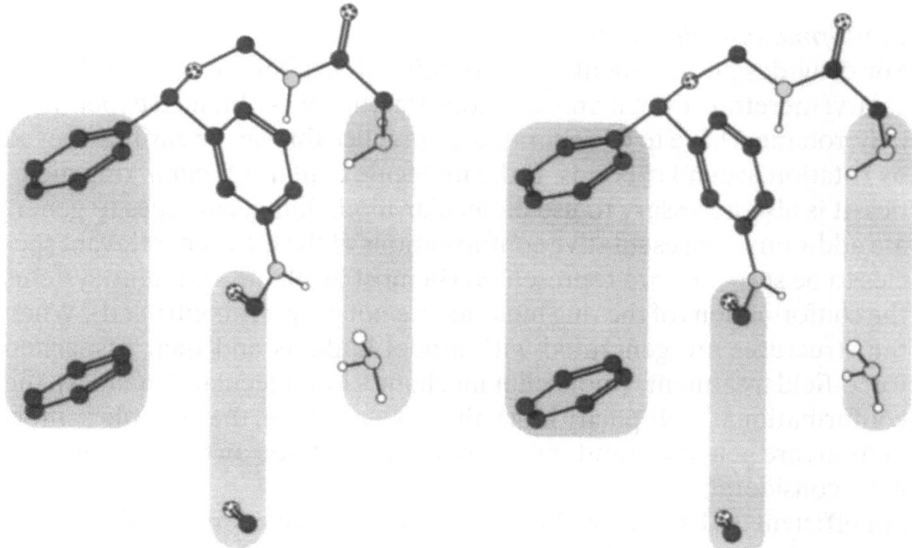

Fig. 5
Stereo view of the structure in Fig. 3f superimposed on the pharmacophore example in Fig. 1. Atom patterns: dark grey, Carbon; light grey, Nitrogen; white, Hydrogen; dotted pattern, Oxygen. Hydrogen atoms on carbons are omitted.

For example, from the pharmacophore shown in Figure 1 it would be desirable to get a solution such as that represented in Figure 2. Other types of solutions are also possible (see the structures represented in Figure 3). The strong advantage of 3-D searching relies in its potential capacity to reveal a broad range of chemically unrelated possible solutions to the problem posed. Despite the three-dimensional structural diversity that they present, they all conform to the structural 3-D requirements of the pharmacophore. This is visualized for two solutions in Figures 4 and 5.

In summary, lead structures are either generated (the construction approach) or retrieved from existing databases (the database approach). Both methods are discussed in the following sections.

3.5.1 The database approach: sources of small molecules in 3-D

The 3-D structure of small molecules can be obtained from various sources. The molecular geometries generally derive either from experimental methods (X-ray crystallography, NMR spectroscopy), or from theoretical calculations (molecular modelling). Atomic coordinates from both sources can be stored in databanks for subsequent computerized treatments. Table 2 indicates various ways of obtaining the conformational information for small molecules needed for 3-D searching.

Conformational flexibility

For drug-design treatments conformational flexibility is absolutely necessary; therefore, even if only one conformation was obtained experimentally, rotamers have to be generated. In practice this can be easily achieved by rotation around σ-bonds. If the molecule contains flexible ring moieties, it is also necessary to use molecular-modelling techniques to generate additional representative conformations of the different relevant species to be sure they are represented (in most available searching systems the conformations of the ring moieties are not properly controlled). When the structures are generated with model builders and their associated force-field treatments (molecular mechanics or molecular dynamics), the conformational multiplicity is usually not a problem, the possible conformations are generated and can afterwards be filtered on the basis of energetic considerations.

An efficient 3-D search will be complete when all energetically permissible conformations of the molecules are considered. If all conformations of every molecule are to be stored in the database, the sheer volume of the informational content will, of course, greatly prolong search operations. Compromise solutions such as storing a limited number of conformations in the database are not satisfactory: in general any such selec-

Table 2.
Sources of 3-D structures for searching

A: Crystallographic databases

	Ref.	
Cambridge Structural Database	33	CSD
Corporate Databases		INDUSTRY

B: Commercially available databases

	Ref.	Abbreviation	Company
Chapman & Hall Dictionary of Chemicals	34	CHDC	Chapman & Hall
Chemical Abstracts Service	35	CAST-3D	Chemical Abstracts
Chemical Abstracts Service Registry	36	CAS-RF	Chemical Abstracts
Fine Chemicals Directory	37	FCD-3D	Molecular Design
Ltd.			
Comprehensive Medicinal Chemistry	38	CMC-3D	Molecular Design
MACCS Drug Data Report	39	MDDR-3D	Molecular Design
ChemDBS-3D	40	CHEMDBS3D	Chemical Design Ltd.
UNITY	41	UNITY	Tripos Associates
POMONA	42	POMONA-92C	Daylight
TRIAD	43	TRIAD	Molecular Simulations

C: Computerized model-builders (2D-3D converters)

	Ref.	Features[a]
ATCOOR	44	S, M
CONCORD	45	S
MOLGEO	46	S
AIMB	47	S, F
COBRA	48	S, F, M, AI
WIZARD	49	S, F, M, AI
CORINA	50	S
CHEM-X	51	S, F
ALCOGEN	52	S
Catalyst	14	S
SCRIPT	53	S, M, F
CONVERTER	54	S, M, DG
DBMAKER	55	S, M
3DGEN	138	M

[a] S: stereochemistry preserved; M: multiple conformations are generated; F: library of 3-D fragments used; DG: distance geometry algorithm; AI: artificial intelligence algorithm.

tion will be out of all proportion to the actual number of possible conformations the molecules can adopt, and the risk of not identifying the relevant conformations is therefore extremely high. Methods that use more chemical knowledge have been explored: for example, ALADDIN [67] and EMBED [56] use distance-geometry concepts that represent conformational multiplicity within the framework of a distance-bounds matrix. Along these lines, multiple interatomic distances ranges are used to implicitly define conformational flexibility. This approach has been shown to give encouraging results in matching molecules of a database to the requirements of a 3-D query [57]. More recently, new systems have been exploring the possibilities that flexible conformations are generated 'on the fly', in which case the storage of only one conformation of the molecule considered is generally sufficient. Although this approach appears very promising, it is too early to say whether it will lead to an important breakthrough in this area.

3.5.2 The database approach: How leads are retrieved from databanks

Pharmacophores are often a starting point in drug design. They can be used as queries in 3-D databases to search for known structures that match the targeted structural elements. Database 3-D substructure searching is actually a computerized form of screening aimed at identifying new lead structures; it is an extension of the well-known 2-D searching already used in chemistry for several decades. The more recent availability of tools for molecular modelling permitted the upgrade of current systems from 2-D to 3-D. Today, powerful model builders can convert existing 2-D databases (the most popular 3-D databases are mentioned in Table 2). One of the limitations of some of the first generation of converters is that they aimed at the generation of only one conformation per molecule. As already mentioned, the strategy for dealing with conformational multiplicity in structure searching is not yet definitively established; however most recent model builders are functioning beyond the one-conformation capability.

From the conceptual point of view, 2-D and 3-D searching are very similar: the only difference is that in the latter the connectivity table is no longer the sole information needed to search for matches; the relative location of the atoms in the 3-D space is also required. The search can be conducted for an exact match or for a certain degree of similarity (defined by the value of a similarity coefficient). In more recent systems, not only rigid 3-D matching is considered, but also conformational flexible searching (CFS) [40, 41, 64]. The query consists of a 2-D diagram or a 3-D model

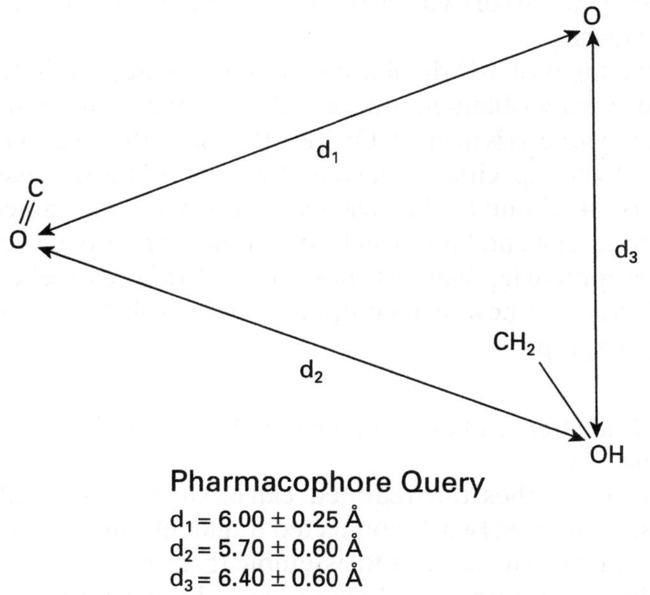

Fig. 6
Example of a pharmacophore query: pharmacophore for the protein-kinase C receptor (see text). Reproduced with permission from ref. 58 (Wang S., Zaharevitz D.W., Sharma R., Marquez V.E., Lewin N.E., Du L., Blumberg P.M. and Milne G.W.A.: The Discovery of Novel, Structurally Diverse Protein-Kinase C Agonists through Computer 3D-Database Search. Molecular Modelling Studies. J. Med. Chem. *37*, 4479–4489 (1994)).

described with the aid of a molecular-graphics system. Geometrical objects are then selected (points, lines, planes, centroids, spheres), and their desired 3-D relationships are defined (distances, angles, dihedral angles, etc.) with tolerance values associated to each. Such systems are generally easy to use, and when applied on relatively small databases they give very reasonable computing times. Figure 6 shows an example of such a query, defined for protein-kinase C (PK-C) agonists [58]. The database used (the NCI 3-D database [59]) contained more than 200,000 structures, and it required approximately one week of computer time on an Iris Indigo workstation. In Figure 7 are displayed the 11 most potent hits obtained out of the 165 compounds actually selected for the PK-C binding assays. It is worth mentioning that molecular modelling studies revealed additional features associated with the pharmacophore. These results were confirmed by synthetic modifications of two inactive compounds leading to two active series of derivatives.

One of the advantages of 3-D database searching is that candidate molecules might be rapidly obtained and tested, avoiding additional delays when a chemical synthesis is needed. On the other hand the solutions might be either biased by the specific "molecular diversity" of the database concerned, or overlooked due to the absence of a new type of molecule in the database. Although database structure searching has proved very useful, construction approaches have also been shown to afford excellent tools for the identification of new lead compounds. This will be presented in the following paragraph.

3.5.3 How lead structures are generated with construction approaches

In construction approaches, the treatment can be simply described as follows. Given a set of at least two disconnected fragments, the problem consists of finding appropriate spacers to assemble these moieties in a single molecule. Multiple solutions are likely to occur, because many connections with different combinations of spacers are possible. In construction approaches, the spacers are either generated atom by atom (Linkor [60]) or using elementary units such as library-spacers, single-atoms, and fusering spacers (Newlead [61]). The solutions are expected to conform to the following three criteria: they must be chemically plausible, geometrically valid and energetically acceptable.

The conceptual frame used in such treatments is visualized in Figure 8. As already mentioned, the construction approach offers the advantage of not being biased or dependent on a given databank in providing the structural diversity necessary to allow a synthetic target to be chosen as a first lead for further optimization. The major benefit of these automatic linking programs is that they show many alternatives for positioning the same key fragments.

3.5.4 Programs that propose molecules conforming to pharmacophores

Several programs were developed in the field of pharmacophore-based drug design. They create new molecules from initial 3-D pharmacophores. The majority of them are database-oriented, whereas those based on construction approaches are relatively rare and still under development. A list of programs that create new molecules from pharmacophores is given in Table 3. The specific features of each program are also mentioned in

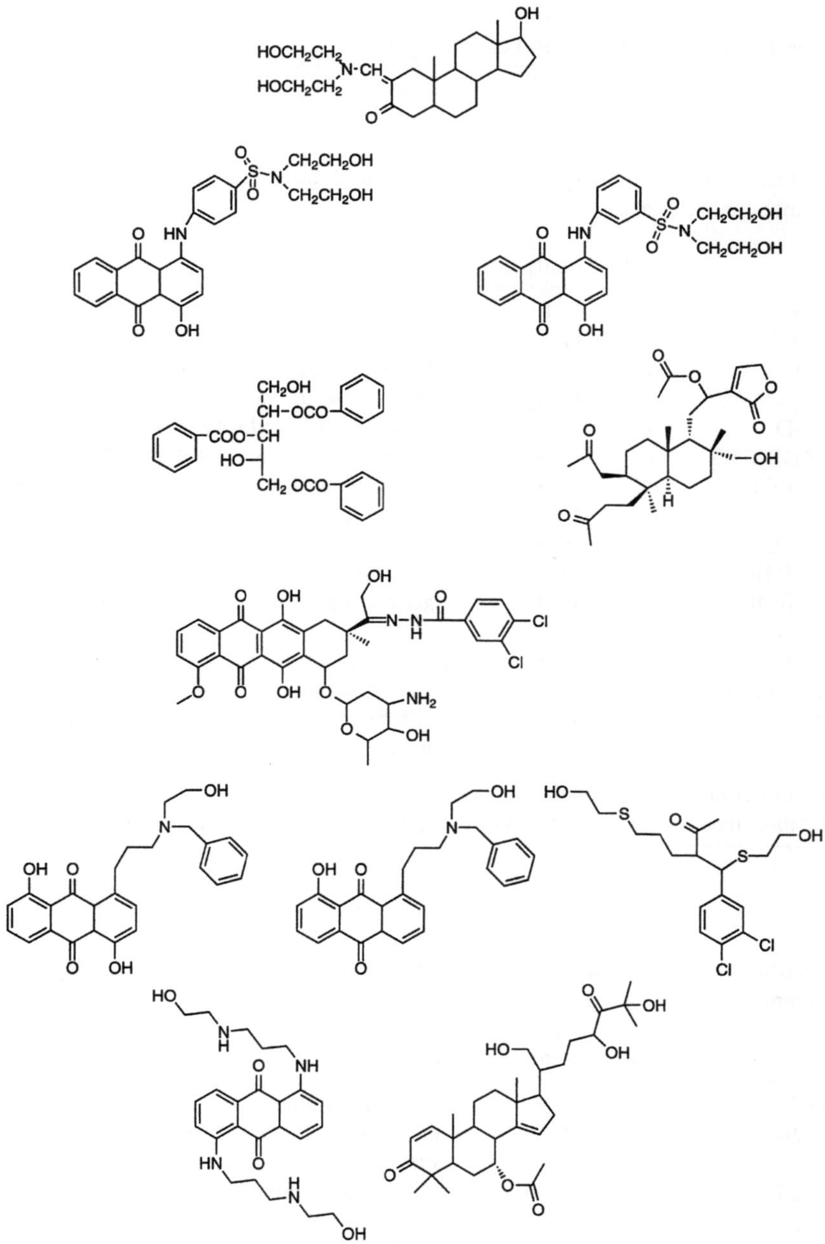

Fig. 7
Solutions obtained with the query shown in Fig. 6. Reproduced with permission from ref. 58 (Wang S. et al.: The Discovery of Novel, Structurally Diverse Protein-Kinase C Agonists through Computer 3D-Database Search. Molecular Modelling Studies. J. Med. Chem. *37*, 4479–4489 (1994)).

Table 3.
Programs in pharmacophore-based drug design

A: Database approaches: programs that extract candidate structures conforming to a pharmacophore query.

	Ref.	Features[a]	Comments
CAVEAT	62	V, J	Retrieves rigid ring systems from the CSD
MACCS-3D	63	G, S, F	Torsional-optimization technique
ISIS-3D	64	G, S, F	Torsional-optimization technique
UNITY	41	G, S, F	"Directed-tweak" approach
CAST-3D	35	G, S	"Fuzzy match" similarity search
CHEMDBS-3D	40	G, S, F	Rule-based conformational analysis
3DSEARCH	65	G, S	Topological and substructural 3-D searches
Iditis	66	G, S, F	Search engine for the Brookhaven databank
ALADDIN	67	G, S	Automated modification of hit structures
MENTHOR	68	G, S	Biological data integrated in the searches
LEAPFROG	69	F, D	A genetic algorithm used for automated docking
QUEST3D and VISTA	70	G, S	Query software for the CSD
THREEDOM	71	G, S	Icosahedron-mapping algorithm
LUDI	72	D	Positions several small fragments in the cavity
DOCK	73	D	Docking of database molecules

[a] V: query defined as vector pairs; G: geometric search; S: structure/substructure search; F: flexible structures; J: hits joined to the query fragments; D: automated docking.

B: Construction approaches: programs that construct new molecules assembling the 3-D elements of a pharmacophore

	Ref.	Features[b]	Comments
NEWLEAD	61	T, V	Connects fragments of a pharmacophore
LINKOR	60	A	Creates new structures based on reference molecules
SPROUT	74	T, AI	Structure generation with A.I. techniques
HOOK	75	T, V	Grows into receptor from starting points ("hooks")
SPLICE	76	T	Combines large number of templates
RING-BRACING	77	T, F	Rings generated after attaching linear spacers

[b] A: one atom at a time added; T: library of templates used; F: flexible spacers; V: vector matching; AI: artificial-intelligence algorithm

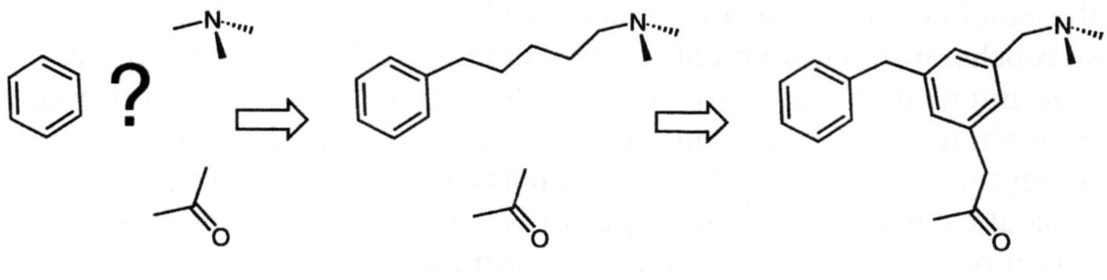

Fig. 8
The conceptual frame used to create a structure by a construction approach. For clarity, the structures are represented in 2-D; in reality all the treatments are made in 3-D.

in Table 3. The specific features of each program are also mentioned in the table.

4 Receptor structure-based drug design

The specificity and the affinity of a ligand for a protein receptor is controlled by the principles of molecular recognition. Over the last few years, an increasing number of protein structures have been elucidated to atomic resolution using X-ray crystallography and nuclear magnetic resonance spectroscopy. Advances were made in molecular biology, in protein-purification methods, in the control of the overexpression of biological systems, in data-collection techniques in protein crystallography, and in molecular modelling and have all contributed to the emergence of the nowadays so-called "structure-based drug design" approach in rational drug design.
If a protein constitutes a key element in the development of a disease to be cured, the information carried in the three-dimensional structure of this protein, alone or complexed with a ligand, is then of paramount importance for drug design. The strategies currently considered in receptor structure-based drug design are reviewed in the following sections.

4.1 How lead structures are obtained

As in pharmacophore-based drug design, in receptor structure-based approaches lead structures can be either generated (the construction approach) or retrieved from existing databases (the database approach). The new situation created by the knowledge of the 3-D structure of the macromolecular receptor introduces an additional level of complexity:

the candidate molecule is expected to take advantage of the precise 3-D stereochemical requirements of the binding site, both in terms of favorable interactions and also to avoid steric repulsions that could occur between the candidate prototype and the surface of the receptor.

Receptor-structure-based drug design has widened the horizons of pharmaceutical research. It not only affords a means for the rational optimization of a given molecule, but also permits the *de novo* design of new chemical entities. Several years ago, this was a pure dream, but nowadays most research groups have remarkable examples of successful design conducted along these lines. The complexity of such treatments should not be underestimated: photographs of a river do not reveal how to build a bridge across it [78]. The physicochemical forces regulating biological processes involve the subtle contribution of a whole set of forces, including hydrophobic and electrostatic effects, within a complex network of anchorage points comprising hydrogen bonds or others structural interactions. The state of the art both in the database approach and the approach based on construction algorithms will be reviewed and discussed in the following sections.

4.1.1 The database approach: How leads are retrieved from databanks

The database approach consists of searching in 3-D databases for ligands that are complementary to the cavity of a given receptor. The database systematically searches for interesting potential candidates. Stewart et al. [79] validated this approach by showing in the case of inhibitors of chymotrypsin that they were able to correctly identify the two best known inhibitor structures within a series of more than one hundred compounds. The objective of such a method is to identify interesting hits showing activities at the micromolar range and then optimize them. In order to increase the binding to the nanomolar range, it is necessary to introduce chemical groups that are designed on the basis of the 3-D-modelled complex and expected to produce additional favorable attractions with the receptor. There is a large collection of 3-D structures currently available for treatments of this type (see Table 2). The Cambridge Data base is the most popular of the experimentally available structures, but its application remains limited. Although it can serve to identify chemical moieties that are accepted by the cavity, the use of other databases, even if their structures were not determined experimentally, is more attractive (corporate databanks or databases containing compounds that are commercially accessible), because the compounds are more readily available for performing binding tests. In this field, speeding up the optimization step becomes a determining factor. The concepts underlying the database approach are simple, as when a locksmith tries to open a door using the various sets of keys he has accumulated over the years. As far as computerized approaches are concerned, for lead finding it is not a major issue: the user can well afford to wait a day or two before he gets the answer, provided the resultant hits appear to have a high informational content. This database approach can be easily combined with screening techniques; in particular, it can be expected that the use of advanced screening techniques such as combinatorial chemistry will provide a powerful complement to the rational approach.

Several years ago, attempts were made to identify non-peptidic inhibitors of the HIV-1 protease. The 3-D structure of the enzyme was used as a screen in order to identify small molecules with shapes complementary to the active site. The DOCK program [73] generated a negative image of the active site, consisting of a cylinder composed of 34 overlapping spheres. A template of these spheres was then used to screen in the Cambridge Structural Database [33]. From the list of the 200 best-fit solutions, haloperidol was selected as a possible lead. The compound was tested for inhibitory efficacy and exhibited a moderate affinity (125 μM) for the HIV-1 protease. Attempts were made to increase the affinity of this reference molecule by introducing additional reactive groups in order to obtain new irreversible inhibitors [80]. The authors were able to increase the affinity of some analogs by as much as 1,000-fold. X-ray analyses of complexes with the HIV-1 protease revealed that in fact two distinct binding modes were present in the active site of the enzyme (one corresponding to that expected and the other rotated by 80 degrees and translated 4.8 Å away from the predicted mode). This study indicates that complications can arise in predicting the binding of small molecules to large target sites in which multiple binding modes may be possible. In this example, the most active compounds showed significant cytotoxicity; however the haloperidol story has shown that it was possible to identify a non-peptidic lead with moderate affinity, and analogs of haloperidol were designed and shown to be much more potent than the initial lead. Meanwhile, the DOCK [73] program has been improved, in that the complementarity to the macromolecular cavity is not only based on shape fitting, but also relies on a well-conceived scoring function [73d]. More recently, Kuntz et al. used the improved DOCK program to explore the minor and major grooves of A-, B- and Z-type DNA dodecamers [81]. They used the same methodology as described above and searched in a subset of the Cambridge Crystallographic Database. One of the molecules that scored best in terms of the new DOCK algorithm was actually CC-1065, a potent anti-

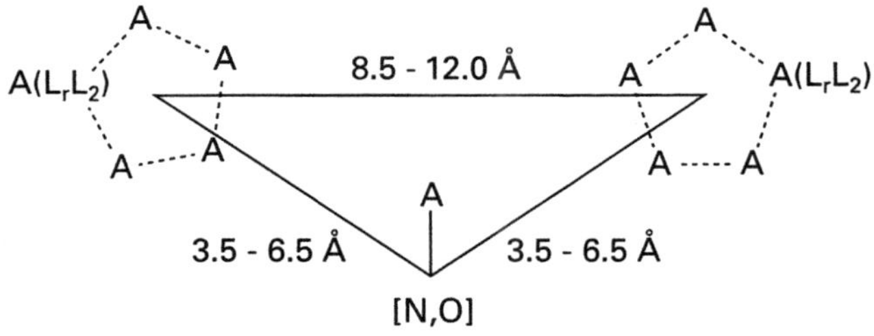

Fig. 9
The pharmacophore model used to search the Cambridge database for potential ligands for the HIV-1 protease. Reproduced with permission from ref. 82 (Lam P.Y.S. et al.: Rational Design of Potent, Bioavailable, Nonpeptide Cyclic Ureas as HIV Protease Inhibitors. Science *263*, 380–384 (1994)).

tumor agent known to bind the minor groove of B-DNA. The chemical diversity of the various hits obtained in this study confirms the advantage of such an approach. Many of the leads identified may serve as a starting point for a chemical program to design more potent and more specific ligands.

Another spectacular design [82] was published by the DuPont group. They were among the first to successfully design non-peptide inhibitors of the HIV-PR protease. Looking for orally bioavailable HIV-PR inhibitors this group began with structural information available from published X-ray crystal structures of HIV-PR inhibitor complexes [83] showing the presence of a tetracoordinated structural water molecule linking the bound inhibitor to the enzyme. Assuming that the incorporation of the binding features of this structural water molecule in a non-peptidic mimic would be beneficial because its displacement should be energetically favorable, they adopted a database strategy in order to find potent non-peptide inhibitors.

A simple pharmacophore model was used, based on two key intramolecular distances between two hydrophobic groups, designated P1 and P1' (see Figure 9) that occupy corresponding enzyme pockets, S1 and S1'. A 3-D database search gave initial hits that were progressively modified and eventually allowed the discovery of cyclic urea molecules active in the nanomolar range. Figure 10 shows one representative of this series, DMP-323, which is also the first molecule selected for clinical trials in this family (IC_{50} = 36 nM). Crystal structures of complexes with various

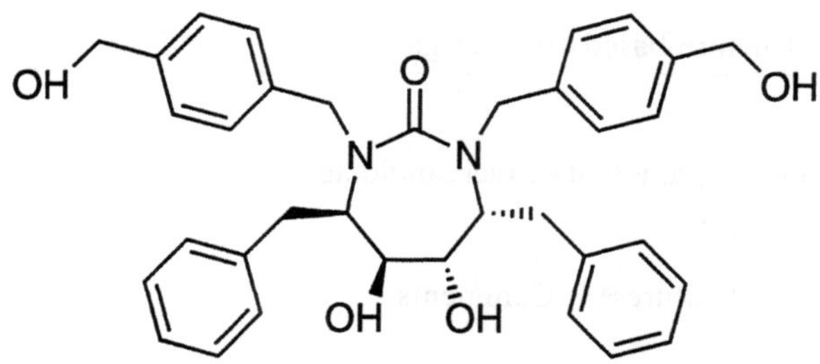

Fig. 10
The structure of DMP-323, a potent inhibitor of the HIV-PR enzyme, discovered following a database strategy (see text).

cyclic urea-HIV-PR complexes proved the validity of the approach. Although oral bioavailability stymied the first clinical compound from this series, the research team is currently looking for analogs with improved properties.

4.1.2 *How lead structures are generated with construction approaches*

Construction approaches in receptor structure-based design constitute one of the most stimulating challenges in rational drug design. *De novo* structures are constructed, and every time a new atom or group of atoms is added, it is dynamically chosen in order to achieve an optimal fit with the receptor. The actual shapes of sub-pockets, hydrogen bonds, and coulombic forces between the ligand and the receptor are fully exploited to achieve the best attraction between ligand and receptor. This approach can be used either to build a new-lead scaffold from scratch [89], or to extend the structure of a starting chemical frame [74]. In this case, additional structural moieties will be explored to obtain extended structures with higher binding energies. The growth can take place without assumptions, or with optional parameters under the control of the user. Scoring functions are currently used to discriminate between several alternatives, they generally rely on molecular mechanics force-fields, sometimes including a solvation [95] and also an entropic [135] component.

Table 4.
Programs in receptor structure-based drug-design

A: Database approaches: programs that extract candidate structures that fit into the active sites of a protein

	Ref.	Features[a]	Comments
DOCK	73, 92	S, Q, D	First automated docking program
AUTODOCK	84	S, Q, F	Simulated annealing algorithm
LUDI	85	S, Q, J, E	Can be used with large databases or libraries
ADAM	86	S, Q, F	Flexible docking program
EVE	87	S, Q, F	Allows the use of ADAM with large databases
FOUNDATION	88	S	Flexible, complex user-defined queries
SPLICE	76	S, J	Combines hits from FOUNDATION to form new ligands

[a] S: steric fit; Q: electrostatic complementarity; F: ligands treated as flexible; J: hits combined to form new molecules; D: desolvation; E: scoring of rotational entropy.

B: Construction approaches: programs that construct new molecules that fit into the active site of a protein

	Ref.	Features[b]	Comments
LEGEND	89	A	Generation of ligands with force field energy refinement
ADAM	86	F	Automatic generation of alternative binding modes
GROW	90	T, F, D	Grows a peptide in the active site
GROWMOL	91	A	Metropolis sampling on complementarity scores
LUDI	85	T, V, E	Finds optimal binding of small fragments
SPLICE	76	T, S	Joins a large number of templates
CONCEPTS	92	A, SM	Ensemble of pseudo-atoms as ligand model
MCDNLG	93	A, SM	Ensemble of pseudo-atoms as ligand model
CLIX	94	T, S	Concept of chemical fit
SPROUT	74	T, AI, E	Structure generation with A.I. techniques
HOOK	75	T, V	Multicopy-simulation search approach
GROUPBUILD	95	T, D	Ligand generated by joining fragments from a library
GenStar	96	A	Grows tetrahedral atoms in the active site

[b] A: one atom at a time added; T: library of templates used; F: flexible templates; V: vector matching; S: shape, steric complementarity; AI: artificial-intelligence algorithm; SM, statistical mechanics/dynamics methods used; D: desolvation; E: scoring of rotational entropy.

4.1.3 Programs that propose molecules fitting into active sites

Several systems have been developed in the last few years based on either the database or the construction approach. They are being continuously further developed (for example, the DOCK program, initially conceived in the early eighties to dock a known ligand, has evolved through the years and is now used to find novel lead compounds from a large database). Some of these programs are indicated in Table 4. Although some efforts are being made by commercial companies to offer products of this type, up to now the use of such systems has mainly been restricted to the specialists.

4.2 Data currently used in receptor structure-based drug design

X-ray crystallography and macromolecular modelling provide the most detailed possible view of drug-receptor interactions. The Brookhaven Protein Databank is the central database *par excellence*. In 1990, it contained more than 300 structures of proteins and nucleic acids, and there are now [139] more than 3000 full-release atomic coordinate entries (2,869 proteins, enzymes and viruses; 212 DNA, RNA and tRNA; 10 carbohydrates; 31 NMR entries), including several ligand-macromolecule complexes. This expansion clearly shows the revolution that has taken place in the field of structural biology during the past few years, resulting in an enormous increase in the number of laboratories engaged in structural studies of biological macromolecules. This is due to improvements in crystallographic techniques and the availability of new proteins through recombinant DNA approaches.

5 Analysis and treatment of the solutions obtained

5.1 Visual representations

As far as the computer representation is concerned, molecules consist of sets of atoms with their corresponding connectivities and 3-D coordinates. They are ready to be visualized using any molecular modelling system. Interactive molecular graphics representations have proved very useful to medicinal chemists for revealing the essential chemistry of the structures considered. The visualization of molecular structures and interactions allows them to calibrate their chemical intuition and develop a 'feel' for how structural variations will change the properties of interest [97].

5.2 Modifying the solutions

However sophisticated the software algorithms, it is up to the synthetic chemists to make the final decision. The structures that appear in the successive computerized treatments are only candidate scaffolds showing how the prototype compounds conform optimally to the desired structural requirements. How beautiful is the art of the medicinal chemist when he decides to modify the initial theoretical prototype in order to have a makeable molecule! When this stage is reached the theoretical model is no longer volatile and is already on its way into the real world. Ten years ago, it was not so easy to find success stories showing the utility of such approaches. Nowadays, no review of the field can ever be exhaustive. To give an idea of areas where success stories were reported, we have listed some of them in Table 5.

5.3 Energy and scoring functions

The estimation of the binding between a ligand and a protein must be attempted at some level of approximation by any program in receptor structure-based drug design. Due to the computational demand made by fully fledged molecular-mechanics calculations, most investigators resort to scoring functions, algorithms that assign a numerical score to a given structure inside a ligand. The score should ideally give a measure of the ligand-protein binding constant. Discrete grids of points are generally used to represent the protein surface.

Full utilization of the structural information requires proper evaluation of the free energy of binding of the prototype ligands considered. Calculation of this quantity is crucial in a structure-based approach to drug design. The important limitations currently existing in the ability to calculate such energies also explains the difficulties of developing reliable scoring algorithms. The binding of a ligand to a protein is a complex process in which the surfaces of both protein and ligand have to be progressively desolvated until the approach of the ligand is completed and a complex is formed with the protein. In this process, the geometrical changes of both protein and ligand are energetically driven in order to allow the proper conformation and orientations of the two interacting partners. Efforts are now being made to allow the calculation of some of the components of the free energy, such as the calculation of the changes in free energy of hydration, the loss of conformational, translational, and rotational entropy upon binding, the enthalpy change of forming the protein-ligand complex, etc. For example,

Table 5.
Some typical examples of successful discovery of lead structures

Design of inhibitors or antagonists or mimics of	Therapeutic area	Method[a]	Ref.
Dihydrofolate Reductase	Anticancer	R	98
HIV-1 Protease	AIDS	R	82, 93, 99
Thromboxane	Antithrombotic	P	100
Thrombin	Antithrombotic	R	101
Thymidylate Synthase	Anticancer	R	102
Dopamine Receptor	Antipsychotics	P	103
Purine Nucleoside Phosphorylase	T-Cell proliferation	R	104
Carbonic Anhydrase	Antiglaucoma	R	105
Neutrophil Elastase	Emphysema	R	106
Angiotensin II	Hypertension	P	107
Substance P	Anxiolytic	P	108
Renin	Hypertension	R	109
Phopholipase A2	Inflammation	R	110
Phopholipase A2	Inflammation	P	111
Thermolysin	Model system	R	112
Aromatase	Anticancer	P	113
Elastase	Arthritis, Emphysema	R	114
Neutral Endopeptidase	Hypertension	R	115
DNA	Anticancer	R	81
Serine & Cysteine Proteases	Antiparasitics	R	116
Sialidase	Antibody Mimic	R	117
Cyclophilin	Immunosuppressant	R	118
Influenza Virus Sialidase	Antiviral	R	119
Rotamase	Immunosuppressant	R	120
Opioid Kappa	Analgesic	P	121
HIV-1 Reverse Transcriptase	AIDS	P	122
Potassium-Channel Openers	Hypertension	P	123
Cholecystokinin	Obesity	P	124
GABA-Uptake Inhibitors	Parkinson	P	125
Benzodiazepine Receptor	Anxiety	P	126
Serotonin Receptor	Anxiolytic, Antidepressants	P	127
Aldose Reductase	Diabetes Mellitus	P	128
Protein-kinase C	Anticancer	P	58, 129
Cardiac Glycoside Receptor	Cardiotonics	P	130
Peptides	Peptidomimetics	P	131

[a] P: pharmacophore-based; R: receptor-based.

desolvation is considered by DOCK, GROW, and GroupBuild; rotational entropy is scored in LUDI and SPROUT.

Goodford's program GRID [132] builds surfaces describing favorable interaction sites for biologically important groups such as amino groups, carbonyl groups, etc. The interaction is represented by a simple scoring function containing a Lennard-Jones potential for van der Waals interactions, a simple Coulombic electrostatic term, and a distance dependent H-bond term that is also of the Lennard-Jones type. Water is treated as a neutral entity with no dipole capable of donating up to two Hydrogens and to accept up to two Hydrogens in H-bond formation. GREEN [133], a program for interactive docking, represents the receptor cavity as a grid of points to each of which an interaction potential is assigned. The electrostatic and van der Waals terms are similar to the approach discussed previously. The H-bond term simply returns a code number for the type of interaction (acceptor, donor, or ambivalent), if one is found. The outcome of the program is a visual rendering of the strength and type of the interaction based on color coding. The DOCK program [73d] uses a scoring function to dock existing ligands from a database into a protein cavity. The terms are similar to Goodford's except for a more complex electrostatic contribution derived from the DelPhi potential [134]. An approximation allows the separation of the ligand from the protein contributions to the interaction, so that the protein contributions can be precalculated and represented as a discrete grid of points. The score for each ligand is given by combining the contributions from each atom on the ligand and the contribution from the nearest grid point. GROW [90] builds peptide ligands inside a protein. The ligand is grown by adding one aminoacid fragment at a time. A complex scoring function is used to choose the best conformations as the chain grows. A special term depends on the conformation of each new fragment, based on extensive tabulated data for each amino acid. Such exhaustive treatment is possible because only a limited number of building blocks (natural amino acids) are being used. GroupBuild [95] also builds ligands inside a protein cavity, based on fragment-building blocks. The scoring function estimates solvent effects from the difference of the solvent-accessible surface of the ligand-protein complex and the sum of the areas of the isolated structures. A weighting factor for polar atoms is used, to provide an extra energetic reward for burying non-polar atoms inside the protein cavity. A completely numerical scoring function is used in the GrowMol program [91], which builds ligands atom by atom inside a protein cavity. A relatively fine grid of 0.25 Å mesh defines the cavity in terms of binding-site zones, such as lipophilic surfaces and H-bond sites. When an atom from the growing ligand structure falls next to a grid point it is assigned an integer number depending on its complementarity with the binding site zone. The outcome of the growth depends on the numerical score and on a statistical weighting function. A recent paper by Böhm [135] describes a scoring function that can qualitatively reproduce actual protein-ligand binding constants, yet is fast enough to be used in structure-generation programs such as LUDI [85]. The H-bond and ionic terms are discontinuous functions that give constant positive (unfavorable to binding) contributions for short distances, variable contributions for intermediate distances, and null contributions after a cutoff distance. A similar dependence on the angles is also introduced. The lipophilic contacts are estimated from contact surfaces, which are approximated by grids of points. There is also an entropic term proportional to the number of rotatable bonds of the ligand. This accounts for the loss of binding energy due to the freeze of rotational degrees of freedom in the ligand. All the terms contain adjustable parameters, and an extra constant term is added to account for all the contributions neglected. The parameters and the additive constant are determined by fitting the binding constants of protein-ligand complexes of known structures.

6 Future perspectives

In the past, drugs were designed with almost total naïveté from the point of view of the underlying molecular mechanisms. More recently, considerable efforts have been made to gain an understanding of the diseases in molecular terms. The recent emergence of rational drug design has clearly revealed the critical importance of 3-D aspects in molecular recognition and discrimination processes. Recognition of these aspects has played a determinant role in bringing molecular modelling from its infancy to maturity. By considering molecules in three rather than in two dimensions, medicinal chemists have contributed to the acceleration of the entire process of pharmaceutical research. This perception is useful not only for small molecules, but also for very large macromolecules: two proteins can have very different primary sequences and yet possess overall 3-D functional similarities.

The above-mentioned progress was due to the move from 2-D to 3-D representation in the perception of molecular entities. More recently, it has become apparent that a new process has started and is refining the previous one by adding another dimension to the perspectives. The numerous efforts to characterize chemical fragments not merely by their 3-D atomic locations, but also on the basis of their corresponding contributions to local and global 3-D physicochemical properties show the nature of this new dimension. In this context, attempts to define a more general "pharmacophore language" based on a broader description of functional groups are noteworthy. For example, with a view to revealing functionally equivalent, but structurally different compounds, Greene et al. have proposed that the definition of chemical functions should be generalized [136]. They started to work on relevant structural properties such as hydrogen bonding capabilities, hydrophobicity, and charged groups.

The last decade has witnessed the development of useful approaches. However, they were essentially of an analytical nature: they were oriented towards the modelling of known candidate structures, studied to verify how well they conform to the desired requirements. The second generation has produced more creative methods whereby candidate new lead structures are now proposed by the computer.

Prediction of the binding constant of a given compound is still far beyond the scope of current computational techniques and theoretical simulation precision, largely because of the ubiquitous effects of water [137]. Our imperfect understanding of intermolecular interactions is, in current practice, compensated for by an efficient iterative scheme in which the creativity, ingenuity, and experience of the members of the research team are optimally combined. The new developments and achievements in the field would have appeared incredible just a few years ago. Major milestones have now been achieved, and future prospects in this rapidly evolving field look very promising. Current efforts are directed towards integrated methods with even higher levels of computer automation, rationalization, quantification, and, eventually, the design of useful novel molecules. The aim of this article has been to review and discuss existing approaches in the design of new lead structures. We have tried to present the important trends that have already taken place in their correct perspectives. The coverage of the literature is far from being exhaustive, and for that we express our apologies to colleagues whose excellent contributions in the area have not been mentioned.

References

1 Cohen N.C.: Rational Drug Design and Molecular Modeling. Drug Future *10*, 311–328 (1985).
2 Asp, distributed by Oxford Molecular Ltd., Oxford, England, U.K.
3 Sanz F., Manaut, F., Rodriguez, J., Lozoya, E. and Lopez-de-Brinas, E.: MEPSIM: A Computational Package for Analysis and Comparison of Molecular Electrostatic Potentials. J. Comput.-Aided Mol. Des. *7*, 337–347 (1993).
4 (a) Van Geerestein V.J., Perry N.C., Grootenhuis P.D.J. and Haasnot C.A.G.: 3D Database Searching on the Basis of Ligand Shape Using the SPERM prototype Method. Tetrahedron Comput. Methodol. *3*, 595–613 (1990). (b) Mellema J.R. and Van Geerestein V.J.: 3-D Shape Similarity Ranking in Combination with Conformationally Flexible Pharmacophore Searching. 12th Annual Conference of the Molecular Graphics Society, Interlaken, Switzerland, June 7–11, 1993; Abstract O29.
5 Hermann R.B. and Herron D.K.: OVID and SUPER: Two Overlap Programs for Drug Design. J. Comput.-Aided Mol. Des. *5*, 511–524 (1991).
6 Kato Y., Itai A. and Iitaka, Y.: A Novel Method for Superimposing Molecules and Receptor Mapping. Tetrahedron *43*, 5229–52236 (1987).
7 Kato Y., Inoue A., Yamada M., Tomioka N. and Itai A.: Automatic Superposition of Drug Molecules Based on their Common Receptor Site. J. Comput.-Aided Mol. Des. *6*, 475–486 (1992).
8 (a) Martin Y.C., Bures M.G., Danaher E.A., DeLazzer J., Lico I.; Pavlik P.A.: A Fast New Approach to Pharmacophore Mapping and its Application to Dopaminergic and Benzodiazepine Agonists. J. Comput.-Aided Mol. Des. *7*, 83–102 (1993). (b) DISCO, distributed by Tripos Associates, St. Louis, MO, USA.
9 (a) Cramer R.D. III, Patterson D.E. and Bunce J.D.: Comparative Molecular Field Analysis (CoMFA). 1. Effect of Shape on Binding of Steroids to Carrier Proteins. J. Amer. Chem. Soc. 110, 5959–5967 (1988). Kaminski J.J.: Computer Assisted Drug Design and Selection. Adv. Drug Design Reviews *14*, 331–337 (1994). c) CoMFA, distributed by Tripos Associates, St. Louis, MO, USA.
10 (a) Nakamura H., Komatsu K., Nakagaura S. and Umayama H.: Visualization of Electrostatic Recognition by Enzymes for their Ligands and Cofactors. J. Mol. Graphics *3*, 2–11 (1985). (b) BIOCES, distributed by Kissei-Comtec, Matsumoto-City, Japan.
11 Chan S.L., Chau P.-L. and Goodmann J.M.: Ligand Atom Partial Charges Assignment for Complementarity Electrostatic Potentials. J. Comput.-Aided Mol. Des. *6*, 461–474 (1992).
12 Kellog, G.E. and Abraham, D.J.: KEY, LOCK, and LOCKSMITH: Complementarity Hydropathic Map Predictions of Drug Structure from a Known Receptor-Receptor Structure from Known Drugs. J. Mol. Graphics *10*, 212–217 (1992).
13 Kearsley S.K. and Smith G.M.: An Alternative Method for the Alignment of Molecular Structures: Maximizing Electrostatic and Steric Overlap. Tetrahedron Comput. Methodol. *3*, 615–633 (1990).
14 Sprague P.W.: CATALYST: A Computer-Aided Drud Design System Specially Designed for Medicinal Chemists. In: Recent Advances in Chemical Information, Proceedings of the 1991 Chemical Information Conference (Coller H., ed.), pp. 107–111, Royal Society of Chemistry, London (1991). (b) Catalyst, distributed by Molecular Simulations, Burlington, MA, USA.

15 (a) Golender V. and Vorpagel E.R.: Computer-Assisted Pharmacophore Identification. In: 3D QSAR in Drug Design – Theory, Methods and Applications (Kubinyi H., ed.), pp. 137–149, ESCOM, Leiden (1993). (b) Apex-3D, distributed by Biosym Technologies, Inc., CA, USA.
16 Furet P., Sele A. and Cohen N.C.: 3D Molecular Lipophilicity Potential Profiles: A New Tool in Molecular Modeling. J. Mol. Graphics *6*, 182–200 (1988).
17 (a) Vedani A., Zbinden P. and Snyder J.P.: Pseudoreceptor Modeling: A New Concept for the Three-Dimensional Construction of Receptor Binding Sites. J. Recept. Res. *13*, 163–177 (1993). (b) Vedani A., Zbinden P., Snyder J.P. and Greenidge P.: Pseudoreceptor Modeling: The Construction of Three-Dimensional Receptor Surrogates. J. Amer. Chem. Soc. (submitted). (c) Yak, distributed by Swiss Institute for Alternatives to Animal Testing (SIAT), Basel, Switzerland.
18 Marshall G.R., Barry C.D., Bosshard H.E., Dammkoehler R.A. and Dunn D.A.: The Conformational Parameter in Drug Design: The Active Analog Approach. In: Computer-Assisted Drug Design (Olson E.C. and Christoffersen R.E., eds.), pp. 205–226, ACS Symposium Series 112; American Chemical Society, Washington, DC (1979).
19 (a) Sheridan R.P., Nilakantan R., Dixon J.S. and Venkataraghavan R.: The Ensemble Approach to Distance Geometry: Application to the Nicotinic Pharmacophore. J. Med. Chem. *29*, 899–906 (1986). (b) Crippen G.M.: Distance Geometry Approach to Rationalizing Binding Data. J. Med. Chem. *22*, 988–997 (1979). (c) DGEOM: distance geometry, distributed by Quantum Chemistry Program Exchange, program number 590, Department of Chemistry, Indiana University, Bloomington, Indiana, USA.
20 Labanowski J., Motoc I., Naylor C.B., Mayer D. and Dammkoehler R.A.: Three-Dimensional Quantitative Structure-Activity Relationships. 2. Conformational Mimicry and Topological Similarity of Flexible Molecules. Quant. Struct.-Act. Relat. *5*, 138–152 (1986).
21 Struthers R.S., Rivier J. and Hagler A.T.: Design of Peptide Analogs. In: Conformationally Based Drug Design: Peptides and Nucleic Acids as Templates or Targets (Vida J.A. and Gordon M., eds.), pp. 239–261, ACS Symposium Series 251; American Chemical Society, Washington, DC (1984).
22 Cohen N.C.: Beyond the 2-D Chemical Structure. In: Computer Assisted Drug Design (Olson E.C. and Christoffersen R.E., eds.), pp. 371–381, ACS Symposium Series 112; American Chemical Society, Washington, DC (1979).
23 Crippen G.M.: Quantitative Structure-Activity Realtionships by Distance Geometry: Systematic Analysis of Dehydrofolate Reductase Inhibitors. J. Med. Chem. *23*, 599–606 (1980).
24 Danziger D.J. and Dean P.M.: The Search for Functional Correspondences in Molecular Structure Between Two Dissimilar Molecules. J. Theor. Biol. *116*, 215–224 (1985).
25 Dean P.M. and Chau P.L.: Molecular Recognition: Optimized Searching Through Rotational 3-Space for Pattern Matches on Molecular Surfaces. J. Mol. Graphics *5*, 152–158 (1987).
26 Navasivayan S. and Dean P.M.: Statistical Methods for Surface Pattern-Matching Between Dissimilar Molecules: Electrostatic Potentials and Accessible Surfaces. J. Mol. Graphics *4*, 46–50 (1986).
27 Dean P.M., Callow P. and Chau P.L.: Molecular Recognition: Blind Searching for Regions of Strong Structural Match on the Surfaces of Two Dissimilar Molecules. J. Mol. Graphics *6*, 28–34 (1988).

28 (a) Hopfinger A.J.: A QSAR Investigation of Dihydrofolate Reductase Inhibition by Baker Triazines Based Upon Molecular Shape Analysis. J. Amer. Chem. Soc. *102*, 7196–7206 (1980). (b) Hopfinger A.J.: Inhibition of Dehydrofolate Reductase; Structure-Activity Correlation of 2,4 Diamino-5-benzylpyramidines Based Upon Molecular Shape Analysis. J. Med. Chem. *24*, 818–822 (1981). (c) Hopfinger A.J.: Theory and Application o Molecular Potential Energy Fields in Molecular Shape Analysis: A Quantitative Structure-Activity Relationship Study of 2,4-Diamino-5-benzylpyrimidines. J. Med. Chem. *26*, 990–996 (1983). (d) Hopfinger A.J.: Computer Assisted Drug Design. J. Med. Chem. *28*, 1133–1139 (1985).

29 Itai A., Kato Y., Tomioka N., Iitaka Y., Endo Y., Hasegawa M., Shudo K., Fujiki H. and Sakai S.I.: A Receptor Model for Tumor Promoters: Rational Superposition of Teleocidines and Phorbol Esters. Proc. Natl. Acad. Sci. U.S.A. *85*, 3688–3692 (1988).

30 DePriest S.A., Mayer D.M., Naylor C.B. and Marshall G.R.: 3D-QSAR of Angiotensin-Converting Enzyme and Thermolysin Inhibitors: A Comparison of CoMFA Models Based on Deduced and Experimentally Determined Active Site Geometries. J. Amer. Chem. Soc. *115*, 5372–5384 (1993).

31 Prendergast K., Adams K., Greenlee W.J., Nachbar R.B., Patchett A.A. and Underwood D.J.: Derivation of a 3D Pharmacophore Model for the Angiotensin-II Site One Receptor. J. Comput.-Aided Mol. Des. *8*, 491–512 (1994).

32 Brint A.T. and Willet P.: Pharmacophore Pattern Matching In Files of 3D Chemical Structures: Comparison of Geometric Searching Algorithms. J. Mol. Graphics *5*, 49–56 (1987).

33 (a) Allen F.H., Bellard S., Brice M.D., Cartwright B.A., Doubleday A., Higgs H., Hummelink T., Hummelink-Peters B.G., Kennard O., Motherwell W.D.S., Rogers J.R. and Watson D.G.: The Cambridge Crystallographic Data Centre: Computer-Based Search, Retrieval, Analysis and Display of Information. Acta Cryst. B*35*, 2331–2339 (1979). (b) Allen F.H., Davies J.E., Galloy J.J., Johnson O., Kennard O., Macrae C.F., Mitchell E.M., Mitchell G.F., Smith J.M. and Watson D.G.: The Development of Versions 3 and 4 of the Cambridge Structural Database System. J. Chem. Inf. Comput. Sci. *31*, 187–204 (1991). (d) Cambridge Structural Database, distributed by Cambridge Crystallographic Data Centre, Cambridge, England, U.K.

34 Chapman and Hall Dictionary of Chemicals; available from Chapman & Hall, London, England, U.K., and Chemical Design Ltd., Oxford, England, U.K.

35 CAST-3D, distributed by Chemical Abstract Services, Columbus, OH, USA.

36 Fisanick W., Cross K.P., Forman J.C. and Rusinko A.I.: Experimental System for Similarity and 3D Searching of CAS registry Substances. 1. 3D Substracture Searching. J. Chem. Inf. Comput. Sci. *33*, 548–559 (1993). (b) CAS-RF, distributed by Chemical Abstract Services, Columbus, OH, USA.

37 FCD-3D, distributed by Molecular Design Ltd., San Leandro, CA, USA.

38 Compounds described in the multivolume textbook "Comprehensive Medicinal Chemistry" available form Molecular Design Ltd., San Leandro, CA, USA.

39 MDDR-3D, distributed by Molecular Design Ltd., San Leandro, CA, USA.

40 (a) Murral N.W. and Davies E.K.: Conformational Freedom in 3D Databases. 1. Techniques. J. Chem. Inf. Comput. Sci. *30*, 312–316 (1990). (b) ChemDBS, distributed by Chemical Design Ltd., Oxford, England, U.K.

41 UNITY, distributed by Tripos Associates, St. Louis, MO, USA.

42 POMONA, distributed by Daylight Chemical Information Systems, Irvine, CA, USA.

43 Bartlett P. A., Lauri G. and Weiss, G.: CAVEAT, ILIAD & TRIAD: 3D Searching for Molecule Design. 12th Annual Conference of the Molecular Graphics Society, Interlaken, Switzerland, June 7–11, 1993; Abstract O32.

44 Nordlander J.E., Bond A.F. IV and Bader M.: ATCOOR: A Program for Calculation and Utilization of Molecular Atomic Coordinates from Bond Parameters. Comp. Chem. *9*, 209–235 (1985).

45 (a) Rusinko A., Sheridan R.P., Nilakantan R., Haraki K.S., Bauman N., Venkataraghavan R.: Using CONCORD To Construct a Large Database of Three-Dimensional Coordinates from Connection Tables. J. Chem. Inf. Comput. Sci. *29*, 251–255 (1989). (b) CONCORD, distributed by Tripos Associates, St. Louis, MO, USA.

46 Gordeeva E.V., Katrizky A.R., Shcherbulchin V.V. and S Z.N.: Rapid Conversion of Molecular Graphs to Three-Dimensional Representations Using the MOLGEO Program. J. Chem. Inf. Comput. Sci. *33*, 102–111 (1993).

47 (a) Wipke W.T. and Hahn M.A.: Analogy and Intelligence in Model Building. In: Artificial Intelligence Applications in Chemistry (Pierce T.H. and Hohne B.A., eds.), pp. 136–146, ACS Symposium Series 306; American Chemical Society, Washington, DC (1986). (b) Wipke W.T. and Hahn M.A.: AIMB: Analogy and Intelligence in Model Building. System Description and Performance Characteristics. Tetrahedron Comput. Methodol. *1*, 141–167 (1988).

48 (a) Leach A.R. and Smellie A.S.: A Combined Model-Building and Distance Geometry Approach to Automated Conformational Analysis and Search. J. Chem. Inf. Comput. Sci. *32*, 379–385 (1992). (b) Leach A.R. and Prout K.: Automated Conformational Analysis: Directed Conformational Search Using the A* Algorithm. J. Comput. Chem. *11*, 1193–1205 (1990). (c) Cobra, distributed by Oxford Molecular Ltd., Oxford, England.

49 Dolata D.P., Leach A.R. and Prout K.: WIZARD: AI in Conformational Analysis. J. Comput.-Aided Mol. Des. *1*, 73–85 (1987).

50 Gasteiger J., Rudolph C. and Sadowski J.: Automatic Generation of 3D-Atomic Coordinates for Organic Molecules. Tetrahedron Comput. Methodol. *3*, 537–547 (1990).

51 Chem-X, distributed by Chemical Design Ltd., Oxford, England, U.K.

52 ALCOGEN, distributed by Chemical Concepts, Weinheim, Germany.

53 Cohen N.C., Colin P. and Lemoine G.: SCRIPT: Interactive Molecular Geometrical Treatments on the Basis of the Computer-Drawn Chemical Formula. Tetrahedron *37*, 1711–1721 (1981).

54 InsightII, distributed by Biosym Technologies Inc., San Diego, CA, USA.

55 Ho C.M.W. and Marshall G.R.: DBMAKER: A Set of Programs to Generate Three-Dimensional Databases upon User-Specified Criteria. J. Comput.-Aided Mol. Des. *9*, 65–86 (1995).

56 Kuntz I.D. and Crippen G.M.: EMBED, Department of Pharmaceutical Chemistry, University of California, San Francisco, San Francisco CA, USA.

57 Clark D.E., Willet P. and Kenny P.W.: Pharmacophoric Pattern Matching in Files of Three-Dimensional Chemical Structures: Use of Bounded DIstance Matrices for the Representation and Searching of Conformationally Flexible Molecules. J. Mol. Graphics *10*, 194–204 (1992).

58 (a) Wang S., Zaharevitz D.W., Sharma R., Marquez V.E., Lewin N.E., Du L., Blumberg P.M. and Milne G.W.A.: The Discovery of Novel, Structurally Diverse Protein Kinase C Agonists through Computer 3D-Database Search. Molecular Modeling Studies. J. Med. Chem. *37*, 4479–4489 (1994). (b) Wender P.A. and Cribbs C.M.:

Computer Assisted Molecular Design Related to the Protein Kinase C Receptor. Advances in Medicinal Chemistry *1*, 1–53 (1992).
59 Milne G.W.A., Nicklaus M.C., Wang S. and Zaharevitz D.W.: The NCI Drug Information System 3D Database. J. Chem. Inf. Comput. Sci. *34*, 1219–1224 (1994).
60 Inoue A., Kanazawa T., Takeda M., Tomioka N. and Itai A.: unpublished.
61 Tschinke V. and Cohen N.C.: The NEWLEAD Program: A New Method for the Design of Candidate Structures from Pharmacophoric Hypotheses. J. Med. Chem. *36*, 3863–3870 (1993).
62 (a) Bartlett P.A., Shea J.T., Telfer S.J. and Waterman S.: CAVEAT: A Program to Facilitate the Structure-Derived Design of Biologically Active Molecules. Spec. Publ.-R. Soc. Chem. 78 Molecular Recognition in Chemical and Biological Problems (Roberts S.M. ed.), 182–196 (1989). (b) CAVEAT, distributed by Molecular Simulations Inc., Burlington, USA.
63 Moock T.E., Christie B. and Henry D.: MACCS3D: A New Database System for Three-Dimensional Molecular Models. In: Chemical Information Systems: Beyond the Structure Diagram (Bawden D. and Mitchell E.M., eds.), pp. 42–49, Ellis Horwood, Chichester (1990).
64 (a) Moock T.E., Henry D.R., Ozkabak A.G. and Alamgir M.: Conformational Searching in ISIS/3D Databases. J. Chem. Inf. Comput. Sci. *34*, 184–189 (1994). (a) Isis, distributed by Molecular Design Ltd., San Leandro, CA, USA.
65 Sheridan R.P., Nilakantan R., Rusinko A., Bauman N., Haraki K.S. and Venkataraghavan R.: 3DSEARCH: A System for Three-Dimensional Substructure Searching. J. Chem. Inf. Comput. Sci. *29*, 255–260 (1989).
66 Iditis, distributed by Oxford Molecular, Oxford, England, U.K.
67 (a) Van Drie J.H., Weiniger D. and Martin Y.C.: ALADDIN: An Integrated Tool for Computer-Assisted Molecular Design and Pharmacophore Recognition from Geometric, Steric, and Substructure Search of 3D Molecular Structures. J. Comput.-Aided Mol. Des. *3*, 225–251 (1989). (b) ALADDIN, distributed by Daylight Chemical Information Systems, Irvine, CA, USA.
68 Martin Y.C., Danaher E.B., May C.S. and Weininger D.: MENTHOR, A Database System For The Storage and Retrieval of Three-Dimensional Molecular Structures in Associated Data Searchable by Substructural, Biologic, Physical, or Geometric Properties. J. Comput.-Aided Mol. Des. *2*, 15–29 (1988).
69 LEAPFROG, distributed by Tripos Associates, St. Louis, MO, USA.
70 Quest3D, VISTA, distributed by Cambridge Crystallographic Data Centre, Cambridge, England, U.K.
71 Bladon P.: THREEDOM: A Program for Three-Dimensional Database Searching. QCPE Bullettin *14*(3), 48 (1994).
72 Böhm H.-J.: On the Use of LUDI to Search the Fine Chemical Directory for Ligands of Proteins of Known three-Dimensional Structure. J. Comput.-Aided Mol. Des. *8*, 623–632 (1994).
73 (a) DesJarlais R.L., Sheridan R.P., Dixon J.S., Kuntz I.D. and Venkataraghavan R.: Docking Flexible Ligands to Macromolecular Receptors by Molecular Shape. J. Med. Chem. *29*, 2149–2153 (1986). (b) DesJarlais R.L., Sheridan R.P., Seibel G.L., Dixon J.S., Kuntz I.D. and Venkataraghavan R.: Using Shape Complementarity as an Initial Screen in Designing Ligands for a Receptor Binding Site of Known Three-Dimensional Structure. J. Med. Chem. *31*, 722–729 (1988). (c) DesJarlais R.L., Seibel G.L., Kuntz I.D., Furth P.S., Alvarez J.C., Ortiz de Montellano P.R., DeCamp D.L. and Craik C.S.: Structure-Based Design of Non-Peptidic Inhibitors Specific for the

Human Immunodeficiency Virus 1 Protease. Proc Natl Acad Sci USA 87, 6644–6648 (1990). (d) Meng E.C., Shoichet B.K. and Kuntz I.D.: Automated Docking with Grid-Based Energy Evaluation. J. Comput. Chem. *13*, 505–524 (1992).

74 Gillet V., Johnson A.P., Mata P., Sike S. and William P.: SPROUT: A Program For Structure Generation. J. Comput.-Aided Mol. Des. *7*, 127–153 (1993).

75 (a) Eisen M.B., Wiley D.C., Karplus M. and Hubbard R.E.: HOOK: A Program for Finding Novel Molecular Architectures That Satisfy the Chemical and Steric Requirements of a Macromolecule Binding Site. Proteins *19*, 199–221 (1994). (b) HOOK, distributed by Molecular Simulations, Burlington, MA, USA.

76 (a) Ho C.M.W. and Marshall G.R.: SPLICE: A Program to Assemble Partial Query Solutions from Three-Dimensional Database Searches into Novel Ligands. J. Comput.-Aided Mol. Des. *7*, 623–647 (1993). (b) SPLICE, distributed by Center for Molecular Design, Washington University, St. Louis, MO, USA.

77 Leach A.R. and Lewis R.A.: A Ring-Bracing Approach to Computer-Assisted Ligand Design. J. Comput. Chem. *15*, 233–240 (1994).

78 Dixon J.S.: Computer-Aided Drug Design: Getting the Best Results. TIBTECH *10*, 357–363 (1992).

79 Stewart, K.D., Bentley, J.A. and Cory, M.: DOCKing Ligands into Receptors: The Test Case of a-Chymotrypsin. Tetrahedron Comput. Methodol. *3*, 713–722 (1990).

80 Rose J.R. and Craik C.S.: Structure-Assisted Design of Nonpeptide Human Immunodeficiency Virus-1 Protease Inhibitors. Am. J. Respir. Critical Care Med. *150*, No. 6, Pt. 2, S176–S182 (1994).

81 Grootenhuis P.D.J., Roe D.C., Kollman P.A. and Kuntz I.W.: Finding Potential DNA-Binding compounds by using Molecular Shape. J. Comput.-Aided Mol. Des. *8*, 731–750 (1994).

82 Lam P.Y.S., Jadhav P.K., Eyermann C.J., Hodge C.N., Bacheler L.T., Meek J.L., Otto M.J., Rayner M.M., Wong Y.N., Chang C.-H., Weber P.C., Jackson D.A., Sharpe T.R. and Erickson-Viitanen S.: Rational Design of Potent, Bioavailable, Nonpeptide Cyclic Ureas as HIV Protease Inhibitors. Science *263*, 380–384 (1994).

83 Wlodawer A. and Erickson J.: Structure-Based Inhibitors of HIV-1 Protease. Annu. Rev. Biochem. *62*, 543–585 (1993).

84 (a) Goodsell D.S. and Olson A.J.: Automated Docking of Substrates to Proteins by Simulated Annealing. Proteins *8*, 195–202 (1990). (b) AUTODOCK is available to the public through its authors.

85 (a) Böhm H.J.: The Computer Program LUDI: A New Method for the De Novo Design of Enzyme Inhibitors. J. Comput.-Aided Mol. Des. *6*, 61–78 (1992). (b) Böhm H.J.: LUDI: Rule-based Automatic Design of New Substituents for Enzyme Inhibitor Leads. J. Comput.-Aided Mol. Des. *6*, 593–606 (1992). (c) LUDI, distributed by Biosym Technologies Inc., San Diego, CA, USA.

86 (a) Yamada M. and Itai A.: Development of an Efficient Automated Docking Method. Chem. Pharm. Bull. *6*, 1200–1202 (1993). (b) Yamada M. and Itai A.: Application and Evaluation of the Automated Docking Method. Chem. Pharm. Bull. *6*, 1203–1205 (1993).

87 Mitzutani Y. and Itai A.: unpublished.

88 (a) Ho C.M.W. and Marshall G.R.: FOUNDATION: A Program to Retrieve all Possible Structures Containing a User-Defined Minimum Number of Matching Query Elements from Three-Dimensional Databases. J. Comput.-Aided Mol. Des. *7*, 3–22 (1993). (b) FOUNDATION, distributed by Center for Molecular Design, Washington University, St. Louis, MO, USA.

89 (a) Nishibata Y. and Itai A.: Automatic Creation of Drug Candidate Structures Based on Receptor Structure. Starting Point for Artificial Lead Generation. Tetrahedron *47*, 8985–8990 (1991). (b) Nishibata Y. and Itai A.: Confirmation of Usefulness of a Structure Construction Program Based on Three-Dimensional Receptor Structure for Rational Lead Generation. J. Med. Chem. *36*, 2921–2928 (1993). (c) LEGEND, distributed by Molecular Simulations Inc., Burlington, USA.

90 Moon J.B. and Howe W.J.: Computer Design of Bioactive Molecules: A Method for Receptor-Based de Novo Ligand Design. Proteins *11*, 314–328 (1991).

91 Bohacek R.S. and McMartin C.: Multiple Highly Diverse Structures Complementarity to Enzyme Binding Sites: Results of Extensive Application of a de Novo Design Method Incorporating Combinatorial Growth. J. Amer. Chem. Soc. *116*, 5560–5571 (1994).

92 Pearlman D.A and Murcko M.A.: CONCEPTS: New Dynamic Algorithm for De Novo Drug Suggestion. J. Comput. Chem. *14*, 1184–1193 (1993).

93 Gehlhaar D.K., Moerder K.E., Zichi D., Sherman C.J., Ogden R.C. and Freer S.: De Novo Design of Enzyme Inhibitors by Monte Carlo Ligand Generation. J. Med. Chem. *38*, 466–472 (1995).

94 Lawrence M.C. and Davis P.C.: CLIX: A Search Algorithm for Finding Novel Ligands Capable of Binding Proteins of Known Three-Dimensional Structure. Proteins *12*, 31–41 (1992).

95 (a) Rotstein S.H. and Murcko M.A.: GroupBuild: A Fragment-Based Method For De Novo Drug Design. J. Med. Chem. *36*, 1700–1710 (1993). (b) GroupBuild, distributed by Molecular Simulations Inc., Burlington, USA.

96 Rotstein S.H. and Murcko M.A.: GenStar: A Method For De Novo Drug Design. J. Comput.-Aided Mol. Des. *7*, 23–43 (1993).

97 Gund T.: Molecular Modeling of Small Molecules; Chapter 3, Guidebook on Molecular Modeling in Drug Design, (Cohen N.C. Ed.), Academic Press, (to be published).

98 Kuyper L.F., Roth B., Baccanari D.P., Ferone R., Beddell C.R., Champness J.N., Stammers D.K., Dann J.G., Norrington F.E.A., Baker D.J., and Goodford P.J.: Receptor-Based Design of Dihydrofolate Reductase Inhibitors: Comparison of Crystallographically Determined Enzyme Binding with Enzyme Affinity in a Series of Carboxy-Substituted Trimethoprim Analogues. J. Med. Chem. *25*, 1120–1122 (1982). (b) Kuyper L.F., Roth B., Baccanari D.P., Ferone R., Beddell C.R., Champness J.N., Stammers D.K., Dann J.G., Norrington F.E.A., Baker D.J. and Goodford P.J.: Receptor-Bound Design of Dihydrofolate Reductase Inhibitors: Comparison of Crystallographically Determined Enzyme Binding with Enzyme Affinity in a Series of Carboxy-Substituted Analogues. J. Med. Chem. *28*, 303–311 (1985). (c) Roth B.: Design of Dihydrofolate Reductase Inhibitors from X-ray Crystal Structures. Federation Proceedings *45*, 2765–2772 (1986).

99 (a) Vara Prasad J.V.N., Para K.S., Lunney E.A., Ortwine D.F., Dunbar Jr. J.B., Ferguson D., Tummino P.J., Hupe D., Tait B.D., Domagala J.M., Humblet C., Bhat T.N., Liu B., Guerin D.M.A., Baldwin E.T., Erickson J.W. and Sawyer T.K.: Novel Series of Achiral Low Molecular Weight, and Potent Hiv-1 Protease Inhibitors. J. Am. Chem. Soc. *116*, 6989–6990 (1994). (b) Thaisrivongs S., Tomich P.K., Watenpaugh K.D., Chong K.-T., Howe W.J., Yang C.-P., Strohbach J.W., Turner S.R., McGrath J.P., Bohanon M.J., Lynn J,C., Mulichak A.M., Spinelli P.A., Hinshaw R.R., Pagano P.J., Moon J.B., Ruwart M.J., Wilkinson K.F., Rush B.D., Zipp G.L., Dalga R.J., Schwende F.J., Howard G.M., Padbury G.E., Toth L.N., Zhao Z., Koeplinger K.A., Kakuk T.J., Cole S.L., Zaya R.M., Piper R.C. and Jeffrey P.: Structure-Based

Design of HIV Protease Inhibitors: 4-Hydroxycoumarins and 4-Hydroxy-2-pyrones as Non-peptidic Inhibitors. J. Med. Chem. *37*, 3200–3204 (1994). (c) Lunney E.A., Hagen S.E., Domagala J.M., Humblet C., Kosinski J., Tait B.D., Warmus J.S., Wilson M., Ferguson D., Hupe D., Tummino P.J., Baldwin E.T., Bhat T.N., Liu B. and Erickson J.W.: A Novel Nonpeptide HIV-1 Protease Inhibitor: Elucidation of the Binding Mode and its Application in the Design of Related Analogs. J. Med. Chem. *37*, 2664–2677 (1994).

100 (a) Bhagwat S.S., Gude C., Cohen D.S., Lee W., Furness P. and Clarke F.H.: Thromboxane Receptor Antagonism Combined with Thromboxane Synthase Inhibition. 1.(+/–)(3-Pyridinylbicycloheptyl) alkanoic Acids. J. Med. Chem. *34*, 1790–1797 (1991). (b) Ezumi K., Yamakawa M. and Narisada M.: Computer-Aided Molecular Modeling of a Thromboxane Receptor Antagonist S-145 and Its Related Compounds. J. Med. Chem. *33*, 1117–1122 (1990).

101 Tapparelli C., Metternich R., Ehrhardt C. and Cook N.S.: Synthetic Low-Molecular Weight Thrombin Inhibitors: Molecular Design and Pharmacological Profile. TIPS *14*, 366–376 (1993).

102 (a) Appelt K., Bacquet R.J. Bartlett C.A.., Booth C.L.J., Freer S.T., Fuhry M.A.M., Gehring M.R., Herrmann S.M., Howland E.F., Janson C.A., Jones T.R., Kan C.-C., Kathardekar V., Lewis K.K., Marzoni G.P., Matthews D.A., Mohr C., Moomaw E.W., Morse C.A., Oatley S.J., Ogden R.C., Reddy M.R., Reich S.H., Schoettlin W.S., Smith W.W., Varney M.D., Villafranca J.E., Ward R.W., Webber S., Webber S.E., Welsh K.M. and White J.: Design of Enzyme Inhibitors Using Iterative Protein Crystallographic Analysis. J. Med. Chem. *34*, 1925–1934 (1991). (b) Webber S.E., Bleckman T.M., Attard J., Deal J.G., Kathardekar V., Welsh K.M., Webber S., Janson C.A., Matthews D.A., Smith W.W., Freer S.T., Jordan S.R., Bacquet R.J., Howland E.F., Booth C.L.J., Ward R.W., Hermann S.M., White J., Morse C.A., Hilliard J.A. and Bartlett C.A.: Design of Thymidylate Synthase Inhibitors Using Protein Crystal Structures: The Synthesis and Biological Evaluation of a Novel Class of 5-Substituted Quinazolinones. J. Med. Chem. *36*, 733–746 (1993). (c) Reich S.H., Nguyen D., Varney M.D., Marzoni G.F., Welsh K.M., Webber S., Bartlett C.A., Booth C.L.J., Herrmann S.M., Howland E.F., Morse C.A., Ward R.W. and White J.: Novel Angular Tricyclic Inhibitors of Thymidylate Synthase. Med. Chem. Res *2*, 195–207 (1992).

103 (a) Olson G.L., Cheung H.-C., Morgan K.D., Blount J.F., Todaro L., and Berger L.: A Dopamine Receptor model and Its Applications in the Design of a New Class of Rigid Pyrrolo[2,3-g]isoquinoline Antipsychotics. J. Med. Chem. *24*, 1026–1034 (1991) (b) Martin Y.C.: 3D Database Searching in Drug Design. J. Med. Chem. *35*, 2145–2154 (1992).

104 (a) Ealick S.E., Babu Y.S., Bugg C.E., Erion M.D., Guida W.C., Montgomery J.A. and Secrist III J.A.: Application of Crystallographic and Modeling Methods in the Design of Purine Nucleoside Phosphorylase Inhibitors. Proc. Natl. Acad. Sci. U.S.A. *88*, 11540–11544 (1991). (b) Guida W.C., Elliott R.E., Thomas H.J., Secrist III J.A., Babu Y.S., Bugg C.E., Erion M.D., Ealick S.E. and Montgomery J.A.: Structure-Based Design of Inhibitors of Purine Nucleoside Phosphorylase. 4. A Study of Phosphate Mimics. J. Med. Chem. *37*, 1109–1114 (1994) and references cited.

105 Baldwin J.J., Ponticello G.S., Anderson P.S., Christy M.E., Murcko, M.A., Randall W.C., Schwam H., Sugrue M.F., Springer J.P., Gautheron P., Grove J., Mallorga P., Viader M.-P., McKeever B.M. and Navia M.A.: Novel Topically Active Carbonic Anhydrase Inhibitors fot the Treatment of Glaucoma. J. Med. Chem. *32*, 2510–2513 (1989).

106 Firestone R.A., Barker P.L., Pisano J.M., Ashe B.M., and Dahlgren M.E.: Monocyclic Beta-Lactam Inhibitors of Human Leukocyte Elastase. Tetrahedron *46*, 2255–2262 (1990).

107 (a) Duncia J.V., Carini D.J., Chiu A.T., Johnson A.L., Price W.A., Wong P.C., Wexler R.R. and Timmermans P.B.M.W.M.: The Discovery of DuP-753, a Potent Orally Active Nonpeptide Angiotensin II Antagonist. Med. Res. Rev. *12*, 149–191 (1992). (b) Bioorganic & Medicinal Chemistry Letters 4 (1), (1994): Special Symposia Issue on: Recent Advances in the Design of Angiotensin II Receptor Antagonists, (W.J. Greenlee and N.B. Mantlo Ed.), Symposia-In-Print Number 9 (1994). (c) DERWENT, Global Research Trends on Angiotensin II Receptor Antagonists, Special Edition, August 1993.

108 Schilling W., Bittiger H., Brugger F., Criscione L., Hauser K., Ofner S., Olpe H.-R., Vassout A. and Veenstra S.: Approaches Towards the Design and Synthesis of Nonpeptidic Substance-P Antagonists. In: Perspectives in Medicinal Chemistry (B. Testa, E. Kyburz, W. Fuhrer and R. Giger Eds.), pp. 207–220, Verlag Helvetica Chimica Acta, Basel (1993).

109 (a) Williams P.D., Perlow D.S., Payne L.S., Holloway M.K., Siegl P.K.S., Schorn T.W., Lynch R.J., Doyle J.J., Strouse J.F., Vlasuk G.P., Hoogsteen K., Springer J.P., Bush B.L., Halgren T.A., Richards A.D., Kay J. and Veber D.F.: Renin Inhibitors Containing Conformationally Restricted P1-P1' Dipeptide Mimetics. J. Med. Chem. *34*, 887–900 (1991). (b) Lunney E.A., Hamilton H.W., Hodges J.C., Kaltenbronn J.S., Repine J.T., Badasso M., Cooper J.B., Dealwis C., Wallace B.A., Lowter W.T., Dunn B.M. and Humblet C.: Analyses of Ligand Binding in Five Endothiapepsin Crystal Complexes and their Use in the Design and Evaluation of Novel Renin Inhibitors. J. Med. Chem. *36*, 3809–3820 (1993). (c) Wittenberger S.J., Baker W.R., Donner B.G. and Hutchins C.W.: The Design and Synthesis of Cyclic Renin Inhibitors. Tetrahedron Lett. *32*, 7655–7658 (1991). (d) de Laszlo S.E., Bush B.L., Doyle J.J., Greenlee W.J., Hangauer D.G., Halgren T.A., Lynch R.J., Schorn T.W. and Siegl P.K.S.: Synthesis and Use of 3-Amino-4-phenyl-2- piperidones and 4-Amino-2-benzazepin-3-ones as Conformationally Restricted Phenylalanine Isosteres in renin Inhibitors. J. Med. Chem. *35*, 833–846 (1992). (e) Greenlee W.J.: Renin Inhibitors, Medicinal Research Reviews *10*, 173–236 (1990).

110 Ripka W.C., Sipio W.J. and Blaney J.M.: Molecular Modeling and Drug Design: Strategies in the Design and Synthesis of Phospholipase A2 Inhibitors. Lect. Heterocycl. Chem. *9*, S95 (1987).

111 Pisabarro M.T., Ortiz A.R., Palomer A., Cabre F., Garcia L., Wade R.C., Gago F., Mauleon D. and Carganico G.: Rational Modification of Human Synovial Fluid Phospholipase A2 Inhibitors. J. Med. Chem. *37*, 337–341 (1994).

112 Morgan B.P., Holland D.R., Matthews B.W. and Bartlett P.A. Structure- Based Design of an Inhibitor of the Zinc Peptidase Thermolysin J. Am. Chem. Soc. *116*, 3251–3260 (1994).

113 (a) Furet P., Batzl C., Bhatnagar A., Francotte E., Rihs G. and Lang M.: Aromatase Inhibitors: Synthesis, Biological Activity and Binding Mode of Azole-Type Compounds. J. Med. Chem. *36*, 1393–1400 (1993). (b) Lang M., Batzl C., Furet P., Haeusler A. and Bhatnagar A.: New Aromatase Inhibitors: Synthesis, Biological Activity and Molecular Modeling. In: Perspectives in Medicinal Chemistry (B. Testa, E. Kyburz, W. Fuhrer and R. Giger Eds.), pp. 87–97, Verlag Helvetica Chimica Acta, Basel (1993).

114 (a) Veale C.A., Bernstein P.R., Bryant C., Ceccarelli C., Damewood Jr. J.R. Earley R., Feeney S.W., Gomes B., Kosmider B.J., Steelman G.B., Thomas R.M., Vacek

E.P., Williams J.C., Wolanin D.J. and Woolson S.: Nonpeptidic Inhibitors of Human Leukocyte Elastase. 5. Design, Synthesis and X-ray Crystallography of a Series of Orally Active 5-Aminopyrimidin-6-one Containing Trifluoromethyl Ketones. J. Med. Chem. *38*, 98–108 (1995). (b) Edwards P.D., Meyer E.F., Vijayalakshmi J., Tuthill P.A., Andisik D.A., Gomes B. and Strimpler A.: Design, Synthesis and Kinetic Evaluation of a Unique Class of Elastase Inhibitors, the Peptidyl alfa-Ketbenzoxazoles, and the X-ray Crystal Structure of the Covalent Complex between Porcine Pancreatic Elastase and Ac-Ala-Pro-Val-2-Benzoxazole. J. Am. Chem. Soc. *114*, 1854–1863 (1992).

115 MacPherson L.J., Bayburt E.K., Capparelli, M.P., Bohacek R.S., Clarke F.H., Ghai R.D., Sakane Y., Berry C.J., Peppard J.V. and Trapani A.J.: Design and Synthesis of an Orally active Macrocyclic Neutral Endopeptidase 24.11 Inhibitor. J. Med. Chem. *36*, 3821–3828 (1993).

116 Ring C.S., Sun E., McKerrow J.H., Lee G.K., Rosenthal P.J., Kuntz I.D. and Cohen F.E.: Structure-Based inhibitor Design by Using Protein Models for the Development of Antiparasitic Agents. Proc. Natl. Acad. Sci. USA *90*, 3583–3587 (1993).

117 Smythe M.L. and von Itzstein M.: Design and Synthesis of a Biologically Active Antibody Mimic Based on an Antibody-Antigen Crystal Structure. J. Am. Chem. Soc. *116*, 2725–2733 (1994).

118 Alberg D.G. and Schreiber S.L.: Structure-Based Design of a Cyclophilin-Calcineurin Bridging Ligand. Science *262*, 248 (1993).

119 Von Itzstein M., Wu W.-Y., Kok G.B., Pegg M.P., Dyason J.C., Jin B., Phan T.V., Smythe M.L., White H.F., Oliver S.W., Colman P.M., Varghese J.N., Ryan D.M., Woods J.M., Bethell R.C., Hotham V.J., Cameron J.M and Penn C.R.: Rational Design of Potent Sialidase-Based Inhibitors of Influenza Virus Replication. Nature *363*, 418–423 (1993).

120 Holt D.A., Luengo J.I., Yamashita D.S., Oh H.-J., Konialian A.L., Yen H.-K., Rozamus L.W., Brandt M., Bossard M.J., Levy M.A., Eggleston D.S., Liang J., Schultz L.W., Stout T.J. and Clardy J.: Design, Synthesis and Kinetic Evaluation of High-Affinity FKBP Ligands and the X-ray Crystal Structures of Their Complexes with FKBP12. J. Am. Chem. Soc. *115*, 9925–9938 (1993).

121 Higginbottom M., Nolan W., O'Toole J., Ratcliffe G.S., Rees D.C. and Roberts E.: The Design and Synthesis of Kappa Opioid Ligands based on a binding Model for Kappa Agonists. Biorganic & Medicinal Chemistry Letters *3*, 841–846 (1993).

122 Schafer W., Friebe W.-G., Leinert H., Mertens A., Poll T., von der Saal W., Zilch H., Nuber B. and Ziegler M.L.: Non-Nucleoside Inhibitors of HIV-1 Reverse Transcriptase: Molecular Modeling and X-ray Structure Investigations. J. Med. Chem. *36*, 726–732 (1993).

123 Koga H., Ohta M., Sato H., Ishizawa T. and Nabata H.: Design of Potent K+ Channel Openers by Pharmacophore Model. Biorganic & Medicinal Chemistry *3*, 625–631 (1993).

124 (a) van der Bent A., Blommaert A.G.S., Melman C.T.M., Ijzerman A.P., van Wijngaarden I. and Soudijn W.: Hybrid Cholecystokinin-A Antagonists Based on Molecular Modeling of Lorglumide and L-364,718. J. Med. Chem. *35*, 1042–1049 (1992). (b) Freidinger R.M., Whitter W.L., Gould N.P., Holloway M.K., Chang R.S.L. and Lotti V.J.: Novel Glutamic Acid Derived Cholecystokinin Receptor Ligands. J. Med. Chem. *33*, 591–595 (1990).

125 N'Goka V., Schlewer G., Linget J.-M., Chambon J.-P. and Wermuth C.-J.: GABA-Uptake Inhibitors: Construction of a General Pharmacophore Model and Suc-

cessful Prediction of a New Representative. J. Med. Chem. *34*, 2547–2557 (1991).

126 Fryer R.I. and Gu Z.-Q.: The Rational Design and Synthesis of Haptens Having Specific Activity as Full Agonists or Full Antagonists at the Benzodiazepine Receptor. Life Sciences *47*, 833–840 (1990).

127 (a) Hibert M.F., Gittos M.W., Middlemiss D.N., Mir A. and Fozard J.R.: Graphics Computer-Aided Receptor Mapping as a Predictive Tool for Drug Design: Development of Potent, Selective, and Stereospecific Ligands for the 5-HT1A Receptor. J. Med. Chem. *31*, 1087–1093 (1988). (b) Griffith R.C., Gentile R.J., Robichaud R.C. and Frankenheim J.: Cis-1,3,4,6,7,11b-Hexahydro-2methyl-7phenyl-2H-pyrazino[2,1-a] isoquinoline: A New Atypical Antidepressant. J. Med. Chem. *27*, 995–1003 (1994).

128 Butera J., Bagli J., Doubleday W., Humber L., Treasurywala A., Loughney D., Sestanj K., Millen J. and Sredy J.: Computer- Assisted Design and Synthesis of Novel Aldose Reductase Inhibitors. J. Med. Chem. *32*, 757–765 (1989).

129 Wender P.A., Koehler K.F., Sharkey N.A., Dell'Aquila M.L. and Blumberg P.M.: Analysis of the Phorbol Ester Pharmacophore on Protein Kinase C as a Guide to the Rational Design of New Classes of Analogs. Proc. Natl. Acad. Sci. U.S.A. *83*, 4214–4218 (1986).

130 Rakhit S., Marciniak G., Leclerc G. and Schwartz J.: Computer Assisted Pharmacophore Search in a Series of Non Steroidal Cardiotonics. Eur.J. Med. Chem. Chim. Ther. *21*, 511–515 (1986).

131 For a recent review: Adang A.E.P., Hermkens P.H.H., Linders J.T.M., Ottenheijm H.C.J. and van Staveren C.J.: Case Histories of Peptidomimetics: Progression from Peptides to Drugs. Recl. Trav. Chim. Pays-Bas *113*, 63–78 (1994).

132 Goodford P.J.: A Computational Procedure for Determining Energetically Favourable Binding Sites on Biologically Important Macromolecules. J. Med. Chem. *28*, 849–857 (1985).

133 (a) Tomioka N., Itai A. and Iitaka Y.: A Method for Fast Energy Estimation and Visualization of Protein-Ligand Interaction. J. Comput.-Aided Mol. Des. *1*, 197–210 (1987). (b) Tomioka N. and Itai A.: GREEN: A Program Package for Docking Studies in Rational Drug Design. J. Comput.-Aided Mol. Des. *8*, 347–366 (1994).

134 Klapper I., Hagstrom R., Fine R., Sharp K. and Honig B.: Focusing of the Electrostatic Fields in the Active Site of Cu-Zn Superoxide Dismutase: Effects of Ionic Strength and Amino-Acid Modification. Proteins *1*, 47–59 (1986).

135 Böhm H.-J.: The Development of a Simple Empirical Scoring Function to Estimate the Binding Constant for a Protein-Ligand Complex of Known Three-Dimensional Structure. J. Comput.-Aided Mol. Des. *8*, 243–256 (1994).

136 Greene J., Kahn S., Savoy H., Sprague P. and Teig S.: Chemical Function Queries for 3D Database Search. J. Chem. Inf. Comput. Sci. *34*, 1297–1308 (1994).

137 Verlinde C.L.M.J. and Hol W.G.J.: Structure-Based Drug Design: Progress, Results and Challenges. Structure *2*, 577–587 (1994).

138 Ivanov J., Karabunarliev S. and Mekenyan O.: 3DGEN: A System for Exhaustive 3D Molecular Design Proceeding from Molecular Topology. J. Chem. Inf. Comput. Sci. *34*, 234–243 (1994).

139 Protein Data Bank, Quarterly Newsletter, Release 71, January 1995.

Progress in Drug Research, Vol. 45 (E. Jucker, Ed.)

Natriuretic hormones II

By Elaine J. Benaksas, E. David Murray, Jr., and William J. Wechter
Laboratory of Chemical Endocrinology, Loma Linda University,
Loma Linda, California 92350, USA

1 Introduction

Renal sodium metabolism, an important determinant of blood pressure, is regulated with great precision by a variety of endocrine, autocrine, and neuronal factors. Although these factors regulate sodium metabolism by affecting the rate of tubular sodium reabsorption, the molecular mechanisms by which they act are poorly understood. It has been proposed that the antidiuretic agents angiotensin II and norepinephrine and the diuretic agents dopamine and atrial natriuretic peptide (ANP) may achieve their effects through a common pathway that involves a bidirectionally regulated intracellular protein phosphorylation cascade. This in turn modulates the activity of renal tubular Na^+/K^+-ATPase [1]. An exaggerated natriuretic response to acute volume expansion by intravenous saline has been demonstrated in essential [2] as well as borderline hypertension [3]. The overall response to acute volume expansion by intravenous saline has been characterized by a complex humoral pattern which includes the acute suppression of the renin-angiotensin-aldosterone system [4]. Recent studies by Bullivant et al. [5] demonstrate that plasma levels of angiotensin II, prostaglandins, kinins, dopamine, ANP, adrenal hormones, or factors released by the renal nerves are unchanged by renal arterial saline infusion. Thus none of these is directly responsible for the saline induced natriuresis.

Using the classical methods of cross-circulation and isovolemic exchange transfusion of blood, the question of the actual humoral natriuretic stimulus by saline has been addressed [6]. These authors examined the changes in flow rate and pressure in the renal artery, concentration of plasma solutes, GFR and hydrostatic and colloid osmotic pressure, production of hormones, and changes in sodium and chloride concentration. This study concluded that renal arterial saline infusion activates a mechanism that increases sodium excretion by the infused kidney. There is a concurrent release of a natriuretic factor that could be transferred between animals by cross-circulation and passive transfer. Increased sodium concentration in renal arterial blood was the only stimulus found to produce this effect. Furthermore, the observed effects might be due to increased levels of a substance which inhibits sodium absorption or modulated by another factor.

Evidence generated since 1940 correlates increased plasma sodium chloride with a delayed remote indirect action resulting in the volume expansion-induced release of a Na^+, K^+-ATPase inhibitor [7]. This decreases sodium pump activity in the vascular smooth muscle cell, resulting in an increased intracellular sodium concentration followed by an increased intracellular calcium concentration and vasoconstriction. Temporal correlations between the changes in blood pressure and the changes in vascular sodium pump activity during development and reversal of reduced renal mass-saline induced hypertension in rats support the notion of an endogenous pump inhibitor [8].

It is well known that Na^+, K^+-ATPase activities are specifically inhibited by cardiac glycosides. The existence of a specific and conserved binding site for digitalis and the variety of pharmacological effects of these compounds raise the possibility of the existence of unknown endogenous digitalis-like compounds (EDLC), hormone or autocoid, which regulate the activity of the Na^+, K^+-ATPase through its binding site. However, a molecule binding to a single protein that acts as both its receptor and effector at the cell membrane, thereby directly affecting transmembrane ion flux, would be unusual for a hormone or autocoid. As an alternative hypothesis for the evolutionary conservation of the cardiac glycoside binding site, Kelly and Smith [9] suggest that its endogenous ligand may exist within the cell.

Recently, there has been a resurgence of interest in circulating inhibitors of the sodium pump [10]. One reason for this renewed interest is recent evidence linking circulating sodium pump inhibitors to hypertension in humans. In addition, the activity of EDLC's is believed to be increased in some disease states, including end-stage renal failure, active acromegaly, and experimental and essential hypertension [11]. These factors may or may not be the same as those postulated to promote natriuresis frequently associated with volume expanded states.

A number of candidates have been proposed as the circulating EDLC, but none has as yet has been widely accepted as the sole or even major mediator. Indeed, an extraordinary range of molecular species has been proposed, including ouabain, an isomer of ouabain, and digoxin (see discussion below). We believe this confusing array partially reflects the use of criteria that are inadequately stringent. The candidate may or may not be capable of inhibiting Na^+, K^+-ATPase. A correlation between volume status, blood pressure level, and circulating concentration of EDLC in the model selected should be addressed.

2 Cardenolides

Transmembrane sodium and potassium gradients are essentially maintained by the activity of the sodium pump whose energetics and biochemical support is the transmembrane Na^+, K^+-ATPase. This enzyme participates in the control of various cellular processes, including cellular volume, nutrient transport, calcium content, and cellular excitability. Several endogenous substances inhibit Na^+, K^+-ATPase. These include unsaturated fatty acids [12], lysophosphatidylcholines [13], dopamine [14], dehydroepiandrosterone sulphate [15], lignans [16], and ascorbic acid [17]. However, none of these compounds appears to be the natural ligand of the digitalis receptor of Na^+, K^+-ATPase because of their limited specificity and affinity.

The cardiac glycosides are extracted from the dried leaf of the common purple foxglove, *Digitalis purpura*, and the seeds and leaves of some other plants [18]. Cardenolides are steroids with a five-membered, unsaturated lactone ring at C_{17} and a glycosidic bond at C_3. In the animal kingdom, structurally related compounds with cardiotonic activity have been shown, until recently, to exist only in the poison glands of bufonid toads and in the skin of several species of amphibia [19]. Based on the biological properties of digitalis compounds, the methods for detection and isolation of EDLC's are: (1) inhibition of Na^+, K^+-ATPase activity of renal or cerebral preparations; (2) inhibition of ouabain binding to whole tissues, whole cells, or purified Na^+, K^+-ATPase; (3) inhibition of sodium pump activity in various kinds of cells or tissues; (4) inhibition of ^{86}Rb uptake by different types of tissues or cells; and (5) cross-reaction with either antidigoxin or antiouabain antibodies.

2.1 Digoxin
(Figure 1: structure I, shown as the aglycone digoxigenin)

The notion that certain drugs may mimic the action of endogenous ligands at receptor sites has become compelling with the discovery of the endorphins as ligands of the opiate receptor. Much evidence suggests that, by analogy, natural ligands of the digitalis receptor of the sodium pump may exist in the mammalian body [20]. The conservation of a specific binding site for cardiac glycosides through evolution strongly argues for the presence of a natural ligand for the receptor. Many investigators have measured digoxin-like immunoreactivity to identify the putative digitalis-like factors on the assumption that biological substances which bind to the same receptors as drugs may compete with antibodies specific for the drugs. Because many compounds give false positive results, it has become evident that the use of antidigoxin antiserum in RIA systems to detect digitalis-like factors may yield erroneous findings [21].

In a study by Longerich et al. [22], commercially packaged teas and teas prepared from purchased herbs were assayed for digoxin-like factors (DLF) by their cross-reactivity with digoxin antibody and the inhibition of ouabain binding to membrane Na^+, K^+-ATPase. Three packaged and three herbal teas gave Na^+, K^+-ATPase inhibitory DLF values > 30 µg digoxin equivalents/cup. Two packaged and three herbal teas gave immunocross reactive DLF values of > 0.050 µg digoxin equivalents/cup. After ingestion, three of the teas elicited an increase in plasma Na^+, K^+-ATPase inhibitory DLF and two of the teas produced a measurable increase in immunocross reactivity. This suggests that some digoxin-like factors in human plasma may have a dietary source.
The question of dietary source of cardenolides may indeed require testing for such compounds in food. Many essential mammalian nutrients are dietary in origin, these include some amino acids, minerals and vitamins. For example, vitamin D converts to a hormone *in vivo*. Thus, the concept of what is endogenous may cover a range of compounds from the anabolic products of acetate to the subtle metabolism of ingested substances.

2.2 Ouabain (Figure 1, structure II)

The issue of endogenous production of ouabain is controversial. Commercial ouabain is plant derived and bears a ring structure conformation that is quite specific to plants. It has a L-rhamnose side group, a sugar that is only known to be produced in plants. While previous studies have reported the existence of a ouabain-like inhibitor (OLI) or ouabain in human materials and animal tissues, the principal sources for the OLI have been controversial. Previous studies have reported that the adrenal gland is a major source of circulating OLI, since adrenalectomy decreases the plasma levels of immunoreactive OLI, and passaged cultured cells from the human adrenal cortex produce immunoreactive OLI [23]. Kitano et al. [24] have found that orally administered ^3H-ouabain effectively accumulates in the adrenal gland and releases radioactivity into the circulation.
Ouabain produces a marked increase in potassium excretion with little or no change in sodium excretion [25, 40]. The acute IV injection of ouabain (0.5 mg) failed to alter blood pressure or urine sodium excretion over 6 hours, compared to a placebo injection, in 7 healthy males studied under strictly controlled conditions of posture and electrolyte intake [26]. A fur-

ther placebo controlled study of 10 healthy volunteers showed that ouabain (0.3 mg given IV 42 and 18 hours before the study) failed to alter pressor responsiveness to incremental infusions of norepinephrine and angiotensin II. To assess the effect of chronic administration, ouabain was infused IV continuously at 0.25 mg/day into 6 sheep for 3 weeks. There was no change in blood pressure or in pressor responsiveness to incremental angiotensin II despite steady-state plasma ouabain levels of greater than 1 nmol/L. Higher infusion rates were cardiotoxic and often fatal. Short term ouabain administration alters neither blood pressure nor pressor responsiveness in man, and is without effect during chronic infusion in sheep. If endogenous ouabain is present in human plasma, its concentration is less than 5 pmol/L. The present study [27] demonstrates that ouabain has significant, though minor, acute effects on plasma levels of vasoactive hormones. It fails, however, to confirm that ouabain is an acute pressor or natriuretic substance. If it has an important influence on electrolyte and hemodynamic homeostasis, its actions are likely to develop slowly.

In another study, neither ouabain nor ouabagenin (aglycone) caused a sustained increase in blood pressure when infused in equimolar doses during a 30-minute period in rats. Unlike acute administration, the chronic administration of ouabain produced a dose-dependent, sustained elevation of mean blood pressure in both normal and reduced renal mass (RRM) rats [28]. The greater the reduction in renal mass, the greater the increase in blood pressure. It is hypothesized that this is due to the decreased capacity of urinary sodium and water excretion in these RRM rats, resulting in increased volume and elevated endogenous sodium pump inhibitor (SPI). The authors suggest that SPI acting together with exogenously administered ouabain raised the blood pressure to higher levels. Hamlyn and coworkers demonstrated that chronic infusion of ouabain provokes chronic hypertension in rats [29]. Thus the increased plasma immunoreactive ouabain levels in essential hypertension [30] indicate that endogenous ouabain may be a causative factor. Interestingly, it was found that plasma immunoreactive ouabain levels were almost normal after therapy. It is therefore suggested that ouabain may be a part of a compensatory mechanism through its natriuretic effect, which in turn elevates the blood pressure.

It has been shown that ouabain increases plasma atrial natriuretic peptide concentration, thus serving a counterregulatory function given ANP's hypotensive effects [31]. It is believed that ouabain's hypertensive effects are mediated by changes in cytosolic calcium. Both external calcium influx and calcium release from the sarcoplasmic reticulum contribute equally to the rise in calcium.

2.3 Bufodienolides

Digitalis-like compounds (DLC) isolated from toad (*Bufo viridis*) tissues inhibit ATP hydrolysis and ion transport by Na^+, K^+- ATPase [32]. These bufogenins are C_{24} steroids with a six-membered lactone group that differentiates them from the plant's digitalis-like steroids. Although the highest levels of DLC such as bufalin (Figure 1, structure III) and resibufogenin are found in toad skin, they are also detected in plasma and many internal organs. The concentration of these DLC in toad plasma is 30 µM, of which 25–30% DLC is plasma protein bound [33]. The abundant distribution and different levels of DLC in various tissues exclude the possibility that toxicity is the only function of these compounds in the toad and raise the possibility of its participation in the physiological regulation of ion transport in these tissues.
Recent work from the Lichtstein group gives rise to evidence for endogenous mammalian origin of bufodienolides (see section 3.4 below). They hypothesize that the synthesis of six-membered cyclic unsaturated lactone steroids is not restricted to amphibians but is achieved by mammalian tissues as well. Upon photo-oxidation, bufodienolides can be chemically synthesized from digitalis compounds such as digitoxigenin.
Haddy et al. [34] compared the acute and chronic effects of equimolar doses of commercially available bufalin, an aglycone analog of resibufogenin, and ouabain in normal rats. Bufalin infused intravenously into anesthetized rats increased blood pressure, dP/dt, heart rate, urine volume, and urinary sodium excretion. Although equimolar doses of ouabain caused the same directional changes in all parameters except heart rate, the magnitudes of these changes were always less than those produced by bufalin. In fact, ouabain decreased blood pressure at higher doses. Acutely, bufalin raised blood pressure, but ouabain had little effect. In contrast, given chronically, ouabain substantially increased blood pressure in normal rats and in 70% reduced renal mass rats on a salt-free diet. Blood pressure did not increase in normal rats receiving a low dose of bufalin. However rats receiving a higher dose of bufalin or 70% reduced renal rats receiving a low dose of bufalin developed significant increases in blood pressure. Increases in blood pressure were associated with decreases in myocardial Na^+, K^+-ATPase activity and correlated with increased plasma Na^+, K^+-ATPase inhibitory activity. Furthermore, by inhibiting renal tubular cell sodium pump activity and by raising BP, bufalin also causes natriuresis and diuresis. Kaliuresis is induced by the infusion of these inhibitors. This is possibly due to the massive increase in the excre-

tion of sodium, which is then exchanged for potassium in the distal convoluted tubule.

The differences between these two agents could not be attributed to the fact that ouabain is a glycoside and bufalin is an aglycone because ouabagenin, the aglycone of ouabain, was without any effect on any hemodynamic or renal excretory parameter [35]. The ability of ouabain to raise BP when given chronically but not acutely may be due to the fact that the association rate constant for cardiac glycosides such as ouabain is often several-fold less than that of aglycones such as bufalin. Acutely administered ouabain may not act as a vasopressor simply because of slow binding to rat Na^+, K^+-ATPase. Weiland et al. [36] and Kim and Labella [37] point out that certain steroid inhibitors of Na^+, K^+-ATPase, particulary the progesterones, are negatively inotropic when allowed to enter the cardiac cell but positively inotropic when restricted to the cell surface by attaching certain sugars to the molecule. Clearly all Na^+, K^+-ATPase inhibitors do not produce the same hemodynamic and renal effects in rats. Although bufalin is a more potent pressor agent than ouabain when given acutely, ouabain is at least as potent a vasopressor agent as bufalin when given chronically.

3 Endogenous factors

In the search for a substance responsible for the natriuresis that accompanies volume expansion, many groups have isolated materials in various states of purity from a number of sources. These isolates elicit one or more of the following responses believed to be properties of the putative natriuretic hormone, namely pump inhibition, cross-reactivity with anti-digoxin or anti-ouabain antibodies, ^3H-ouabain displacement, pressor activity, and natriuresis. The following discusson is a comprehensive review of the progress being made by these groups. This summary concentrates on those isolates with sufficient reported data to distinguish them from one another. As shown in the summary chart (below), the following information is tabulated on each of the reported isolates: the source of the material; purification methodology; the ultraviolet (UV) characteristics of the material; the molecular weight (MW) of the material; whether it cross-reacts with anti-digoxin antibodies (DLS?); whether it displaces ouabain from free or bound Na^+, K^+-ATPase (ouabain disp?); whether it inhibits cellular or isolated Na^+, K^+-ATPase activity (inhibits Na^+, K^+-ATPase?); whether it shows *in vivo* or other *in vitro* activity (*In Vivo/In Vitro* activity?); other distinguishing characteristics of the material and any coined names for the material (other); and finally the laboratory that has done the isolation work (Lab). Though the summary chart is comprehensive and complete, the following section documents only recent progress. Refer to our first review published in 1990 for discussion of prior progress in the field [38].

3.1 Urine

While it is possible that the putative natriuretic hormone is a sodium pump inhibitor, inhibitory activity does not necessarily lead to natriuresis. It has been the premise of Wechter et al. [38] that the use of search tools based on the binding to and inhibition of Na^+, K^+-ATPase are poor at best for seeking the putative hormone. Consequently, in order to isolate and purify a natriuretic substance, the assay developed and used by Wechter and coworkers measures natriuresis, as well as kaliuresis, diuresis and blood pressure changes *in vivo* [39]. A series of endogenous materials that produce prolonged natriuresis in the normal conscious female rat have been isolated from human uremic urine. Human uremic urine (5800 L) was preprocessed by ultrafiltration (3000 Da cut-off) and lyophilization. The lyophilisate was resuspended and passed over a Sephadex G-25 gel filtration column to obtain the post-salt fraction IV. Fraction IV was lyophilized and then sequentially extracted with isopropanol and diethyl ether. The organic soluble material extracted was subjected to sequential C_{18}-reversed phase high performance liquid chromatography (RP HPLC). The natriuretic isolate designated LLU-α was purified to homogeneity by silica gel HPLC followed by C_{18}-RP HPLC (Summary chart, Entry 1) [40, 41]. A total of 1.8 mg of LLU-α was isolated for an overall yield of ~1.3×10^{-8}% from 1400 L of uremic urine. This would indicate a minimum concentration in urine of 5 nM. This pure material was analyzed by nuclear magnetic resonance (NMR), infrared spectroscopy (IR), and mass spectrometry (MS). The molecular weight of 264.1368, determined by EI-MS, best fit the molecular formula $C_{15}H_{20}O_4$; the ultraviolet spectral analysis (UV) suggested an extended conjugated system or an aromatic ring (λ_{max} 205 and 294 nm); and FTIR indicated the presence of a non-conjugated carboxy group, a hydroxyl group, and a vinyl ether, in addition to the conjugated double bonds. COSY, HMQC, DEPT, ^1H-NMR and ^{13}C-NMR experiments yielded the structural information to identify LLU-α as (S)-2,7,8-trimethyl-2-(β-carboxylethyl)-6-hydroxy-chroman (figure 1, structure IV), a probable oxidative metabolite of γ-tocopherol. This structure was unequivocally confirmed by the unambiguous synthesis of racemic LLU-α from 2,3-dimethyl-1,4-hydroquinone and γ-methyl-γ-vinyl-butyrolactone catalyzed by BF_3. This compound when administered to slightly hydropenic conscious rats induced prolonged natriuresis without kaliuresis and no effect on arterial blood pressure at 4 μg/kg. It displays a narrow and biphasic natriuretic dose response curve. In addition, LLU-α does not inhibit Na^+, K^+-ATPase, utilizing the bioassay of rubidium uptake in MDBK cells. It has also been isolated from normal human urine. A second natriuretic material, designated LLU-γ, was isolated from the above organic extracts of Fraction IV (Summary chart, Entry 2). Further purification by C_{18}-HPLC yielded a chemically unstable material that exhibits UV absorbances at 220 and 268 nm. The mass spectrometric techniques, LC-MS and LC-MS-MS, are currently being employed in an attempt to further elucidate the structure. LLU-γ does not influence arterial blood pressure or induce kaliuresis *in vivo*, and it does not inhibit Na^+, K^+-ATPase *in vitro*.

Whether any one of these isolates is the "natriuretic hormone" has yet to be determined. It is possible that one or more of these compounds could be involved in the multifactorial control of extracellular fluid volume.

Goto and coworkers [42] have isolated two candidates for endogenous digitalis-like factors from human urine based on the inhibition of ^3H-ouabain binding to intact human erythrocytes. Isolation of the two ouabain displacing compounds (ODC-1 and ODC-2) from the urine of healthy males was based on adsorption in chromatographic step 1 (Amberlite XAD2), reversed-phase chromatography in steps 2–6 (C_{18} columns), and both gel filtration and adsorption in steps 7–8 (Diol-60 column). The more polar ODC-1 closely resembled ouabain in biological, physicochemical, and chromatographic properties (Summary chart, Entry 3). It lacked a characteristic UV absorption peak between 190 and 300 nm. Anti-ouabain IgG dose-dependently neutralized the action of ODC-1. ODC-1 showed a weak interaction with anti-digoxin antibody. The rise in cystolic free calcium concentration in cultured vascular smooth muscle cells (VSMC) induced by the polar ODC-1 tended to be slower in onset and more sustained than that induced by arginine vasopressin [43]. Goto and group have also confirmed the presence of identical ODC-1 in mammalian plasma [44] and rat hypothalamus. The less polar ODC-2 behaved identically to digoxin in three analytical HPLC and thin layer chromatography systems and UV absorption (220 nm) (Summary chart, Entry 4). FAB MS (protonated ion m/z 781.6) and ^1H NMR support the notion that ODC-2 may be indistinguishable from digoxin. Approximately 7.9 μg ODC-2 was obtained from 9×10^4 L urine (purification factor of 3×10^7 based on dry weight), thus the concentration in the original urine may be 10–50 pM. ODC-2 displayed prominent digoxin-like immunoreactivity and the dose-response curve was almost parallel to that of digoxin [45]. It was not vasoactive.

Tamura, Inagami, and coworkers [46] have purified to homogeneity an endogenous sodium pump inhibitor, coined uroxin, from normal pig urine. A crude extract was prepared from 88.6 L of urine using Amberlite XAD-2 adsorption chromatography. Reversed phase C_{18} LPLC was used as a second step of purification for preparative fractionation of activities. Seven distinct activity peaks were isolated. The peak showing dose-dependent inhibition of and time-dependent binding to Na^+, K^+-ATPase that appeared to be sensitive to extracellular potassium concentration, and cross-reactivity to anti-ouabain antibodies was further purified by a series of HPLCs. Preparative amino, ODS, and phenyl columns were used to isolate a homogeneous material with a UV absorption of 214 nm and molecular weight of m/z 626 determined by fast atom bombardment mass spectrometry (FAB MS) (Summary chart, Entry 5). Uroxin was not fully soluble in water. Acid and alkaline treatment of uroxin resulted in the destruction of inhibitory activity. Size exclusion chromatography, crude ^{1}H-NMR, and HPLC clearly indicate that uroxin is different from the cardiotonic steroids, including the toad toxins, unsaturated fatty acids, and a number of other known inhibitory compounds. Heat treatment and enzymatic digestion of uroxin did not affect its inhibitory activity, suggesting that the isolate is neither peptidic nor nucleotidic. A total of 10 μg of uroxin was isolated, a purification factor of 11 million fold.

The slope of the dose-response curve for Na^+, K^+-ATPase binding of uroxin was nearly parallel with that of ouabain at a range of 10^{-9}–10^{-7} M. Inhibition of 50% of Na^+, K^+-ATPase activity was obtained with 89 nM uroxin and 200 nM ouabain. The binding of ^{3}H-ouabain to the purified rat brain ATPase was almost completely inhibited by 0.5 μM uroxin and ouabain. A 50% displacement was observed with 53 nM uroxin and 30 nM ouabain. Uroxin fully cross-reacted with anti-ouabain specific antibodies (0.1–100 nM). Inhibition of rubidium uptake into intact human erythrocytes by uroxin markedly diminished with increasing potassium concentration. Uroxin had no significant effect on Ca^{2+}-ATPase activities from sarcoplasmic reticulum membrane or plasma membrane, or on the Mg^{2+}-ATPase activities from erythrocyte plasma membrane or brain synaptosomal membrane. In conclusion, uroxin is functionally very similar to ouabain, yet is structurally different from any of the known cardiotonic steroids.

Two major forms of cardiac peptides have been established: CDD/ANP-1-126, a prohormone of 126 amino acids from the endocrine heart and CDD/ANP-99-126, circulating in blood plasma. Forssmann and coworkers [47] have implemented the same methodology used to isolate the circulating form of cardiodilatin from human blood to detect and analyze the biologically active, predominant form of the same polypeptide family excreted by the kidneys. Each step of the isolation procedure was bioassayed using an *in vitro* vascular smooth muscle relaxation test and a highly specific RIA against cardiodilatin (CDD-99-126). The acidified polypeptides excreted in 1000 L of normal human urine were adsorbed to 2.5 kg of alginic acid. After elution with 0.2 M HCl and lyophilization, the isolate was processed on a G-25 Sephadex column. The crude polypeptide fractions were subjected to ion-exchange chromatography followed by four HPLC steps. The amino acid analysis and gas phase sequence analysis showed that the main form of urinary cardiodilatin is a 32 amino acid peptide containing CDD-95-126; the molecule is N-terminally extended (Summary chart, Entry 6). This vasorelaxant peptide, coined urodilatin, was synthesized using the Merrified solid-phase process. Synthetic urodilatin exhibited a strong relaxant effect on aorta smooth muscle strips, and intravenous application in animals resulted in strong diuresis. It is postulated that urodilatin is a polypeptide produced in the kidney itself and is differentially processed from the same prohormone. Secreted into the tubular lumen, urodilatin exerts a paracrine effect on more distally located luminal receptors, initiating a strong diuresis. This introduces a new concept of kidney function with a primarily internal regulation.

From the urine of salt-loaded healthy men, Kramer and coworkers have isolated a natriuretic factor (NF) [48] and a ouabain-like factor (OLF) [49]. Twenty four-hour urines were collected during high sodium intake (> 30 g NaCl/ day), lyophilized, acidified, and subjected to Sephadex G-25 chromatography. The isolates of interest eluted in the post-salt fraction IV and were then separated on Sephadex G-10. Natriuretic factor (Summary chart, Entry 7) was subjected to further purification by affinity chromatography using an anti-digoxin antibody. Subsequent RP HPLC revealed a small peptide composed of Asp, Glu, Gly, Ser with a molar ratio of 1:1:2:2 and a molecular weight of ~640 Da. This peptide elutes from Dowex 1W-X4 between pH 6.5 and 4.0 and moves on high voltage thin layer gel electrophoresis toward the cathode as a ninhydrin-negative compound with an isoelectric point at ~pH 5. The natriuretic activity is destroyed by chymotrypsin. Amino acid sequence analysis revealed protection of the amino terminal end probably by acetylation. Since the physiological significance of ANF is still debated, the endogenous NF of noncardiac origin, a small acidic peptide, may have important implications in mammalian regulation of salt and water balance.

The small molecular weight fractions from the above Sephadex G-10 chromatography were subjected to RP HPLC and resulted in an inhibitory fraction eluting at 18% acetonitrile (Summary chart, Entry 8). OLF significantly inhibited Na^+, K^+-ATPase from hog cerebral cortex *in vitro* and cross-reacted weakly with digoxin antibodies. Further purification by two-dimensional TLC resulted in a single compound with potent dose-dependent Na^+, K^+-ATPase inhibition of up to 85% at 10^{-5} M, in parallel to ouabain. This concentration of OLF caused a rapid 3-fold rise in internal calcium concentration in cultured rat vascular smooth muscle cells (VSMC). Ouabain (10^{-5} M) causes a rise in internal calcium concentration of similar magnitude as OLF but with a markedly slower onset. Results from infrared and mass spectroscopy were compatible with a ouabain (γ-strophanthin)-like inhibitor. However, final identification with NMR resulted in an endogenous urinary apolar compound that is not identical with ouabain.

Cloix and coworkers have continued their search for an endogenous digitalis-like compound (EDLC), coined endalin, using the urine of hypertensives and their normotensive offspring [50]. EDLC was purified to apparent homogeneity by chromatography using a variety of reversed-phase and anion exchange columns. The compound was isolated according to its digitalis-like biological properties. The isolate specifically and reversibly inhibits dog kidney Na^+, K^+-ATPase activity; its inhibition of Na^+, K^+-ATPase is reversed by potassium; it is a competitive inhibitor of ouabain binding to Na^+, K^+-ATPase; it binds to the E_2P form of the enzyme; it inhibits Na^+, K^+-ATPase noncompetitively with ATP; its binding to the enzyme was maximal in the presence of Mg^{2+} and P_i; it inhibits Na^+ pump activity in human red blood cells; it inhibits serotonin uptake by human platelets; it induces diuresis and natriuresis without kaliuresis in a rat bioassay; and it cross-reacts with antidigoxin antibodies. Analysis by nuclear magnetic resonance and mass spectrometry revealed that EDLC might be a glucurosteroid with a molecular mass close to 500 Da. (Summary chart, Entry 9). Determination of EDLC activity in rat tissue extracts suggests that the pituitary gland, hypothalamus, and adrenal glands contain the highest amounts of this compound [51].

Urodiolenone was isolated by Chayen [52] and coworkers from the urine of a large number of subjects with neurocirculatory asthenia, labile hypertension, and adrenal hyperplasia (Summary chart, Entry 10). Urodiolenone is a dihydroxy derivative of the sesquiterpene nootkatone, a constituent of grapefruit. It has a molecular weight of 252 and a UV maximum at 240 nm. Urodiolenone inhibits oubain-sensitive Na^+, K^+-ATPase in guinea pig kidney tissue in a dose dependent fashion at concentrations below 0.5 pg/ml [53]. Such inhibition was observed in cells of the distal and proximal tubules, and in the thick ascending limb of Henle, as shown by a cytochemical bioassay. This finding raises the question whether the presence of urodiolenone in urine is a direct result of diet, or from the metabolism of nootkatone which may be specific in hypertensive people, or is produced endogenously by hypertensives. Urodiolenone and steroids share a common biogenetic pathway deriving from farnesyl pyrophosphate. It appears that ACTH stimulation moves the equilibrium toward steroidogenesis, whereas suppression of ACTH by dexamethasone allows the formation of urodiolenone. Urodiolenone was not found to be natriuretic or kaliuretic *in vivo*. Potassium administration or angiotensin infusion in patients with hypertension cause a dose response increase in the excretion of urodiolenone by 30–100-fold under strict dietary conditions. Excretion of elevated amounts of urodiolenone is exhibited by hypertensives and not by normotensive subjects. It has been postulated that the role of urodiolenone may be a reaction to stress.

Garay and coworkers [54] have isolated a potent inhibitor of the Na-K-Cl cotransport system from the urine of salt-loaded rats. Cotransport inhibitory factor (C.I.F.) was partially purified by ether extraction of acidified urine from male Wistar rats orally loaded with 2% saline (Summary chart, Entry 11). The ether phase was further extracted with flux media at pH 10–11, which was then removed and neutralized to pH 7.4. By ultrafiltration, C.I.F. is believed to have a molecular weight lower than 500 Da. C.I.F. potently inhibited cotransport fluxes in MDCK cells and in human erythrocytes, inhibited sodium-dependent chloride/bicarbonate exchange with 2–3 times less potency than cotransport, but showed no immunoreactive digoxin activity. It strongly increased natriuresis (400–700% after 90–120 min) and diuresis (250–350% after 90–120 min) after intravenous infusion into conscious rats. No kaliuresis was observed.

In an interesting study, Tamura, Inagami and coworkers [55] have demonstrated that most of the Na^+, K^+-ATPase inhibitory activity detected in the urine from normotensive and experimentally hypertensive rats is derived from diet. When their diet was switched to one which contains all synthetic nutrients or purified nutrient ingredients, most of the sodium pump inhibitory activities in the rat urine disappeared within one week. Pig urine derived OLI, described above (Summary chart, Entry 5), does not decrease in excretion level even 3 weeks after switching to an inhibitor-free synthetic diet. This observation suggests that the OLI detected in rat urine is possibly of endogenous origin, although the continuous appearance of the inhibitory activity may only reflect slow clearance.

Two sodium pump inhibitors, A and B, detected in the urine of reduced renal mass (RRM) rats on normal diet were individually purified to homogeneity by a combination of adsorption chromatography (Amberlite XAD-2) and RP HPLC. Inhibitors A and B were subsequently identified as a stereoisomer of the strophanthidine derivative, convalloside, and a monorhamnoside of periplogenin or its stereoisomer, respectively (Summary chart, Entry 12 and 13). Liquid secondary ion mass spectrometric studies provided a single deprotonated dominant ion peak at *m/z* 711 for isolate A and *m/z* 535 for isolate B. Both materials exhibited UV absorbance maxima at 218 nm, characteristic of cardenolides. The ^{1}H NMR of inhibitor A and from convalloside purified from the plant *C. majalis* were very similar but not superimposable, differing only in the carbohydrate signals. Inhibitor A could be neoconvalloside, a stereoisomer of convalloside differing only in the configuration of the glycosidic bond between the two sugars. On the basis of mass spectral evidence, the aglycone of inhibitor B is periplogenin. With the site of attachment presumed to be the 3 hydroxyl group, isolate B is believed to be the monorhamnoside of periplogenin.

No significant differences were observed in the pump inhibitory potencies between isolates A and B. Dose-response curves parallel to those of ouabain were observed in the rubidium uptake in erythrocytes and ^{3}H-ouabain-displacement assays. In addition, both inhibitors cross-reacted with specific anti-ouabain and anti-digoxin antibodies, although the dose-response curves were not parallel to those of ouabain or digoxin. Isolates A and B from diet are functionally and immunologically identical to those from urine, suggesting that the dietary inhibitors are not metabolized or modified in the rat body under the condition of RRM.

3.2 Plasma

Ludens and coworkers [56] have isolated an endogenous ouabain-like compound (OLC) from human plasma that interacts with the cardenolide receptor on the sodium pump and whose mechanism of inhibition is strikingly similar to that of the digitalis glycosides. From 75 donors irrespective of sex or blood pressure status, 300 L of human plasma was obtained by plasmapheresis and dialyzed against 10 mM ammonium actetate using cellulose acetate membranes (6000–8000 Da). The dialysate was passed over an Amberlite XAD-2 column and the methanol eluates were subjected to two preparative runs of C_{18}-RP HPLC. The pump inhibitory materials were subjected to enzyme affinity extraction using partially purified lamb kidney Na^+, K^+-ATPase. Post affinity chromatography using a phenyl semiprep column followed by a C_{18} semiprep column yielded a highly purified material with a strong absorbance at 220 nm (Summary chart, Entry 14). Representing purification on a dry weight basis of greater than 0.6 billion-fold, 300 L of human plasma yielded 31 µg (53 nmol, < 30%) of OLC.

This material was selected for further study based on its ability to exhibit time-dependent binding to Na^+, K^+-ATPase that appeared to be sensitive to extracellular potassium ions, i.e. digitalis-like. OLC inhibited the transport and hydrolytic activities of the Na^+, K^+-ATPase and blocked the binding of ^3H-ouabain to the enzyme. Based on its effects on evoked tension in guinea pig left atria and aortic rings, OLC has cardiotonic and vasotonic actions qualitatively and quantitatively similar to those observed with ouabain [57]. An ELISA was used to estimate the levels of immunoreactive OLC in blood and tissue extracts of several mammals [58]. The antisera demonstrated a high degree of specificity for ouabain and closely related cardenolides such as strophanthidin, ouabagenin, digitoxin, and digoxin. OLC cross-reacted poorly with dihydro-ouabain antibodies, indicating that the butenolide ring of ouabain is an essential structural component [59]. Plasma levels were similar in humans, dogs, and rats, and most tissues that contained ouabain immunoreactivity. The specific content of the adrenals was ~500-fold greater than the plasma level in the rat. This gland may be a source for the circulating OLC. Plasma immunoreactive OLC was increased 1.6-fold in uninephrectomized rats drinking 0.9% saline and 9-fold in hypertensive DOCA-treated uninephrectomized rats. In plasma drawn from dogs before and 30 and 120 minutes after massive volume expansion with isotonic saline, OLC levels did not change whereas sodium excretion was significantly elevated [60]. Because renal exposure to OLC did not change with saline loading, it is unlikely that any portion of the profuse natriuresis in these animals could be attributed to OLC.

Based on the following evidence, OLC from human plasma is structurally, biologically, and immunologically ouabain or an isomer of ouabain. In four HPLC systems including one utilizing a cyclodextrin solid support useful for resolving geometric, stereo, and structural isomers, OLC and ouabain were found to have identical retention times or to comigrate [61]. Fast atom bombardment mass spectrometry (FAB MS) of OLC yielded a protonated molecular ion of m/z 585.295; the theoretical value for ouabain is 585.291. Linked-scan MS/MS was used to analyze the daughter ion fragments of the m/z 585 peak for OLC and ouabain. Both spectra showed a major ion at m/z 439 corresponding to the aglycone of ouabain, indicating that the sugar moiety of OLC, like that of ouabain, is deoxyhexose. Corresponding to the loss of one more water, OLC does show two peaks (*m/z* 495.1, 385.1) not seen in the spectrum of ouabain. Stereoisomerism at C-11 yielding the β-stereochemistry is proposed. By FAB MS, acetylation of OLC with acetic anhydride/pyridine/DMAP yielded a hexaacetate major product and hepta- and octaacetate minor products reflecting the relative reactivity of the six primary or secondary OH groups and two hindered tertiary OH groups found in ouabain. OLC and ouabain cross-reacted indistinguishably with rabbit polyclonal anti-ouabain antibodies, and binding of OLC to Na^+, K^+-ATPase required the same complement of ligands that supports the binding of ouabain to the sodium pump.

Schoner and coworkers [62] had found that an inhibitor of the sodium pump circulates in increased concentrations in serum of patients with uremia. Therefore 6000 L of hemofiltrate, from seven patients of both sexes at the age of 60–70 years with chronic uremia that had not been treated with cardiac glycosides, was concentrated by adsorption to Amberlite XAD-2 (Summary chart, Entry 15). The ouabain-like activity therein was purified 4,250-fold in 0.04% yield by methanol extraction of the Amberlite column, ultrafiltration (MW 1000 cut-off), C_{18}-flash chromatography, and sequential RP HPLC. The ouabain-immunoreactive material did not elute at the position where ouabain elutes, but at a somewhat higher acetonitrile concentration, indicating a greater hydrophobicity than ouabain. Mass spectrometric analysis of the isolate gave a molecular weight of 582 Da. (MW 584.6 for ouabain). The compound inhibited the sodium pump and led, as ouabain did, to an increase of $[Ca^{2+}]_i$ in high- and low-$[Ca^{2+}]_i$ cells of embryonic chick heart cells. This isolate may be a degradation product of endogenously formed ouabain or an oxidized precursor of it. If biosynthesis of ouabain occurs in the adrenal gland, it would be reasonable to believe that formation of intermediates of differing hydrophobicity could occur.

Lichtstein [63] and coworkers have isolated the bufodienolide resibufogenin (hydroxy-14,15-epoxy-20,22-dienolide glycoside) from toad plasma and skin. Following methanol extraction, three sequential HPLC separations using amino and reversed phase chromatography yielded the compound with a UV maximum of 300 nm and a molecular mass of 352 corresponding to the molecular composition of $C_{23}H_{28}O_3$ (Summary chart, Entry 16). The concentration of resibufogenin was found to be 1 μmol/g and 1 nmol/ml for toad skin and plasma, respectively. This endogenous compound inhibited ^3H-ouabain binding to rat brain synaptosomes and inhibited Na^+,K^+-ATPase activity in a rat brain microsomal fraction and increased the force of contraction of atrial muscle. Detailed study of the characterization of these effects with respect to their sensitivity to ionic composition in the medium revealed that they behave almost identically to digitalis. The inhibition of enzyme activity is enhanced by Na^+ and is inhibited by K^+. The positive inotropic effect increases by lowering K^+ or Ca^{2+} and decreases by elevating K^+ or reducing Na^+ in the medium.

Gonick and coworkers [64] have isolated a low molecular weight hypertension-associated protein (HAP) from the plasma of hypertensives. The 12 kDa plasma protein, separated by SDS-PAGE, varies in staining intensity according to effective arterial volume status. It is markedly increased in patients with aldosteronism and essential hypertension and decreased in those with congestive heart failure. Plasma from hypertensive subjects was ultrafiltered (30 KDa cut-off) and the retentate was heated in the presence of 4% β-mercaptoethanol and 1 M formic acid and subsequently ultrafiltered (30 KDa cut-off) resulting in a filtrate containing the 12 kDa protein. A semi-purified preparation of this protein was natriuretic in a rat bioassay, inhibited Na^+, K^+-ATPase, and displaced ^{3}H-ouabain from Na^+, K^+-ATPase binding sites in a dose-dependent manner. A low molecular weight (< 500 Da) compound was dissociated from the 12 KDa HAP by alkalinization to pH 10, and separated from the protein by C_{18}-RP HPLC using a linear acetonitrile gradient. This compound which eluted at 4% acetonitrile, was found to be a potent inhibitor of both the Na^+, K^+-ATPase and K-pNPPase enzyme assay systems in a dose-related manner, similar to ouabain. Plasma Na^+, K^+-ATPase inhibitor (P-NKAI) also bound to both the high and low affinity binding sites on Na^+, K^+-ATPase, similar to ouabain, but failed to cross-react with ouabain-sensitive digoxin antibody. Rechromatography of P-NKAI on a 3 µm C_{18} column monitored electrochemically, yielded two potent Na^+, K^+-ATPase inhibitors (P-NKAI-1 and PNKAI-2) (Summary chart, Entry 17 and 18). Highly purified P-NKAI-1 was shown by FAB MS to have a molecular weight of 408 Da and to possess intrinsic vasoconstrictor activity as well as to potentiate the vasoconstrictor effects of norepinephrine in isolated rabbit femoral arteries. This isolate impaired the ability of potassium to cause relaxation when present in the medium bathing the arterial rings. Functionally, P-NKAI-1 behaved as a Na^+, K^+-ATPase inhibitor in vascular smooth muscle, competetive with potassium. These results suggest that HAP is a carrier protein for two plasma Na^+, K^+-ATPase inhibitors related to hypertension. A urinary inhibitor, U-NKPI, was also isolated from hypertensives. It coelutes on HPLC with

P-NKAI, has a molecular weight < 500 Da, and exhibits similar but not identical physiological behavior as P-NKAI [65].
Plasma from borderline hypertensives was used by Boschi et al. [66] to isolate and partially purify an endogenous Na^+, K^+-ATPase inhibitory material. Boiled (15 min) and untreated plasma samples were subjected to solid phase extraction followed by two HPLC steps. The fractions which showed the highest Na^+, K^+-ATPase inhibitory activity were pooled and subjected to ultrafiltration (1000 Da. cut-off). It is believed that the material of interest has a low molecular weight, < 1000 (Summary chart, Entry 19). This ultrafiltered material inhibited Na^+, K^+-ATPase, ^3H-ouabain binding to Na^+, K^+-ATPase, ouabain sensitive ^{86}Rb uptake, and pNPPase activity. Based on chromatographic retention times, this material is free of lipids, fatty acids, dehydroepiandrosterone sulphate, and ascorbic acid. The isolate is believed to have a polar nature due to the observed greater retention of this material on a polar diol column. Fluorescamine derivatization carried out under conditions typical for peptides showed increased fluorescence. Further studies are necessary to confirm the proposed peptidic nature and structurally characterize this isolate.
In another study [67] published by the Lichtstein group, a new unsaturated fatty acid derivative was isolated from bovine plasma (Summary chart, Entry 20). The purification procedure consisted of organic extractions and batch chromatography followed by three subsequent separations using reversed phase HPLC. The presence of this DLC was monitored by its ability to inhibit ^3H-ouabain binding to rat brain synaptosomes and microsomal Na^+, K^+-ATPase activity. Fifty per cent inhibition was obtained at 10^{-7} M (ouabain equivalents) of fatty acid; this potency in inhibiting Na^+, K^+-ATPase was three orders of magnitude higher than that of linoleic, oleic, or arachidonic acid [68]. The compound was identified as 11,13-dihydroxy-14-octadecaenoic acid by mass spectroscopic analysis. The activity of this compound declined with time with a simultaneous loss of the hydroxyl groups, signifying the biological importance of the hydroxyl groups. Efforts are being made to synthesize this compound in a chemically stable form to enable its biological characterization.
While attempting to isolate the natriuretic factor coined endoxin [69] (Summary chart, Entry 21), Rauch and Buckalew, Jr. isolated a plasma fraction containing predominantly lysophosphatidyl choline (LPC) [70] (Summary chart, Entry 22). Conscious, male, Sprague-Dawley rats were volume expanded with 0.9% saline for 0, 15, 30, 60, and 120 minutes, then rapidly decapitated, and the trunk blood collected and centrifuged. By addition of ethanol to the plasma and centrifugation, the denatured pro-

teins were removed. The solution was applied to a C_{18} column and washed with water and ethanol. The dried ethanol eluate was extracted with an organic solvent and the lipid extract was subjected to thin layer chromatography using silica plates. The phospholipid content was quantitated by spectrophotometric determination of phosphate after the digestion of the extracted isolates with perchloric acid at 180°C. The major phospholipids found in the C_{18} extracts of rat plasma were phosphatidyl choline (PC), LPC, and sphingomyelin (SPM).

LPC levels increased at several time points during the volume expansion. In normal plasma, PC (57.3%) was the most abundant phospholipid, followed by LPC (33.8%) and then by SPM (9.9%). During volume expansion, LPC was the most abundant phospholipid at half of the time points examined (increased 99% from control value at 30 min), PC levels decreased at all the time points except one (42% of control value at 60 min), and SPM levels were not altered. Measuring the ^{3}H-ouabain displacement from erythrocyte ghosts, the EC_{50} for LPC was 1 mM. To obtain this level in their assay system would require 3.6 mL of plasma from a control animal and only 1.9 mL from an animal volume expanded for 30 minutes. LPC produced a displacement of tritiated ouabain that was steeper than that produced by cold ouabain. This is typical for lipids with surfactant activity.

The increase in LPC in volume expanded states indictes that lysophospholipids (LPL) may play a physiological role. LPC and other lysophospholipids are capable of producing a long lasting natriuresis in anesthetized rats at concentrations where LPC does not act as a surfactant [71]. LPC evokes an increase in renal sodium and water excretion with a steep biphasic dose response (maximum effect at 0.1–1.0 ng doses). The natriuretic effect begins within 20 min after a bolus injection, attains its maximum effect within 40–60 min (increase of 20%), and lasts for ~7 hours. LPC does not increase kaliuresis at the threshold dose for the natriuresis. No change in systemic blood pressure was observed. When continuously infused over a 90 min period with myristoyl-LPC (13 pmol/min), the analogue with the greatest natriuretic potency in the bolus experiments above, anesthetized rats exhibited a small fall in systemic blood pressure, a 13% decrease in renal plasma flow without significantly altering glomerular filtration rate, and produced a slightly greater excretion of sodium and water than vehicle controls [72]. In mongrel dogs, LPC was natriuretic when given as a bolus of 3.0 μg/kg (natriuresis began 1 h after injection, peaked after 2 h, and lasted 3 h total) or as a constant infusion at 5 ng/kg/min (natriuresis began 1 h after infusion began, remained elevated for 1 h, then returned to baseline after the infusion was terminated) [73]. The natriuresis and diuresis were not affected when the phospholipid was given as an albumin complex. Natriuretic activity was eliminated by substituting an unsaturated 1-acyl group for the saturated 1-acyl group or by removing the 3-choline group, whereas it was increased by 75% when the 1-fatty acid was shortened to 14 carbons. The natriuretic effect is stereospecific: the natural L-stereoisomer is active and the unnatural D-stereoisomer is inactive. These results suggest the existence of specific tissue binding sites for lysophospholipids that mediate their natriuretic effect.

Though progress has not been made on the chemical characterization of endogenous digoxin-like immunoreactivity (EDLI) since our last review (Summary chart, Entry 23), Poston et al. [74] have continued to study the effects of EDLI in the serum of pregnant women. The serum of women in the third trimester of pregnancy demonstrates cross-reactivity with commercially available antibodies to digoxin. Studies have shown that these immunoreactive substances, which are not detectable in normal adult serum, are further increased in patients with pregnancy-induced hypertension. The compound(s) involved are believed to originate in the fetoplacental unit, since a higher concentration of EDLI is found in cord blood and the immunoreactivity disappears rapidly from the serum of the mother post partum [75]. In the infant, however, EDLI remains detectable for several weeks. It is also possible that the same substance(s) may be involved in the control of sodium excretion in the fetus and the neonate. The suggestion that a fetal natriuretic hormone may be present is supported by the recent evidence that an EDLI-rich fraction of cord blood results in natriuresis when injected into the renal artery of a rat [76].

S. Ghione et al. [77] have found positive correlations in newborn plasma between digoxin-like immunoreactivity and the ability to inhibit rubidium uptake and to displace ^{3}H-ouabain on erythrocyte membranes. Partially purified EDLF from umbilical cord blood was obtained by a procedure that comprised lyophilization, preliminary extraction with methanol, purification on Sep Pak C_{18} cartridges, and final separation on RP HPLC (Summary chart, Entry 24). The elution profile revealed two peaks of inhibitory activity on rubidium uptake. Because the second peak reflected a nonspecific interference of various lipophilic compounds, attention was focused on the first peak which showed dose-response curves for erythrocyte rubidium uptake and for digoxin RIA parallel to ouabain and digoxin, respectively. EDLF reacted with the Na^+, K^+-ATPase activity present in leaky sarcolemma vesicles isolated from rat kidney, heart, and brain. Interestingly, the inhibitory activity of this partially purified factor on rubidium uptake could be neutralized by anti-digoxin antibodies, available as a therapeutic tool in digoxin intoxication (FAB fragments). The authors believe this is direct evidence of an association between digoxin-like immunoreactivity and biological digitalis-like activity.

3.3 Hypothalamus, pituitary, and adrenals

Haupert, Jr., Nakanishi, and coworkers [78] have recently isolated and identified a bovine hypothalamic Na^+, K^+-ATPase inhibitory factor (HIF) by using affinity chromatography combined with HPLC. This inhibitor has a molecular weight of 584 determined by ion-spray mass spectrometry, making it isobaric with ouabain (Summary chart, Entry 27). Glycosidase treatment or acid hydrolysis of HIF released L-rhamnose, the hexose found in ouabain, as detected by chiral GC/MS. Enzymatically generated desrhamnosyl HIF was found to have a molecular weight of 438, as does ouabagenin, the aglycone of ouabain. HIF and its aglycone were indistinguishable from ouabain and ouabagenin, respectively, by RP HPLC. Derivatization of ouabain and HIF with naphthoylimidazole followed by HPLC produced fluorescent penta- and hexa-naphthoylate products. HIF was found to be more chemically reactive than ouabain, suggesting a decrease in steric hindrance or an increase in availablity of reactive hydroxyl groups. Based on through-space coupling of chromophores, CD spectroscopy on the HIF and ouabain naphthoylates confirmed that they were not identical but isomeric cardenolides.

The subtle structural differences between HIF and ouabain have a significant effect on their biological activities. Differing from ouabain, the binding and dissociation of HIF in intact renal tubular cells showed positive cooperativity in binding reactions and a relatively rapid dissociation rate constant. HIF was shown to have positive inotropic effects equipotent with ouabain, but at significantly lower doses. At the same intracellular Ca^{2+} concentration in myocytes, ouabain was toxic and HIF was not. While ouabain was without effect, isolated vascular rings from rat pulmonary artery and aorta were potently and reversibly constricted by HIF *in vitro* [79]. The mechanism involved is believed to be local modulation of the sodium pump-sympathetic neuroeffector interaction. HIF, at a concentration of 30 nM, inhibited Na^+, K^+-ATPase extracellularly in two-sided bifunctional Na^+, K^+-ATPase liposomes [80]. At 75 nM HIF, the reversed pump population was also blocked indicating that the inhibitor either traversed the membrane or was also able to act at the intracellular enzyme side at higher concentrations.

While the abundance and biological properties of HIF suggest its role as an endogenous inhibitor of Na^+, K^+-ATPase, it is not known whether HIF is truly the product of *de novo* mammalian biosynthesis. L-rhamnosides are generally found in plants and enteric bacteria, but the availability of L-rhamnose to mammals may explain its incorporation in HIF. Haupert, Jr. and coworkers feel it is extremely unlikely that HIF is ouabain that has isomerized during the isolation process, since the conditions were intentionally chosen to be mild. This material should be compared with the OLC isolated by Ludens et al. [56] and adrexin C (below) purified by Tarmura, Inagami and coworkers [46] to determine possible identities.

A specific pump inhibitor, designated adrexin C, was isolated from ~120 kg of bovine adrenal glands by Tamura, Inagami and coworkers [46]. Trimmed, ground, and lyophilized, the tissue was delipidated with petroleum ether. The delipidated tissue was extracted with methanol and filtered, and the filtrate was subjected to flash C_{18} chromatography. The fraction which contained the majority of the pump inhibitory activity was lyophilized and passed through a DEAE cellulose weak anion exchange column. C_{18}-LPLC followed by cation exchange chromatography and four RP HPLC steps yielded 10 µg of adrexin C. Based on FAB MS and ultrafiltration, the molecular mass was estimated below 350 Da (Summary chart, Entry 28) [81]. Based on size exclusion chromatography and HPLC using hydrophobic columns, the water-soluble, non-UV absorbing, adrenal derived inhibitor was indistinguishable from ouabain. Acid treatment with 6 N HCl vapor at 115°C had no affect on the pump inhibitory activity of both adrexin C and ouabain, whereas alkaline treatment of these compounds destroyed their bioactivity. In addition, heat and enzymatic treatment of this isolate did not effect pump inhibition, suggesting that it is not peptidic or nucleotidic.

The slope of the dose-response curve for Na^+, K^+-ATPase binding of adrexin C was nearly parallel with that of ouabain in a range of 10^{-9}–10^{-7} M. Inhibition of 50% of Na^+, K^+-ATPase activity was obtained with 263 nM adrexin C and 200 nM ouabain. The binding of ^{3}H-ouabain to the purified rat brain ATPase was almost completely inhibited by 0.5 µM adrexin C and ouabain. A 50% displacement was observed with 41 nM adrexin C and 30 nM ouabain. Adrexin C fully cross-reacted with anti-ouabain specific antibodies. Rubidium uptake into intact human erythrocytes by adrexin C markedly diminished with increasing potassium concentration. This substance has no effect on the Ca^{2+}-ATPase activity or the calcium loading rate into the vesicle prepared from skeletal muscle sarcoplasmic reticulum. These results indicate that the adrexin C purified from bovine adrenal glands is apparently indistinguishable from authentic ouabain. The adrenal glands may in fact be a major source of a humoral Na^+, K^+-ATPase inhibitor.

From bovine posterior pituitary, Inagami and coworkers [82] purified a substance that inhibits rubidium uptake by human erythrocytes. The pituitaries were homogenized and boiled in 1 M acetic acid, 20 mM HCl, and pepstatin A. After centrifugation of the mixture, the supernatant was subjected to batchwise extraction on a C_{18}-silica flash column. The inhibitory eluates were subjected to sequential HPLC until homogeneity was achieved. The inhibitory activity was destroyed completely by papain and partially by trypsin. The amino acid composition of the purified peptide was found to be Asx 2.8, Glx 6.4, Gly 5.2, Arg 2.2, Thr 1.0, Ala 2.0, Pro 3.4, Val 2.0 (Summary chart, Entry 29). The sequence was found to be identical to that of the joining peptide, one of the major derivatives of proopiomelanocortin (POMC), with a molecular mass of 2469 Da. The concentration required for 50% inhibition of rubidium uptake in human erythrocytes was 0.5 mM, very weak compared to ouabain. Intracisternal administration of 1–10 nmol of the joining peptide evoked marked hypertensive and tachycardiac effects in SHR but not WKY rats. These effects were dose-dependent, of rapid onset (20 sec), and maximal 3 minutes after administration. The effects resolved after 20 min. Derivatives of POMC, such as γ-melanocyte stimulating hormone and β-endorphin, have been known to be involved in the regulation of water and electrolyte balance as well as blood pressure. The physiological relevance of joining peptide has not been identified. Though the affinity of this peptide to the human erythrocyte sodium pump appears to be too low to play a physiologically significant role, inhibition of Na^+, K^+-ATPase has been known to potentiate neurotransmitter release. Inagami and coworkers speculate that the area of EDLF action may reside in the central nervous system.

The midbrain has been implicated in the control of circulating Na^+, K^+-ATPase inhibitors. Sancho and coworkers [83] have isolated a factor from tissue extracts of bovine hypothalamus and hypophysis that reversibly blocks the active transepithelial sodium transport across anuran membranes, inhibits Na^+, K^+-ATPase from mammalian kidney, and inhibits the binding of labelled ouabain to its celluar receptor in frog urinary bladder. The isolate coined hypothalamic hypophysary inhibitory factor (HHIF) was purified by extraction and chromatography (Summary chart, Entry 30). It has a UV maximum at 274 nm (water) and maximum fluorescence emission of 305 nm suggesting the presence of a phenol ring

[84]. Charring at 250°C for 2 h and alkaline hydrolysis for 2 h destroys its Na^+, K^+-ATPase inhibitory activity. The activity was unaffected by acid hydrolysis, phospholipase C digestion, or BSA incubation. HHIF is neither peptidic, lipidic, nor any known cardioglucoside or Na^+, K^+-ATPase inhibitor. Preincubation of human red blood cells with HHIF (10U/200 μl) caused 50% inhibition of ouabain-sensitive ^{86}Rb uptake. The calcium pump from the plasma membrane derived from synaptosomes is inhibited by HHIF making it a unique physiological effector of cell contraction and cell proliferation. HHIF did not cross-react with anti-digoxin antibodies at the doses tested. The complete purification of this inhibitor was performed in bovine hypothalamus, hypophysary, adrenal, spleen, pancreatic, brain cortex and kidney tissues in parallel. Its absence in brain cortex and the higher concentrations in hypophysis suggest some form of storage in the latter.

Valdes, Jr. and coworkers [85] hypothesize that mammalian adrenal cortex is the principal tissue source of endogenous digoxin-like immunoreactive factors (DLIF) in plasma. They report the isolation of DLIF from bovine adrenal cortex and plasma into a single highly immunoreactive chromatographic peak using reversed phase HPLC (Summary chart, Entry 31). Spectrophotometric absorbance properties are almost identical with those of the cardiac glycosides strongly supporting the notion that DLIF from these sources are structurally similar to one another and have some degree of structural similarity to digoxin. The physicochemical properties of partition coefficient, heat stability, and binding to Sephadex suggests chemical similarity between the isolates from both sources. Preliminary FAB-MS analysis show the presence of ion peaks consistent with a single species m/z of 790 which upon collision decompose into predominant peaks corresponding to m/z 390 and other peaks likely corresponding to sugar moieties. Based on the ratio of 947 pmol of DLIF per pmol of digoxin-equivalent immunoreactivity, DLIF concentrations in plasma and urine are comparable to other biologically active steroids or hormones found in body fluids.

Ferrandi et al. [86] have extracted a ouabain-like factor (OLF) from the hypothalamus and adrenals of adult Milan hypertensive strain (MHS) and Milan normotensive control (MNS) rats (Summary chart, Entry 32). The tissues were homogenized with methanol and the extracts purified on a Sephadex LH-20 column. Following desalting by ion-exchange chromatography, the extracts were further purified on a reversed phase PEP S C_2/C_{18} HPLC column. OLF was identified by its ability to inhibit ouabain-sensitive ^{86}Rb uptake into human erythrocytes, displace ^{3}H-ouabain binding, and to inhibit purified dog Na^+, K^+-ATPase. Preliminary physicochemical characterization showed OLF to have a molecular weight less than 2500, no ultraviolet absorbance, be unaffected by proteolytic treatment or boiling (110°C, 2 h) and only partially degraded by acid (6 N HCl, 110°C, 2 h) or base (1N KOH, 110°C, 2 h) hydrolysis. It has good solubility in water compared with low-order alcohols. Most of the characteristics of OLF were found to be the same as for ouabain. Both substances coelute on RP HPLC, suggesting similar polarity and they interact with Na^+, K^+-ATPase similarly. OLF does not resemble ouabain in its capacity to inhibit the low-affinity Na^+, K^+-ATPase isoform; OLF is greater. The yield of OLF is greater from MHS than MNS hypothalamic and adrenal extracts [87]. These findings represent the first direct evidence that a higher amount of OLF is present in tissues from genetically hypertensive rats than from their inbred normotensive controls, maintained under the same dietary and environmental conditions. This suggests a role for OLF in the pathogenesis of MHS hypertension.

Peripheral ouabain-like activity (OLA) may explain, in part, effects of dietary sodium on vascular smooth muscle and presynaptic regulation of sympathetic activity. In rats, high concentrations of OLA are present in the hypothalamus and pituitary gland and are higher in SHR vs Wistar-Kyoto control rats [88]. In a study by Leenen and Harmsen, SHR and WKY rats were fed high sodium (1,370 μmol/g) diets for 0, 2, and 4 weeks. After arterial blood pressure was measured, the rats were decapitated and the whole brain was removed. Hypothalamic tissue was obtained by dissection and homogenized. After centrifugation the supernatant was filtered through a Sep-Pak C_{18} column (Summary chart, Entry 33). Quantitation of OLA was performed by an assay for Na^+, K^+-ATPase activity. High sodium intake increased blood pressure in SHRs and not in WKY controls, but increased hypothalamic OLA in both strains.

Two cytochemical techniques have revealed the presence of an unidentified substance in the hypothalamus, urine, and plasma. De Wardener and coworkers [89] have found that the substance reversibly inhibits Na^+, K^+-ATPase activity in the proximal tubule of the guinea pig kidney with a maximal effect at 4–6 min (Summary chart, Entry 34). It also reversibly stimulates glucose-6-phosphate dehydrogenase (G6PD) activity maximally at 2 min. Using the capacity of the substance to stimulate G6PD at 2 min, a precise quantitative assay was validated. The plasma concentration of the cytochemically detectable substance in normal humans and the rat rises with increased salt intake. The highest concentration of the substance in the normal rat is in the hypothalamus. The cytochemically detectable activity survives boiling and acid hydrolysis but is destroyed by base hydrolysis and ashing. It passes through an Amicon UM05 ultrafiltration membrane and it is soluble in water and insoluble in chloroform. The findings on silica gel electrophoresis, high voltage paper electrophoresis, HPLC, synthetic derivatization, and proteolytic digestion on the activity of the hypothalamic substance have yielded a set of physicochemical properties that suggest that the active substance contains a functionality of the quarternary ammonium or immonium type.

3.4 Other

Studies have raised the possibility that a Na^+, K^+-ATPase inhibitor is involved in cataract formation. It is well established that the maintenance of Na^+ and K^+ concentration gradients across the epithelial and fiber cells is obligatory for the preservation of a transparent lens. Furthermore, it was demonstrated that the inhibition of lens Na^+, K^+-ATPase activity by ouabain provokes lens opacification. This may indicate that either the synthesis of DLC in the cataractous lens is increased or that compounds are synthesized in other tissues and are accumulated in the lens during cataractogenesis. Lichtstein [90] and coworkers have isolated two materials from 600 human cataractous lens nuclei (Summary chart, Entry 40). These DLC's were purified by a procedure consisting of organic extractions and batch chromatography followed by filtration through a 3000 Da. cut-off filter and subsequent separations using reversed phase HPLC. These DLC's inhibit dose-dependently ^3H-ouabain binding to rat brain synaptosomes and microsomal Na^+, K^+-ATPase and interact with antibodies directed against digoxin. It is suggested that the material present in the lens and is responsible for the digitalis-like activity is mainly 19-norbufalin (UV_{max} 298, MW 372) and a peptide, (Thr-Gly-Ala)-conjugated 19-norbufalin (UV_{max} 289, MW 603). These compounds resemble some bufodienolides which are normal constituents of toad plasma and skin. These findings imply that the synthesis of six-membered cyclic unsaturated lactone steroids is not restricted to amphibians but is achieved by mammalian tissues as well. Upon photo-oxidation, bufodienolides can be chemically synthesized from digitalis compounds such as digitoxigenin. The possibility should be considered that the endogenous digoxin, ouabain, or their metabolites, when exposed to ultraviolet radiation, in the lens, are converted to bufodienolide. It is also interesting to note that the frequency of cataracts in hypertensive patients is significantly higher than in control populations. This is consistent with the hypothesis that cataractogenesis may be related to the hypertensive process.

When the cells of the medullary thick ascending limb of Henle's loop (mTALH), which are invested with high cytochrome p450 monooxygenase activity and have negligible cyclooxygenase activity, are incubated with radiolabeled [1–^{14}C] arachidonic acid (AA), they form two principal peaks that have been designated by McGiff and coworkers as P_1 and P_2 based on their HPLC retention times (Summary chart, Entries 41 and 42) [91]. The primary action of P_1 is relaxation of isolated blood vessels, whereas P_2 exerts a predominantly Na^+/K^+-ATPase inhibitory effect. The principal components of these isolates have been structurally identified. Mass spectrometric data, lack of UV chromophores, and comparisons with authentic standards were consistent with P_1 containing two principal components: 19-hydroxy-5,8,11,14-eicosatetraenoic acid (19-HETE) and 20-hydroxy-5,8,11,14-eicosatetraenoic acid (20-HETE) and P_2 containing primarily 1,20-eicosa-5,8,11,14-tetraenedioic acid (20-COOH-AA). The biological properties of P_1 and P_2 were compared with those of the authentic standards of 19- and 20-HETE and 20-COOH-AA. P_1 dose dependently relaxed precontracted mesenteric arterial rings, as did authentic (19S)- and (19R)-HETE, whereas 20-HETE relaxed at lower and contracted at higher concentrations. Neither P_2 nor 20-COOH-AA exhibited vasoactivity, but each demonstrated a similar potency in inhibiting rabbit medullary Na^+/K^+-ATPase activity. P_2 and 20-COOH-AA and 20-HETE inhibited oxygen consumption of cultured mTALH cells [92]. The AA metabolites did not inhibit Ba^{2+}-sensitive ^{86}Rb efflux, indicating that they do not act through K^+ channels [93]. The authors further concluded that these isolates have a furosemide-like effect; namely, they act principally to inhibit the Na^+-K^+-$2Cl^-$ cotransporter of the mTALH cells. When infused into the rat kidney, 20-HETE produced a natriuresis and diuresis under conditions in which renal hemodynamic effects are absent, suggesting a direct inhibitory action of 20-HETE on resorptive mechanisms [94]. These AA metabolites may play a role in integrated renal function as their formation can be altered by peptide hormones, such as vasopressin and calcitonin, experimental and genetic forms of hypertension, and modification of dietary potassium. P-450-AA metabolites may participate in receptor mediated signal transduction and act as second messengers [95].

Valdes, Jr. and Graves [96] have shown that amniotic fluid (AF) contains a digitalis-like factor (DLF) which is increased in pregnancy-induced hypertension and is correlated to maternal blood pressure (Summary chart, Entry 43). This DLF was found to inhibit Na^+, K^+-ATPase hydrolysis, ouabain binding to its ATPase binding site, rubidium uptake into vascular smooth muscle (VSM), and to cause direct contraction of VSM at concentrations orders of magnitude lower than that required for ouabain.

Although the very high DLF concentration in amniotic fluid facilitated its isolation, AF as a source has a number of limitations. Through immunochemical profiling with different digoxin antisera, Naomi et al. [97] found that the DLF in serum from patients with renal failure was similar to that found in the serum of pregnant women. Because serum collection is limited and its use is complicated by protein binding, and urine may not contain the factor, peritoneal dialysate from patients with chronic renal failure was used to isolate DLF [98]. Patients were sustained with a liberalized salt and fluid intake so that volume expansion could be quantified and sustained, and that volume status and serum DLF could be related to blood pressure. Processing these patient's dialysates by ultrafiltration (< 1000 Da) and RP HPLC (C_{18}) allowed for the identification of a single elution fraction having volume-sensitive Na^+, K^+-ATPase inhibitory activity (Summary chart, Entry 44). This factor was readily distinguishable from ouabain and digoxin but was similar to the DLF isolated from amniotic fluid. The DLF isolated from peritoneal dialysate (PD) and from amniotic fluid were both chemically unstable, with equivalent half-lives. PD DLF showed a concentration-activity profile similar to that of ouabain in the Na^+, K^+-ATPase assay [99]. PD DLF inhibition of the Na^+, K^+-ATPase was similarly increased by low K^+, high Mg^{2+}, and PO_4^{3-}. It had readily measured digoxin crossreactivity which had a dilution response that paralleled digoxin more so than ouabain. The PD DLF, like the AF DLF, caused direct VSM contraction with a slow onset and inhibition of the VSM sodium pump [100].

Yasuhara and coworkers [101] have isolated hemin (chloroprotohemin IX), a potent inhibitor of Na^+, K^+-ATPase from porcine erythrocytes (Summary chart, Entry 45). From the blood cell fraction, the porcine isolate was extracted with acetonitrile and purified by sequential C_{18}-HPLC. Its maximum absorption is 400 nm and FAB MS revealed a molecular ion peak of m/z 616.1. ^{1}H NMR confirmed that the porcine isolate was indeed hemin, as compared with authentic hemin. Hemin is insoluble in water under neutral or acidic conditions but solubilizes in water as a complex with proteins and is distributed in blood, lymph, and various organs. The isolated inhibitor (IC_{50} 10^{-6} M) and authenitic hemin showed coincident dose dependent curves for the inhibition of Na^+, K^+-ATPase and this curve paralleled that of ouabain. Displacement of ^{3}H-ouabain binding to Na^+, K^+-ATPase by hemin was 1/100 as potent as ouabain itself, with a parallel dose dependent curve. Hemin (> 10^{-5} M), like ouabain (10^{-6} M), evoked a sustained increase in blood pressure in the rat. Unlike ouabain (10^{-9} M), hemin is not cytotoxic to cultured bovine aorta endothelial cells (10^{-5} M). Hemin could be relevant to the regulation of Na^+,

K^+-ATPase activity in every organ through heme/hemin interchange caused by biological oxidation/reduction reactions.

It has been demonstrated that the renal excretion of a certain sodium load given to sodium deficient rabbits or humans was much faster when sodium was administered orally than intravenously [102]. Renal sodium excretion was also found to be faster in spontaneously hypertensive rats (SHR) than in Wistar-Kyoto rats (WKY) after an oral sodium load, but similar after an intravenous load [103]. From these observations the researchers proposed a sodium sensor in the gastrointestinal tract/liver that in some way could influence the renal sodium excretion. Hansson and Lundgren [104] have hypothesized that the small intestine produces a natriuretic substance that is released in response to a sodium load in the small intestine. The intestinal tissue from cats was homogenized in tris buffer, fractionated by ultrafiltration (500–10,000 Da), and separated by gel chromatography (Sephadex G-25) (Summary chart, Entry 46). The fractions containing the water soluble material with an apparent molecular mass of 500–1000 Da augmented renal excretion of sodium and water in anesthetized Sprague-Dawley rats. The natriuretic fractions were further purified by ion exchange chromatography using a cation exchanger. Existing as a positively charged species, the material was adsorbed to a cation exchanger at pH 7.8. The natriuretic activity was eluted from the column at a NaCl concentration of 250 mM. This intestinal isolate did not influence arterial pressure nor potassium excretion *in vivo*. It did not inhibit Na^+, K^+-ATPase from pig kidney *in vitro*. The authors do not exclude the possibility that an intestinal natriuretic factor may decrease Na^+, K^+-ATPase activity *in vivo*, since few hormones influence the particular cellular mechanism directly. Instead the control is exerted via changes of intracellular mediators.

4 Endogenous commercially or synthetically available materials

A number of commercially or synthetically available materials have been evaluated for natriuretic activity *in vivo* as well as sodium pump inhibitory activity *in vitro*. Some were discussed in our review in 1990 [38] (see summary chart). We present here a few interesting studies on available materials pertaining to our discussion of potential endogenous natriuretic factors.

Pregnenolone sulfate, a recently characterized neurosteroid, seems to be an endogenous gamma-aminobutyric acid antagonist which inhibits muscimolstimulated ^{36}Cl uptake in rat brain (Summary chart, Entry 49). Garay et al. [105] have shown that it inhibits Cl^--HCO_3^- exchange in erythrocytes at concentrations not much higher than those reported in the rat forebrain (10^{-7} M). Pregnenolone sulfate (IC_{50} 10^{-6} M) was a more potent anion exchange inhibitor than furosemide (IC_{50} 10^{-5} M). Pregnenolone sulfate was natriuretic by direct administration (2.8 mg/kg) into the anesthetized rat renal artery. It did not modify diuresis and slightly decreased kaliuresis. Perhaps this reflects the higher inhibitory potency against Cl^--HCO_3^- exchange.

Progesterone and certain of its derivatives bind directly to the cardiac glycoside recognition site on Na^+, K^+-ATPase and inhibit the enzyme and the sodium pump. Progesterone, itself, and certain structurally related steroids are predominantly cardiodepressant. As shown by LaBella and coworkers [106], chlormadinone acetate (CMA) and chlormadinol acetate (CMLA, 17 α-acetoxy-6-chloro-3β-hydroxy-pregn-4,6-dien-20-one) are among the hormonal steroids with the highest affinity for Na^+, K^+-ATPase and are cardiodepressant *in vitro* and *in vivo*. The arabinoside, rhamnoside, and glucoside of CMLA are less potent inhibitors of Na^+, K^+-ATPase, but unlike CMLA evoke positive inotropy *in vivo* (Summary chart, Entry 50) [107]. In anesthetized cats, the circulation effects of the arabinofuranoside and the rhamnoside appear to be more favorable than those of the digitalis glycoside, digitoxin. On the other hand, 14β-hydroxyprogesterone is a cardiostimulant (Summary chart, Entry 51). In the guinea pig, the glucoside of 14β-hydroxyprogesterone increased sodium excretion significantly but had no effect on potassium excretion, blood pressure, or creatinine clearance, a response profile opposite to that of ouabain [108]. The actions of the digitaloid pregnanes at sites other than Na^+, K^+-ATPase would seem to underlie certain pharmacological responses that distinguish these compounds from the cardiac glycosides, such as digoxin and ouabain.

Both configuration and substituents determine the affinity of the steroid moiety for the target site mediating myocardial depression. The negative inotropic action related to the inhibition of mitochondrial respiration in the progesterone derivatives CMA and CMLA appears to derive from the *trans* (flat)-junction of the A/B and C/D rings of the steroid nucleus. This effect was circumvented by synthesizing the glycoside derivatives for CMLA. Introduction of a 14β-OH moiety into progesterone converts the C/D junction to the *cis* (bent) configuration and confers a positive inotropic action to that steroid, even in the absence of glycosidation. Contrary to current dogma, the C/D bent junction found in plant steroids is not an indispensable requirement for cardiotonic action.

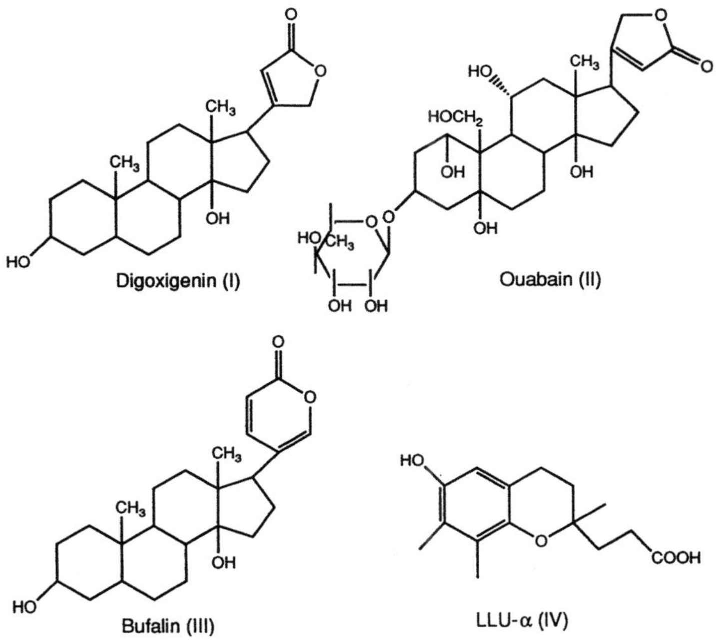

Fig. 1

In conclusion

Much progress has been made since the classic cross-circulation experiments of De Wardener et al. [109] postulated the existence of "natriuretic hormone". The search for natriuretic hormone has led to the discovery of ANF; this discovery, in turn, has led to a reexamination of the mechanisms of plasma volume regulation and to the conclusion that natriuretic hormone is more than one humoral factor. The search for these other factors has led to the identification of the circulating lysophospholipids and the endogenous digitalis-like compounds which may serve as *in vivo* regulators of the sodium pump activity. The isolation of cardenolides of plant origin from mammals has introduced the question of endogenous versus dietary origin. Is ingested plant ouabain epimerized at one or more chiral centers *in vivo* and converted to the isoouabain isolated from man [56] and the cow [78]? Bare in mind the isolation of DLS from tea [22] and cardenolides from common rat chow [55]. Though a change in direction towards the identification of an inhibitor of sodium transport and away from a natriuretic compound has refocused the search, we look forward to the elucidation of the mechanism of sodium regulation with further chemical and physiological characterization of the endogenous isolates summarized in this review.

PUTATIVE NATRIURETIC HORMONES AND/OR PRESSOR FACTORS

Entry	Source	Isolation Methodology	UV	MW	DLS?	Ouabain Disp.?	Inhibits Na^+/K^+-ATPase?	*In Vitro*/ *In Vivo* Activity?	Other	Lab
1	Human uremic urine	F4 (G-25) RP HPLC Silica HPLC	205, 294	264.2	no	no	no	Natriuretic without kaliuresis	**LLU-α** (S)-2,7,8-trimethyl-2-(β-carboxylethyl)-6-hydroxy-chroman	Wechter Murray Kantoci Benaksas (Loma Linda)
2	Human uremic urine	F4 (G-25) RP HPLC Silica HPLC	220, 268	< 500			no	Natriuretic without kaliuresis	**LLU-γ**	Wechter Murray Kantoci Benaksas (Loma Linda)
3	V.E. urine dog plasma	XAD-2 RP HPLC DIOL-60	no	340	weak	yes	yes	not vasoactive	ODC-1 ouabain-like	Goto
4	Normal human urine	XAD-2 RP HPLC DIOL-60	220	780.92	yes	yes	yes	Cardiotonic	ODC-2 **Digoxin** or isomer	Goto
5	Pig urine	XAD-2 RP LPLC RP HPLC	214	626 (FAB)	OLA	yes	yes		**Uroxin** (not a cardiotonic steroid; no 3° Me's by NMR; not peptidic or nucleotidic)	Inagami Tamura Naruse
6	Normal urine	acidification; alginic acid-adsorption; G-25	280	3505.9				Diuretic Vaso-relaxant	**Urodilatin** Residues 95-126 of Pro-ANF; CDD-95-126 Produced in kidney	Forssmann

7	Human urine	F4 (G-25)	280?	~640		yes	yes	Natriuretic	**NF** (Natriuretic Factor)Asx, Glx Gly, Ser (1:1:2:2)	Kramer Meyer-Lehnert
8	Human urine	F4 (G-25) RP HPLC 2D-TLC	220?		weak	yes	yes	$[Ca^{2+}]$ i ↑	**OLF** g-strophanthin-like apolar, not ouabain	Kramer Meyer-Lehnert
9	Hyper-tensive urine	RP and anion exchange chromat.		~500	yes	yes	yes	Natriuretic not kaliuretic	**Endalin** glucurosteroid	Cloix
10	Hyper-tensive urine	Glucuronide Hydrolysis XAD-2	240	252.3			yes	no*	**Urodiolenone** $C_{15}H_{24}O_3$ Gluco-Sesquiterpene (grapefruit)	Chayen
11	V.E. rat urine	Acidification and ether extraction		<500	no		no	inhibits Na/K/2Cl cotransport	**C.I.F.** (cotransport inhibitory factor)	Garay
12	RRM rat urine	XAD-2 RP HPLC	218	711	yes	yes	yes		**Neoconvalloside** (or isomer)	Inagami Tamura
13	RRM rat urine	XAD-2 RP HPLC	218	535	yes	yes	yes		**Monorhamnoside of periplogenin** (or isomer)	Inagami Tamura
14	V.E. human plasma	XAD; HPLC; Batch enzyme affinity extraction	220	584.64	no	yes	yes	Not natriuretic; Cardiotonic	**Ouabain isomer** OLC	Hamlyn Ludens
15	Hemo-filtrate	XAD-2; ultrafiltration; RP HPLC		582		yes	yes	$[Ca^{2+}]$ i ↑	degradation product or precursor of endogenous ouabain	Schoner

16	Toad plasma and skin	methanol extraction; NH_2 and RP HPLC	300 nm	352		yes	yes	increases force of contraction of heart muscle	**Resibufogenin**	Lichtstein
17	Hyper-tensive human plasma	SDS-PAGE alkalinization; RP HPLC		408	no	yes	yes	Vasoconstrictor; Protein bound P-NKAI: natriuretic	**P-NKAI-1**	Gonick
18	Hyper-tensive human plasma	SDS-PAGE alkalinization; RP HPLC		< 500	no	yes	yes	Protein bound P-NKAI: natriuretic	**P-NKAI-2**	Gonick
19	Borderline hyperten-sive plasma	Prep C-18		< 1000		yes	yes		polar molecule Peptide?	Boschi Borghi Ambrosioni
20	Bovine plasma	Extraction; RP HPLC		278		yes	yes		**11,13-dihydroxy-14-octadecenoic acid**	Lichtstein
21†	Human plasma & V.E. dog plasma	Delipidated; RP chromat.			yes	yes	yes		**Endoxin**	Buckalew
22	V.E. rat plasma	C_{18} wash; EtOH extraction; TLC		487	no	yes	yes	constant infusion: bp↓ natriuresis & diuresis	**Lysophosphatidyl-choline (LPC)** (also an article of commerce)	Buckalew
23	Neonatal cord serum; Pre-eclampsia serum	Sep-pack C_{18}	yes	476	yes			Na^+ efflux in leukocytes	Peptide?	Poston, Hilton and Morris

24	Umbilical cord blood	Extraction; RP HPLC			yes	yes	yes	Pump inhibitory activity neutralized by antidigoxin antibodies (FAB fragments	EDLF	Ghione
25†	Human plasma	Deproteinized prep. C_{18}	no	< 2000	yes	yes	yes		3 active peaks	Kelly and Smith
26†	DOCA-salt treated rat plasma	F4 (G-25)			yes		yes			Kojima
27	Bovine-hypothalamus	Extraction; lipophilic gel; affinity chrom	220	584	no	yes	yes	aortic ring contraction; inotropic	**Ouabain isomer** HIF	Haupert Jr. Nakanishi
28	Bovine adrenals	Methanol extraction; RP chromat	no	< 350	yes	yes	yes		**Adrexin C** Ouabain?	Inagami Tamura
29	Bovine posterior pituitary	Extraction; HPLC	214	2469			weak	hypertensive and tachycardiac effects in SHR	**Joining Peptide** (Proopiomelanocortin {POMC} derivative)	Inagami
30	Bovine hypothalamus and hypophysis	Extraction; Sephadex LH-20	274 (H_2O)		no	yes	yes	G6PDH stimulator	**HHIF** (Hypothalamic Hypophysary Inhibitory Factor) non-lipidic	Sancho
31	Bovine adrenals	RP HPLC	215	790 (FAB)	yes				DLIF similar to digoxin	Valdes, Jr.

32	Milan hypertensive & normoten sive rat adrenals	LH20 extraction; C_{18}-chromat.	no	< 2500	no	yes	yes	high affinity for α_1 Na^+/K^+-ATPase	**OLF** nonlipidic; nonpeptidic; hydrophilic	Ferrandi Ferrari Bianchi
33	Rat brain hypothal-amus	SepPak; C_{18}-chromat.	yes		no		yes		**OLA**	Harmsen Leenen
34	Rat hypothal-amus	acetone extraction	no	< 500	yes		yes		stimulates G6PD; $CHCl_3$ insoluble; water soluble; quaternary ammonium or immonium functionality	deWardener Morris
35†	Hypothala-mus; V.E. Urine and Serum	F4 (G-25)		< 1000	yes	yes	yes	natriuretic?	2 tetrapeptides; fluorescent at pH 9	Kramer
36†	Rat brain	Methanol extraction C_{18}-chromat.			yes	yes	yes	increases force of contraction of heart muscle	peptide	Lichtstein
37†	Fetal rat hypothala-mic cells	G-15	280	1468		yes	yes	constricts smooth muscle	**ASTI** peptidic	Mir
38†	Hog adrenals and human urine (Salt-Wasting Syndrome)	Extraction; paper chrom.; synthesis	288	334.5			*no	*no	**SEF** 3β,16α-dihydroxy-5α-pregnan-20-one	Neher Wettstein

39†	Hypothal-amus	Synthesis	288	288.4			*no	*2-OH natriuretic	**Catechol estrogens** (2-hydroxy- and 4-hydroxy-estradiol)	*articles of commerce
40	Human cataract lens nuclei	Organic extraction; RP HPLC	298 289	603 372	yes	yes	yes		**19-norbufalin** (3-OH-14-ene-19-norbufa-20,22-dienolide) 19-norbufalin peptides	Lichtstein
41	mTALH (kidney)	HPLC	no	320	no	no	no	natriuretic	**20-OH-AA** (20 HETE)	M[c]Giff
42	mTALH (kidney)	HPLC	no	344	no	no	yes	inhibits co-porter (Na/K/2Cl); natriuretic	**20-COOH-AA**	M[c]Giff
43	Pre-eclampsia amniotic fluid	Ultrafiltration; C_{18}-chromat.	no	< 1000	yes	yes 10^4 x ouabain	yes	vasoconstrictor	**DLF** neutral; noncovalently protein-bound in serum	Graves
44	Uremic peritoneal dialysate	Ultrafiltration; C_{18}-chromat.		< 1000	yes		yes	vasoconstrictor	**DLF**	Graves and Hollenberg
45	Porcine erythrocytes	CH_3CN extraction; C_{18}-HPLC	400	616.1	yes	yes	yes	Increased blood pressure in rats	**Hemin** $C_{34}H_{32}N_4O_4Fe$	Yasuhara
46	Cat intestine	ultrafiltration; G-25; ion exchange	yes	500–1000			no	Natriuretic, not kaliuretic in rat	positively charged at pH 7.8	Ludgren and Hansson

47†	Human cerebral spinal fluid	ultrafiltration; C_{18}-chromat.		~600		yes	yes		neuro-peptide?	Halperin
48†	Cardiac Atria	C_{18}-chrom.	yes	3080	no	no	no	Natriuretic and depressor	**ANF** short-acting natriuresis; diuresis; decreased arterial b.p.	de Bold
49	Chemical synthesis; commer-cially available			396.55	no	no	no	Natriuretic not kaliuretic; Inhibits Cl^--HCO_3^- exchange	**Pregnenolone sulfate**	Garay
50	Chemical synthesis					yes	yes	inotropic	**Chloramidinol glycosides**	Weiland
51	Chemical synthesis			494		yes	yes	Natriuretic,not kaliuretic; cardio-stimulant	**3β-gluco-14β-OH-progesterone**	LaBella

†Information reported in review: W.J. Wechter and E.J. Benaksas: Progress in Drug Research *34*, 231–260 (1990).
*as evaluated in our laboratories: Loma Linda University School of Medicine, Loma Linda, CA 92350

Acknowledgements

We gratefully acknowledge the sole financial support of Adventist Health Systems, Loma Linda.

References

1 A. Aperia, U. Holtback, M-L. Syren, L-B. Svensson, J. Fryckstedt and P. Greengard: FASEB J. *8*, 436–439 (1994).
2 J. Lowenstein, E.R. Beranbaum, H. Chasis and D.S. Baldwin: Clin. Sci. *38*, 359–374 (1970).
3 F.C. Luft, C.E. Grim and N.S. Fineberg: Am. J. Med. Sci. *283*(3), 119–128 (1982).
4 C. Borghi, S. Boschi, A. Munarini, A. Mussi, F.V. Costa and E. Ambrosioni: Am. J. Hyperten. *3*, 98–104 (1990).
5 A.M.A. Bullivant and D.J.B. Munoz: Am. J. Physiol. *264*, R281–289 (1993).
6 A.M.A. Bullivant and D.J.B. Munoz: Am. J. Physiol. *264*, R268–280 (1993).
7 J. Sancho: J. Cardiovasc. Pharmacol. 22 (Suppl. 2), vii–viii (1993).
8 S.J. Huot, M.B. Pamnani and D.L. Clough: Hypertension *5* (Suppl 1), 94–100 (1983).
9 R.A. Kelly and T.W. Smith: Am. J. Physiol. *256*, C937–C950 (1989).
10 W. Schoner: Prog. Drug Res. *41*, 249–291 (1994).
11 F.J. Haddy: Cardiovasc. Drugs and Therapy *4*, 343–349 (1990).
12 R.A. Kelly, D.S. O'Hara., W.E. Mitch and T.W. Smith: J. Biol. Chem. *261*, 11704–11711 (1986).
13 M. Tamura, T.M. Harris, K. Higashimori, B.J. Sweetman, I.A. Blair and T. Inagami: Biochem. *26*, 2797–2806 (1987).
14 E.M. Clarkson and H.E. De Wardener: Clin. Exp. Hypertens. *7*, 673–683 (1985).
15 S. Vasdev, L. Longerich, E. Johnson, D. Brent and M. Gault: Res. Commun. Chem. Pathol. Pharmacol. *49*, 387–399 (1985).
16 M. Fagoo, P. Braquet, J.P. Robin, A. Esanu and T. Godfraind: Biochem. Biophys. Res. Commun. *134*, 1064–1070 (1986).
17 Y.C. Ng, T. Akera, C.S. Han, W.E. Braselton, R.H. Kennedy, K. Temma, T.M. Brody and P.H. Sato: Biochem. Pharmacol. *34*, 2525–2530 (1985).
18 M.G. Briggs and J. Brotherton in: Steroidal Biochemistry and Pharmacology, London, Academic Press, Inc. pp. 276–285 (1970).
19 K. Meyer and H. Linde in: Venomous Animals and Their Venoms, W. Buhcerl, E. Buckley, eds, London, Academic Press, pp. 521–537 (1970).
20 D. Lichtstein, S. Samuelov, I. Gati and W.J. Wechter: J. Basic Clin. Physiol. Pharmacol. *3* (4), 269–292 (1992).
21 A. Goto, K. Yamada, M Ishii and T. Sugimoto: Nephron *54*, 99–100 (1990).
22 L. Longerich, E. Johnson and M.H. Gault: Clin. Invest. Med. *16* (3), 210–218 (1993).
23 J.H. Ludens M.A. Clark, F.G. Robinson and D.W. DuCharme: Hypertens. *19*, 721–724 (1992).
24 S. Kitano, S. Morimoto, K. Fukuo, S. Yasuda, T. Kaimoto and T. Ogiwara: Ther. Res. *14*, 201–206 (1993).
25 F.S. LaBella, J.F. Templeton, V.P.S. Kumar and D. Bose: Trends in Pharmacol Sci. *10*, 11–14 (1989).

26 G.B. Pidgeon, L.K. Lewis, A.M. Richards and M.G. Nicholls: Meeting of the Council for High Blood Pressure Research, American Heart Association, 75 (1994).
27 G.B. Pidgeon, A.M. Richards, M.G. Nicholls, L.K.Lewis and T.G. Yandle: Clin. Sci. *86*, 391–397 (1994).
28 C. Yuan, P. Manunta, S. Chen, J.M. Hamlyn, F.J. Haddy and M.B. Pamnani: J. Cardiovasc. Pharmacol. *22* (Suppl 2), S10–S12 (1993).
29 P. Manunta, B.P. Hamilton, A.C. Rogowski, E. Pruce and J.M. Hamlyn: J. Hypertens *10* (suppl 4), S 79 (1992).
30 K. Naruse, M. Naruse, A. Tanabe, T. Yoshimoto, Y. Watanabe, F. Kurimoto, N. Horiba, M. Tamura, T. Inagami and H. Demura: Hypertens. *23* (suppl. I), I-102–I-105 (1994).
31 K.D. Bloch, N. Zamir, D. Lichtstein, C.E. Seidman and J.G. Seidman: Am. J. Physiol. *255*, E437–E441 (1988).
32 J.S. Flier, E. Marratos-Flier, J.A. Pallota and D. McIsaac: Nature *279*, 341–343 (1978).
33 D. Lichtstein, I. Gati and H. Ovadia: J. Cardiovas. Pharm. *22* (Suppl 2), S102–S105 (1993).
34 M.B. Pamnani, S. Chen, C.M. Yuan and F.J. Haddy: Hypertension *23* (suppl I), I-106–I-109 (1994).
35 M.B. Pamnani, S. Chen, H.J. Bryant, J.F. Schooley Jr., S.C. Eliades, C.M. Yuan and F.J. Haddy: Hypertension *18*, 316–324 (1991).
36 J. Weiland, K. Schwabe, D. Hubler, W. Schonfeld and K.R. Repke: J. Enzyme Inhib. *2*, 31–36 (1987).
37 R.S. Kim and F.S. Labella: Pharmacol. Ther. *14*, 391–409 (1981).
38 W.J. Wechter and E.J. Benaksas: Prog. Drug Res. *34*, 231–260 (1990).
39 E.J. Benaksas, E.D. Murray, Jr., C.L. Rodgers, T. Pham, A.E. Bigornia, S.A. DeWind, R. Giebel, E.S. Brubacher and W.J. Wechter: Life Sci. *52*, 1045–1054 (1993).
40 E.D. Murray, Jr., D. Kantoci, S.A. DeWind, A.E. Bigornia, D.C. D'Amico, B.H. Levine, M.E. Jung and W.J. Wechter: Life Sciences, in press.
41 W.J. Wechter, D. Kantoci, E.D. Murray, Jr. D.C. D'Amico and M.E. Jung: Proceedings National Academy of Sciences (PNAS), submitted.
42 A. Goto, T. Ishiguro, K. Yamada, M. Ishii, M. Yoshioka, C. Eguchi, M. Shimora and T. Sugimoto: Biochem. Biophys. Res. Commun. *173* (3), 1093–1101 (1990).
43 A. Goto, K. Yamada, M. Ishii , M. Yoshioka, T. Ishiguro, C. Eguchi and T. Sugimoto: Hypertens. *13*, 916–921 (1989).
44 A. Goto, K. Yamada, M. Ishii, M. Yoshioka, T. Ishiguro, C. Eguchi and T. Sugimoto: Biochem. Biophys. Res. Commun. 45 A. Goto, K. Yamada, M. Ishii , T. Sugimoto and M. Yoshioka: Biochem. Pharmacol. *41* (8), 1261–1263 (1991).
46 M. Tamura, M. Naruse, M. Sakakibara, T. Inagami, T. Fitzgerald, P.J. Horton, J. Nelson and E. Price, Jr.: Biochem. Biophys. Acta *1157*, 15–22 (1993).
47 P. Schultz-Knappe, K. Forssmann, F. Herbst, D. Hock, R. Pipkorn and W.G. Forssmann: Klin. Wochenschr. *66*, 752–759 (1988).
48 H.J. Kramer, A. Bäcker, H. Michel, H. Meyer-Lehnert: XIIth Internat. Congress Nephrol. *526* (1993).
49 H.J. Kramer, A. Bäcker, G. Krampitz, H. Meyer-Lehnert and H. Michel: Am. J. Hypertens. *6* (5), 81A (1993).
50 J.-F. Cloix, M. Crabos, M.-L. Grichois, P. Guicheney and P. Meyer: Klin. Wochenschr. *65* (Suppl VIII), 146–153 (1987).
51 J.-F. Cloix: NIPS *5*, 204–207 (1990).

52 R. Chayen, Y. Mazur, H. Wyler, W. Berman, E. Potgieter and S. Goldberg: Phytochem. *27* (2), 369–372 (1988).
53 T. Rosenthal, E. Grossman, S. Goldberg, E. Peleg and R. Chayen: Am. J. Hypertens. *2*, 449–452 (1989).
54 A. Soler, J.O. Alda, I. Gimenez, C. Garcia, C. Nazaret, I. Pares and R.P. Garay: Pflugers Arch. *426*, 357–359 (1994).
55 M. Tamura, T.M. Harris, D. Phillips, I.A. Blair, Y.F. Wang, C.G. Hellerqvist, S.K. Lam and T. Inagami: J. Biol. Chem. *269*, 11972–11979 (1994).
56 J.H. Ludens, M.A. Clark, D.W. DuCharme, D.W. Harris, B.S.Lutzke, F. Mandel, W.R. Mathews, D.M. Sutter and J.M. Hamlyn: Hypertens. *17*, 923–929 (1991).
57 S. Bova, M.P. Blaustein, J.H. Ludens, D.W. Harris, D.W. DuCharme and J.M. Hamlyn: Hypertens. *17*, 944–950 (1991).
58 J.M. Hamlyn, M.P. Blaustein, S. Bova, D.W. DuCharme, D.W. Harris, F. Mandel, W.R. Mathews and J.H. Ludens: Proc. Natl. Acad. Sci., USA *88*, 6259–6263 (1991).
59 D.W. Harris, M.A. Clark, J.F. Fisher, J.M. Hamlyn, K.P. Kolbasa, J.H. Ludens and D.W. DuCharme: Hypertens. *17*, 936–943 (1991).
60 J.H. Ludens, M.A. Clark, K.P. Kolbasa and J.M. Hamlyn: J. Cardiovasc. Phamacol. *22* (Supp 2), S38–S41 (1993).
61 W.R. Mathews, D.W. DuCharme, J.M. Hamlyn, D.W. Harris, F. Mandel, M.A. Clark and J.H. Ludens: Hypertension *17*, 930–935 (1991).
62 W. Schoner, E. Heidrich-Lorsbach, U. Kirch, B. Ahlemeyer and B. Sich: J. Cardiovasc. Pharmacol. *22* (Suppl 2), S29–S31 (1993).
63 D. Lichtstein, S. Kachalsky and J. Deutsch: Life Sci. *38* (14) , 1261–1270 (1986).
64 H.C. Gonick, E.W.J. Weiler, F. Khalil-Manesh, B.A. Prins, R.E. Purdy, D.K. Sensharma: XIIth Internat. Congress Nephrol. 526 (1993).
65 H.C. Gonick, E.W.J. Weiler, B.A. Prins and R.E. Purdy: J. Cardiovasc. Pharmacol. *22* (suppl 2), S69–S71 (1993).
66 S. Boschi, C. Borghi, A. Munarini, F.V. Costa, L. Shuoren, D. deVries and E. Ambrosioni: Biochem. Biophys. Res. Commun. *169* (2), 360–368 (1990).
67 D. Lichtstein, S. Samuelov, I. Gati, A.M. Felix, T.F. Gabriel and J. Deutsch: J. Endocrinol. *128*, 71–78 (1991).
68 D. Lichtstein, S. Samuelov, J. Deutsch, H. Xu and S.S. Chernick: Klin. Wochen. *65*, 40–48 (1987).
69 A.L. Rauch and V.M. Buckalew, Jr.: Biochem. Biophys. Res. Commun. *150* (2), 648–654 (1988).
70 A.L. Rauch and V.M. Buckalew, Jr.: Life Sci. *42*, 1189–1197 (1988).
71 A.L. Rauch and V.M. Buckalew, Jr.: Am. J. Physiol. *254*, F824–F827 (1988).
72 R.K. Handa and V.M. Buckalew, Jr.: Life Sci. *51*, 1571–1575 (1992).
73 V.M. Buckalew, Jr., J. W. Strandhoy and R.K. Handa: J. Cardiovasc. Pharmacol. *22* (Suppl 2), S79–S81 (1993).
74 L. Poston, J.F. Morris, C.D. Wolfe and P.J. Hilton: Clin. Sci. *77*, 189–194 (1989).
75 J.F. Morris, L. Poston, C.D. Wolfe and P.J. Hilton: Clin. Sci. *75*, 577–579 (1988).
76 H. Ebara, S. Suzuki, K. Nagashima and T. Karoume: Life Sci. *42*, 303–309 (1988).
77 S. Ghione, S. Balzan, S. Decollogne, A. Paci, L. Pieraccini and U. Montali: J. Cardiovasc. Pharmacol. *22* (Suppl 2), S25–S28 (1993).
78 A.A. Tymiak, J.A. Norman, M. Bolgar, G.C. DiDonato, H. Lee, W.L. Parker, L.-C. Lo, N. Berova, K. Nakanishi, E. Haber and G.T. Haupert, Jr.: Proc. Natl. Acad. Sci., USA *90*, 8189–8193 (1993).

79 S.P. Janssens, C. Kanchoris, W.L. Parker, C.A. Hales and G.T. Haupert, Jr.: J. Cardiovasc. Pharmacol. *22* (suppl 2), S42–S46 (1993).
80 B.M. Anner and G.T. Haupert, Jr.: J. Cardiovasc. Pharmacol. *22* (suppl 2), S51–S53 (1993).
81 M. Tamura, T-T. Lam, T. Inagami, T. Fitzgerald and E. Price, Jr.: Biochem. *27*, 4244–4253 (1988).
82 T. Hamakubo, H. Furuta, M. Ichimura, M. Appalsamy, R. Mosqueda-Garcia, D. Robertson and T. Inagami: Biochem. Biophys. Res. Commun. *189* (2), 691–696 (1992).
83 M. Illescas, M. Ricote, E. Mendez, R. G-Robles and J. Sancho: FEBS *261* (2), 436–440 (1990).
84 J.M. Sancho, E. Garcia-Martin, R. Garcia-Robles, R. Santirso, W. Villa, C. Gutierrez-Merino and M. Ricote: J. Cardiovas. Pharm. *22* (Suppl 2), S32–S34 (1993).
85 I.M. Shaikh, B.W.C. Lau, B.A. Siegfreid and R. Valdes, Jr.: J. Biol. Chem. *266* (21), 13672–13678 (1991).
86 M. Ferrandi, E. Minotti, S. Salardi, M. Florio, G. Bianchi and P. Ferrari: Am. J. Physiol. *263*, F739–F748 (1992).
87 M. Ferrandi, E. Minotti, S. Salardi, M. Florio, G. Bianchi and P. Ferrari: J. Cardiovascular Pharmacol. *22* (2), S75–S78 (1993).
88 F.H.H. Leenen, B.S. Huang and E. Harmsen: J. Cardiovasc. Pharmacol. *22* (suppl 2), S72–S74 (1993).
89 H.E. de Wardener, S. Holland, J. Alaghband-Zadeh, H.R. Morris, M. Panico and A. Etienne: J. Cardiovasc. Pharmacol. *22* (Suppl 22), S109–S111 (1993).
90 D. Lichtstein, I. Gati, S. Samuelov, D. Berson, Y. Rozenman, L. Landau and J. Deutsch: Eur. J. Biochem. *216*, 261–268 (1993).
91 M.A. Carroll, A. Sala, C.E. Dunn, J.C. McGiff and R.C. Murphy: J. Biol. Chem. *266* (19), 12306–12312 (1991).
92 B. Escalante, D. Erlij, J.R. Falck and J.C. McGiff: Adv. Prostaglandin Thromboxane Leukotriene Res. *21*, 209–212 (1990).
93 B. Escalante, D. Erlij, J.R. Falck and J.C. McGiff: Am. J. Physiol. *266*, C1775–1782 (1994).
94 K. Takahashi, J. Capdevila, A. Karara, J.R. Falck, H.R. Jacobson and K.F. Badr: Am. J. Physiol. *258*, F781–789 (1990).
95 J.C. McGiff: Annu. Rev. Pharmacol. Toxicol. *31*, 339–369 (1991).
96 R. Valdes, Jr. and S.W. Graves: J. Clin. Endocrinol. Metab. *60*, 1135–1143 (1985).
97 S. Naomi, S. Graves, M. Lazarus, G.H. Williams and N.K. Hollenberg: Am. J. Hypertens. *4*, 795–801 (1991).
98 S.W. Graves, K.A. Glatter, J.M. Lazarus, G.H. Williams and N.K. Hollenberg: J. Cardiovasc. Pharmacol. *22* (suppl 2), S54–S57 (1993).
99 K.A. Glatter, S.W. Graves, N.K. Hollenberg, P.A. Soszynski, Q.F. Tao, G.J. Frem, G.H. Williams and J.M. Lazarus: Am. J. Hypertens. 7, 1016–1025 (1994).
100 C. Hamilton, S. Naomi, S.W. Graves and N.K. Hollenberg: J. Cardiovasc. Pharmacol. *22* (suppl 2), S119–S121 (1993).
101 T. Yasuhara, M. Mori, K. Wakamatsu and K. Kubo: Biochem. Biophys. Res. Commun. *178*, 95–103 (1991).
102 R.J. Lennane, R.M. Carey, T.J. Goodwin: Clin. Sci. Mol. Med. *49*, 437–440 (1975).
103 G.C. Hansson, J.Y. Mu and O. Lundgren: J. Cardiovasc. Pharmacol. *22* (Supp 2), S60–S62 (1993).
104 O. Lundgren and G.C. Hansson: Acta Physiol. Scand. *141*, 19–25 (1991).

105 R.P. Garay, C. Nazaret, D. Mesangeau and G. Moinet: J. Hypertens. *9* (suppl 6), S288–S289 (1991).
106 F.S. LaBella, I. Bihler, J. Templeton, R.-S. Kim, M. Hnatovich and D. Rohrer: Fed. Proc. Fed. Am. Soc. Exp. Biol. *44*, 2806–2811 (1985).
107 J. Weiland, K. Schwabe, D. Hubler, W. Schönfeld and K.R.H. Repke: J. Enz. Inhib. *2*, 31–36 (1987).
108 D.D. Smyth, J.F. Templeton, V.P. Sashi Kumar, Y. Yan, W. Widajewicz and F.S. LaBella: Can. J. Pharmacol. *70*, 723–727 (1992).
109 H.E. De Wardener, I.H. Mills, W.F. Clapham and C.J. Hayter: Clin. Sci. *21*, 249–258 (1961).

Progress in Drug Research, Vol. 45 (E. Jucker, Ed.)

Recent developments in the chemotherapy of osteoporosis[1]

By Indra Dwivedy and Suprabhat Ray

Medicinal Chemistry Division, Central Drug Research Institute, Lucknow 226001, India

1 CDRI communication No. 5399

1 Introduction

Osteoporosis has been defined [1] as a disease characterized by a low bone mass, microarchitectural deterioration of bone tissue leading to enhanced bone fragility and a consequent increase in fracture risk. This condition is also known as osteopenia. Bones which generally suffer fracture are of the vertebra, hip and forearm. Bone damage, particularly at an elderly age, could be fatal or render an individual invalid permanently or at least for a long duration, thus affecting his or her quality of life. Hence checking osteoporosis has become a research area of considerable importance.

The two most common forms of primary osteoporosis are postmenopausal osteoporosis in women and senile osteoporosis in both sexes. In senile osteoporosis (in most individuals over 70, or in women 20 years after menopause), the skeletal mass begins to shrink. This is also called type II [2] osteoporosis. It is a slow process and is an age-related disease. In postmenopausal osteoporosis, a faster rate of bone loss sets in. This is possibly due to estrogen deficiency. It is an accelerated process related to menopause and is referred to as type I [2] osteoporosis.

A rare form of metabolic bone disease known as juvenile osteoporosis occurs in children between 8 and 14 years of age. It causes bone pain and fractures. Patients usually have hypercalciuria and decreased intestinal absorption of calcium.

There is not much data available on secondary osteoporosis. However, corticoid-induced osteoporosis is relatively common.

Since the common forms of osteoporosis are age related, the proportion of population suffering from this disease is becoming more significant and alarming with the advancement of medical sciences which have helped in increasing life expectancy. Figures quoted for the United States show that there is a probability of 22% of the population to be over the age of 65 years in the year 2030 as compared to 12% in 1990 [3].Although some agents are known to be helpful in the treatment of osteoporosis and some new candidates are being evaluated for the treatment of this disease, a drug of choice which would help to attain the normal level in bone formation or to be used as a preventive measure is yet to be evolved.

Drug development work in osteoporosis can be better followed with an understanding of the process of bone formation and that of osteoporosis.

2 Bone formation and osteoporosis

Bone is one of the hardest tissues of the human body. It is composed of both mineral (70%) and organic components (30%). The mineral is calcium in the form of hydroxyapatite crystals $[Ca_{10}(PO_4)_6(OH)_2]$. The calcium of the matrix is available when required and through blood its appropriate level throughout the body tissues is maintained. The organic component is mostly type I collagen.

There are two major forms of bone. Cortical or compact bone forms the shell of bones and the shaft of long bones. It constitutes 80% of the human skeleton. Trabecular (spongy or cancellous) bone which is only 20% of the skeleton is the major form found in vertebra, distal ends, long bones and flat bones. It is made up of thin plate-like structures which form the inner mesh work of bones. It has a larger surface area and is more prone to bone loss [4]. In a lifetime, women lose about 35% of their cortical bone and 50% trabecular bone, whereas men lose about 2/3rds of these amounts [5, 6].

Bone is a complex and dynamic tissue which undergoes continuous remodeling throughout life. Three types of cells which are involved in the bone remodeling are the following:

i) *Bone lining cells or osteoprogenitor cells*: resting cells about to be used to produce bone and are located on internal bone surfaces.

ii) *Osteoblasts*: bone forming cells present on the surface of the developing bones.

iii) *Osteoclasts*: large multinucleated bone resorbing cells formed by the fusion of osteoprogenitor cells. These are relatively few in number.

Although osteoclasts and osteoblasts are derived from different stem cells, their activity is highly coupled. This is probably achieved under the influence of local coupling factors.

Bone remodeling takes place in a highly ordered manner (Figure 1) by the bone remodeling unit. The first step in this process is activation. Under the influence of bone-resorbing hormones, the lining cells which cover the inactive bone surfaces, release proteolytic enzymes such as collagenase and plasminogen activator [7]. These enzymes uncover the bone surfaces to osteoclastic resorption [8]. Osteoclasts may also find their way to the bone surface through contraction of the lining cells [9]. It has also been shown that osteoblast-like cells in the presence of parathyroid hormones stimulate osteoclastic bone resorption [10]. In the next stage, replication of the osteoclast progenitors and their differentiation, migration and fusion under the control of local and systemic hormones [11] lead to mature osteoclasts. Hydrogen ions produced at this stage in localized areas,

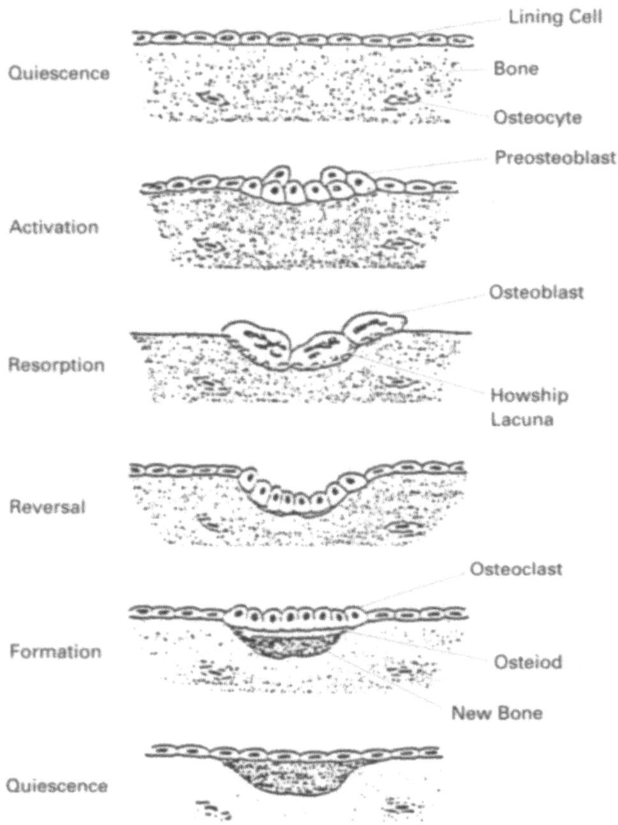

Fig. 1
Bone remodeling sequence (adapted from Marcus [13]

created by the ruffled structure of the osteoclasts, dissolve the bone mineral and lysosomal enzymes which are released, degrade matrix, including collagen at a low pH [12], resulting in the formation of a cavity. On completion of the resorption process, the reversal phase starts. Osteoblast precursors are attracted to the cavity site, and as they mature, they secrete collagen and matrix constituents, known as osteoids which fill the cavity to form new bones [13]. The new bone is then mineralized. This

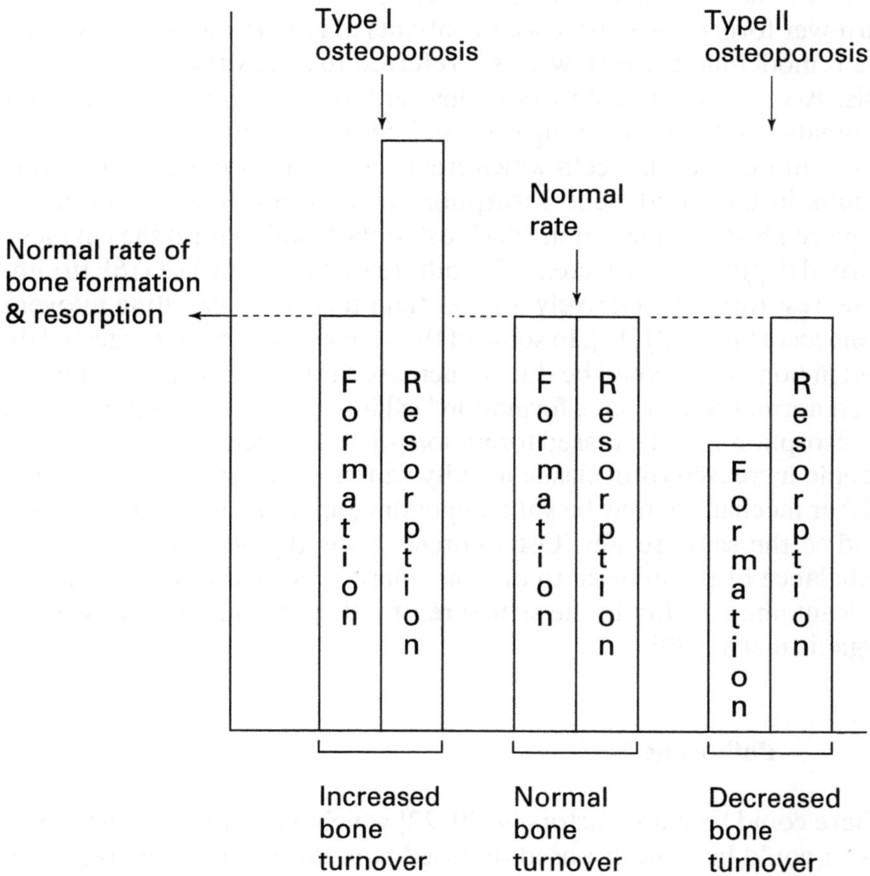

Fig. 2
Bone formation / bone resorption combinations

complex remodeling process takes about 3 to 4 months to complete under the influence of local and systemic factors [14].

In normal growth and development, there is normal bone resorption and increased bone formation which results in a net gain in bone mass. When the two processes are rightly coupled there is no gain in bone mass which generally is the case in normal early adult life. When the bone resorption rate is higher than bone formation, it leads to a net reduction in bone mass.

This situation occurs in osteoporosis. In type I osteoporosis, the overall rate of bone remodeling is high. These patients are said to have a high turnover form of osteoporosis. In patients of type II osteoporosis, where the remodeling rate is slow, this is referred to as low turnover osteoporosis. Accelerated and slow bone loss are associated with two different anomalies of the remodeling process [15]. Accelerated bone loss occurs due to more osteoclast cells which create deeper resorption cavities which results in increased bone resorption. Low turnover is mainly due to impaired bone formation in which osteoblasts fail to refill the cavities of normal depth or even decreased depth created by osteoclast [16]. In either case, resorption is relatively greater than formation resulting in overall bone loss (Figure 2) [17]. In some of the studies it has been suggested that loss in bone mass could be due to increased rate of bone resorption having a normal rate of bone formation [18] but others suggest normal rates of resorption with decreased formation [4]. It has been shown that in older people increased osteoclastic activity causes progressive bone loss [19]. Either mechanism may be valid depending upon the individual and they lead to the same results. Osteoporosis generally does not involve any imbalance of the mineral to organic phase ratio of the bone or any significant abnormality in the structure of either the mineral phase or the organic matrix [20].

3 Pathogenesis

There could be many factors [4, 20–22] which may influence osteoporosis. It could be a predisposed diseased condition, drugs, environmental influences, hormonal imbalance, alcoholism, smoking, dietary conditions, genetic factors etc.

Many systemic and local factors, discussed in the following section have also been identified [14, 23, 24] which affect bone metabolism. A knowledge of these factors is beneficial in understanding the mechanism of the disease, its treatment and the development of new agents for osteoporosis.

3.1 Factors influencing osteoporosis

3.1.1 Hormones effecting bone metabolism

Impaired absorption of calcium resulting in negative calcium balance has been implicated with age-related bone loss. In the absence of an adequate level of calcium, parathyroid hormone (PTH) is released, which promotes bone resorption. Serum concentration of PTH increases with age [25, 26]. However, this increase is not entirely related to a loss in bone mass or an increased incidence of vertebral fractures [27]. Whereas high concentration of PTH inhibits bone formation, in low doses it can increase trabecular bone mass [28]. It has been shown to be helpful in treating vertebral osteoporosis [29]. Its age-related increase affects cortical bone loss resulting in long bone fractures.

1,25-Dihydroxy vitamin D_3 has been found to augment intestinal absorption of calcium in older patients with a lowered serum level of 1,25-dihydroxy vitamin D_3 [30].

Calcitonin is an inhibitor of bone resorption. However, its excess or deficiency in patients does not cause a change in bone mass [31]. Also its level is not lowered in patients suffering from osteoporosis [32]. Decreased levels of calcitonin may be associated with that of testosterone and could be involved in osteoporosis in men [33].

Glucocorticoids exhibit a complex effect on bone metabolism [34]. Under *in vitro* conditions, at low concentrations, glucocorticoids increase osteoblastic collagen synthesis, whereas at high concentrations, bone formation is decreased possibly due to inhibition of replication and differentiation of osteoblast precursors [35]. In *in vivo* situations it causes a decrease in bone formation which may cause osteoporosis.

Insulin has been found to cause stimulation of osteoclastic collagen synthesis [36] and also has an effect on calcium transport and vitamin D metabolism [14]. Studies show a loss in bone mass in type I diabetes [37] but not an increased incidence of osteoporotic fractures [38].

Thyroid hormones decrease bone mass by increasing bone turnover with decreased bone formation [39, 40].

Deficiency of estrogens in women [41] and androgens in men [33, 42] in the development of osteoporosis is well established. Withdrawal of these hormones causes increased bone resorption and lesser increase in bone formation [43]. Progestins may also be involved in bone formation [44]. Stimulation of osteoblast formation [45] and inhibition of PTH could be reasons for the observed effect in reducing bone resorption. Prolactin has also a positive effect in bone formation [46]. The mechanism of estrogen action is described in section 4.5.1.

3.1.2 Effect of bone-derived growth factors in osteoporosis

A number of growth factors have been identified which affect bone metabolism at low concentrations. Most of them are not yet fully characterized. Some of these growth factors are derived from the bone. Among these factors, insulin-like growth factor-I and somatomedin C are important physiologic regulators. IGF-1, which is a low molecular weight peptide, is a potent stimulator of bone cell mitogenesis and differentiated function in bone organ cultures [47, 48] and collagen synthesis [49]. IGF-1 has been shown to increase the production of new bones *in vivo* [50]. There is evidence that growth hormones increase the production of IGF-1 in cartilage [51]. Recently , however , it was found in an *in vivo* study that intermittent administration of IGF-1 may cause bone resorption [52]. The use of insulin-like growth factors in clinical medicine has the potential risk of causing hypoglycemia.

High molecular weight regulatory growth factors found in bone are transforming growth factor β-1 (TGFβ-1) and transforming growth factor β-2 (TGFβ-2) [53, 48, 54, 55]. TGFβ is the key factor involved in the coupling of bone resorption and formation processes both having apparently identical effects. In *in vivo* studies, TGFβ has been found to stimulate osteoblast formation, including precursor proliferation and matrix deposition [56]. It has also been found to enhance prostaglandin (PG) formation which increases osteoclastic bone resorption [57, 58]. However, inhibition of osteoclast activity by TGFβ has also been reported [59, 60]. TGF is present in the bone in a latent complex form [61]. Its release is enhanced by PTH, interleukin-1, 1,25-dihydroxy vitamin D_3 and inhibited by calcitonin.

In addition to these peptides mentioned above, there are a number of other growth factors which influence bone formation. These include fibroblast growth factors present in demineralized bone matrix [62], platelet-derived growth factors [63], bone morphogenic proteins (BMPs) [64] etc. These are all potent mitogens that can affect bone resorption and formation [23]. The BMPs have 6 or more related factors. Their role in normal bone formation and whether all have the same biological effect is not clear. They have been found to be useful in the repair of segmental bone defects and in fracture repair.

Prostaglandins were the first factors to be linked with bone metabolism [65]. Other local factors involved are cytokines and lymphokines, interlukin-1, interferon-α [66, 67–71] etc. which directly or indirectly influence bone metabolism.

Pathogenesis of juvenile osteoporosis is not known. In the case of secondary osteoporosis the situation is more complicated and not much data is available. However, glucocorticoid-induced osteoporosis is caused due to long-term use of glucocorticoids such as prednisone, prednisolone, methyl prednisolone, betamethasone, dexamethasone and triamcinolone drugs. The bone loss is relatively common and more in younger people than older patients and premenopausal women.

4 Chemical control of osteoporosis

4.1 Calcium compounds

Association of calcium (Ca) with bone formation was realized a long way back. Along with phosphorus it forms the principal constituent of bone. Strength of the bone depends upon its supply, absorption, incorporation and withdrawal [72].

Calcium possibly inhibits bone resorption. It appears to be more effective in elderly (type II) osteoporosis particularly at sites which consist of cortical bone [24]. Calcium stabilizes bone loss and may improve mineralization and reverse malfunctioning of bone metabolism. Heaney et al. [73] have observed that the calcium requirement of postmenopausal women (1400 mg/d) is higher compared to premenopausal women (1000 mg/d). This excess requirement is due to less efficient Ca absorption from the gut and poorer Ca reabsorption by the kidney in postmenopausal women. In the case of calcium deficiency, PTH is released, which promotes bone resorption.

Calcium has a protective effect. In a 14-year study carried out by Holbrook et al. [74] it was found that subjects on calcium intake of 765 mg/d had a 60% lower risk of hip fracture compared with subjects with lower intakes. Clinical trials with calcium supplementation have shown reduced rates of bone loss [75]. Calcium absorption from carbonate, acetate, lactate, gluconate and citrate salts and from whole milk is similar in fasting healthy young subjects [76].

4.1.1 Mechanism of action

Calcium is the main requirement in bone mineralization and thus in the formation of bone. Its deficiency leads to bone resorption in an indirect way involving PTH and 1,25-$(OH)_2$ vitamin D_3 discussed under section 4.2.1 [77].

4.1.2 Side effects

The only side effect of calcium therapy is the development of renal stones which is not common in women. It has been shown [78] that calcium citrate inhibits calcium oxalate crystallization in kidney and is therefore a preparation of choice in calcium deficiency.

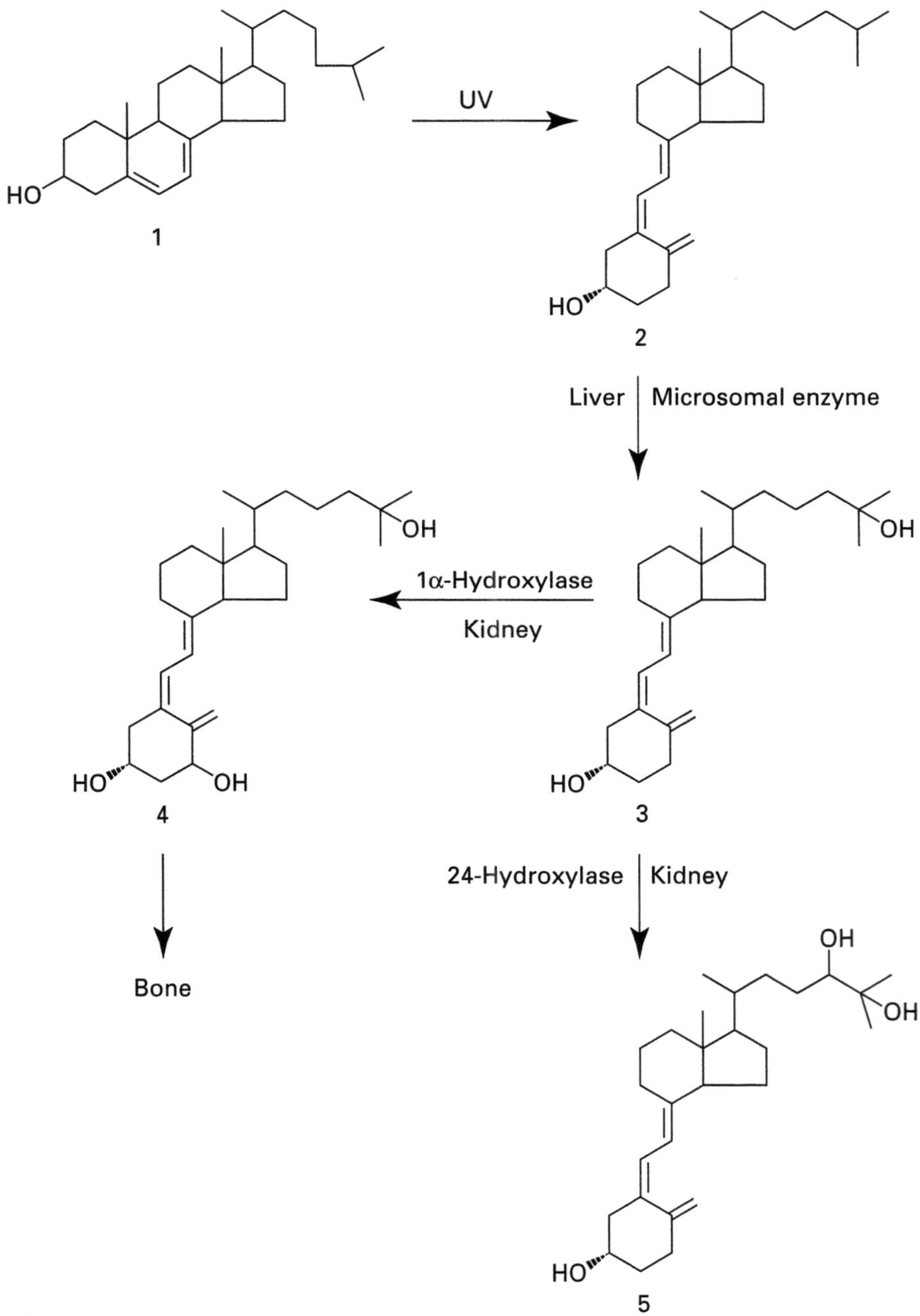
UV
HO
1
HO
2
Liver
Microsomal enzyme
OH
HO
3
1α-Hydroxylase
Kidney
OH
HO
OH
4
24-Hydroxylase
Kidney
Bone
OH
OH
HO
5

Fig. 3

4.2 Vitamin D_3

Deficiency of vitamin D_3 causes diseases of bone abnormalities such as rickets, osteomalacia etc. which are due to deficient mineralization of bone matrix. Owing to this involvement of vitamin D_3 in bone mineralization, its use in osteoporosis appears to be justified. It is commonly used in the treatment of osteoporosis even though its use is not approved by FDA. Vitamin D_3 required by the human body is acquired in two ways: i) the photo-conversion of 7-dehydrocholesterol (**1**) present in the skin by UV irradiation, and ii) through diet such as animal tissues, milk, vegetables etc., the former being the predominant source.
Vitamin D_3 has been found to be beneficial in osteoporotic patients [79, 80]. It promotes mineralization *in vitro*. Vitamin D_3 increases Ca absorption in the gastrointestinal tract and thereby inhibits PTH-mediated bone resorption. It also stimulates bone resorption in an indirect way [see sec. 4.2.1]. In a recent study on a large number of elderly women it was found that supplementation with calcium (1.2 g of elemental Ca) and vitamin D_3 (cholecalciferol 800 1U/day) reduced the risk of hip fractures and other nonvertebral fractures [81]. However, results obtained from use of vitamin D_3 are variable [82].

4.2.1 Mechanism of action

In the liver, vitamin D_3 (**2**) undergoes 25-hydroxylation, mainly through the action of a microsomal enzyme 25-hydroxylase, NADPH, molecular oxygen and Mg ions to give 25-hydroxy vitamin D_3 (**3**). This product **3** undergoes further hydroxylation in the kidney to form the metabolites 1,25-dihydroxy vitamin D_3 (**4**) and 24,25 dihydroxy D_3 (**5**) [83] [see Fig. 3]. Holick et al. [84] identified **4** as the active metabolite of vitamin D_3. It was also found that in elderly persons, there is a decline in the production of **4** [85]. This could be due to impaired vitamin D_3 metabolism with aging [86].
Stimulation of bone growth and mineralization induced by **4** is possibly indirect. It appears that **4** stimulates bone mineralization by increasing intestinal absorption of Ca and P and thereby providing minerals for incorporation into the bone matrix [87].
The bone resorption effect of vitamin D_3 observed in rat is not due to its direct effect on the osteoblast but is caused by its active metabolite **4** which stimulates osteoblastic cells to release a soluble factor that increases osteoclastic bone resorption [88].
1,25-Dihydroxy vitamin D_3 has been shown to increase epidermal growth factor receptors and transforming growth factor β-like activity in a bone-derived cell line [89].

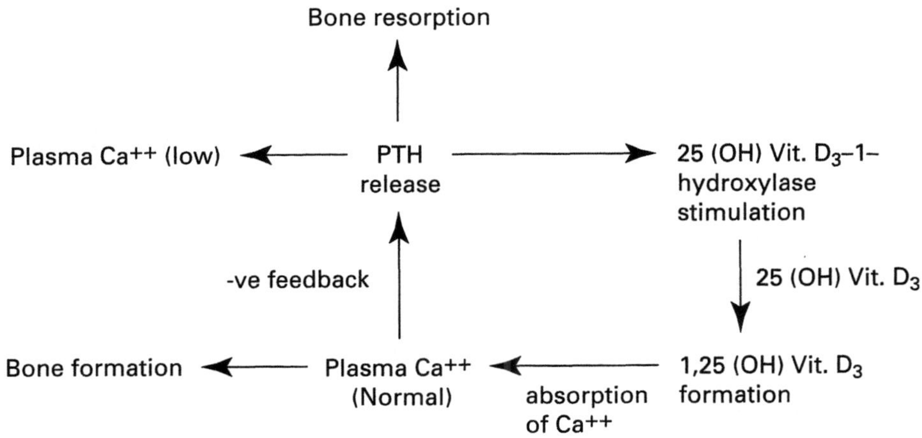

Fig. 4
Calcium regulation

Administration of **4** to rats causes an increase in the number of osteoclasts *in vivo* over a period of several days [90].
Biosynthesis of **4** is regulated by the plasma calcium concentration [91] and also of phosphorus [92] through regulation of the activity of 25(OH)-D_3-1-hydroxylase in the kidney. In this regulation process PTH plays a key role (Fig. 4). Shortage of plasma calcium (hypocalcemia) is sensed by the thyroid gland which secretes PTH. Parathyroid hormones thus produced stimulate 25(OH)vitamin D_3-1-hydroxylase in the kidney to convert 25(OH) vitamin D_3 to the active metabolite **4**; this in turn helps in the absorption of calcium from the intestine. In osteoporotic patients, it has been found that the plasma level of **4** is significantly low as compared to normal. In such cases Ca absorption through the gastrointestinal tract is low and possibly plasma calcium concentration is met with the supply from the skeleton under the influence of PTH.
Some of the studies have shown that there is no clinical benefit in patients with osteoporosis or normal elderly persons from vitamin D_3 [93] or 1,25-$(OH)_2$ vitamin D_3 [94, 95].

4.2.2 Side effects

Some toxicity in the use of vitamin D_3 complicating treatment has been reported [95]. Development of hypercalciuria and hypercalcemia have been observed in osteoporotic patients treated with higher doses of 1,25-$(OH)_2$ vitamin D_3. The side effects are dose related and lower doses of calcitriol up to 0.5 μg/day have been suggested [96]. Use of calcitriol may cause serious nephrotoxicity [97].

4.2.3 *Vitamin D_3 analogues in osteoporosis*

1,25-Dihydroxy-2β-(3-hydroxypropoxy) vitamin D_3 (ED-71, **6**) [Fig. 5] was found to increase plasma Ca level significantly in rats on a Ca-deficient diet [98]. It has been found to have preventive and therapeutic effects on bone mineral loss in ovariectomized rats [99]. It is more effective than **4**. Preparation of an ester of vitamin A with 1-hydroxy vitamin D_3 (**7**) has been reported [100] for the treatment of osteoporosis. Incorporation of vitamin A has presumably been made due to its importance in the distribution and activity of osteoblasts and osteoclasts and thereby, affect the balance between bone resorption and formation [101]. No biological activity data is reported.

Tachibana et al. [102] have reported the preparation of 1α-hydroxy vitamin D_7 (**8**) and D_4 (**9**) as anti-osteoporosis agents. 1α-Hydroxy vitamin D_7 maintains bone density in ovariectomized rats at 2.5 mg/kg/day dose.

1,25R,26-Trihydroxy-22-ene D_3 (**10**) [103] has been reported to be effective in bone loss reversal in type I osteoporosis. This compound at 100 ng/kg dose in beagle dogs was as effective as 15 ng/kg of calcitriol (**4**) in reversing bone loss associated with cessation of ovarian function without the side effects of calcitriol in inducing hypercalcemia.

1α,25-Dihydroxy-22(E)-dehydro vitamin D_3 (**11**) [104] and 1α,24(R)-dihydroxy-22(E)-dehydro vitamin D_3 (**12**) [105] have been recently reported to be effective in the treatment of postmenopausal, senile and steroid-induced osteoporosis.

23(S),25(R)-1,25-Dihydroxy vitamin D_3-26,23-lactone (**13**) at a low dose of 1 μg/kg was found to stimulate bone formation by enhancing bone matrix formation in osteoporotic rats [106].

The cyclopropyl derivative MC 903 (**14**) has been tested in rats and was found to be 100-fold less active than **4** and 1α(OH)D_3 (**16**) in causing hypercalciuria, hypercalcemia and bone calcium metabolism [107].

Preparation of 24,25-dihydroxy vitamin D_3 derivatives for the treatment of osteoporosis has been recently reported [108]. Of these, compound **15** (R = H) showed an increase in bone mass as compared to the control group at 1 n mol/kg doses for 3 weeks in rats. 1α-Hydroxy derivative of vitamin D_3 is a very potent analogue of 1α,25$(OH)_2$ vitamin D_3 and proved to be approximately equal to 1α,25$(OH)_2$ vitamin D_3 in inducing intestinal calcium transport and bone calcium mobilization in normal rats [109].

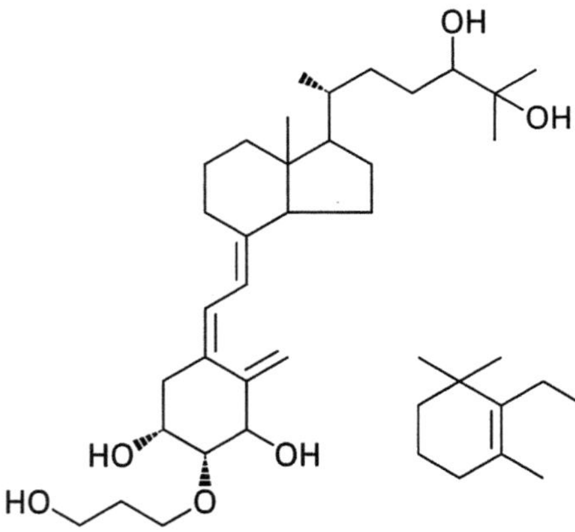

6

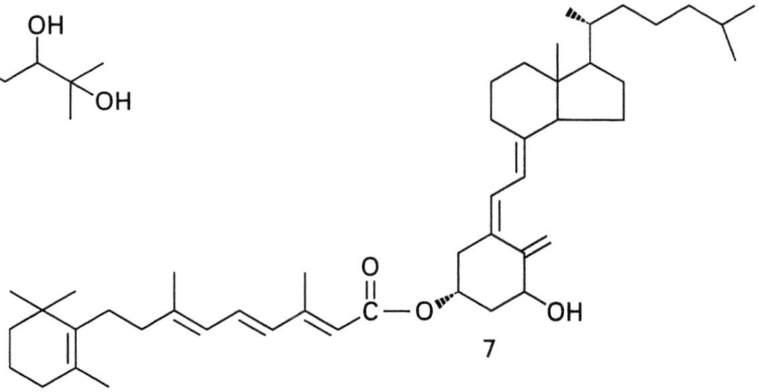

7

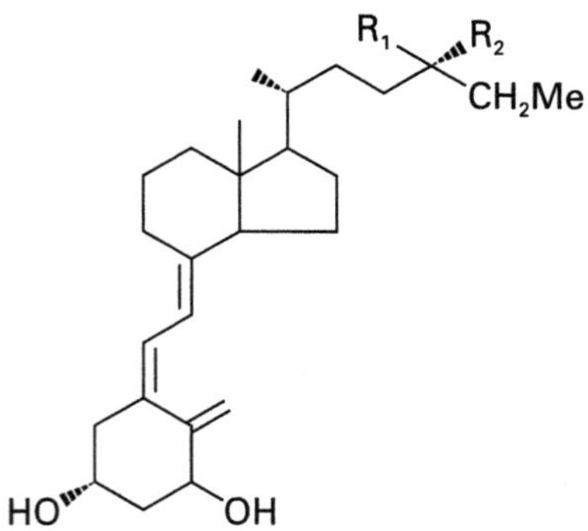

8 R_1=Me, R_2=H
9 R_1=H, R_2=Me

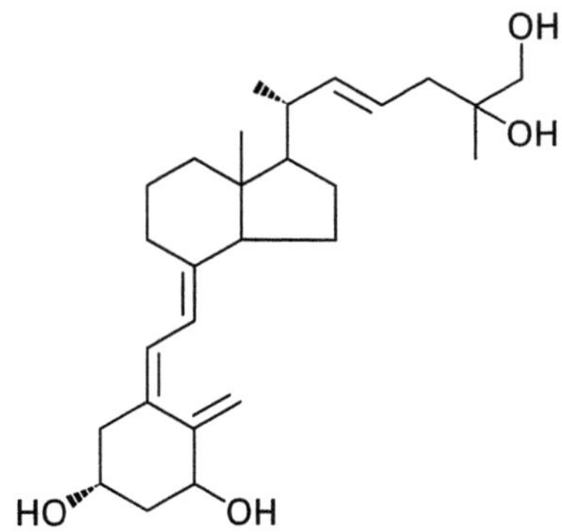

10

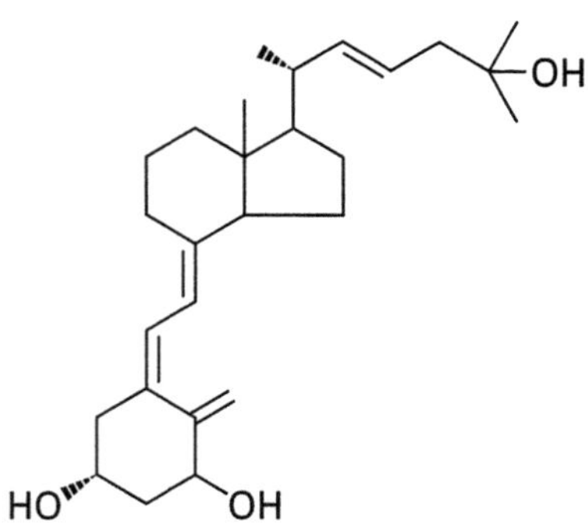

11

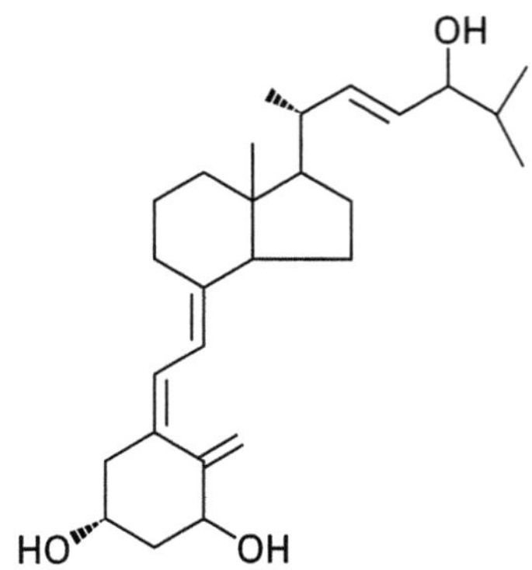

12

Fig. 5

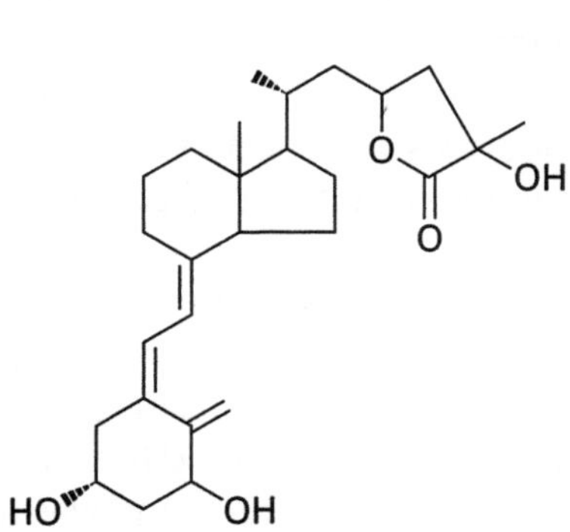

13

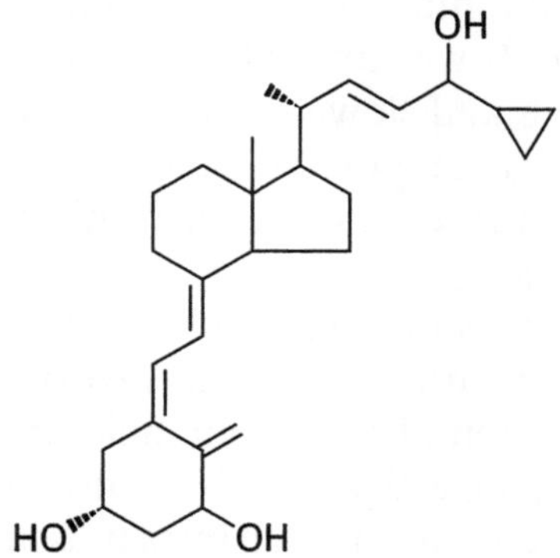

14

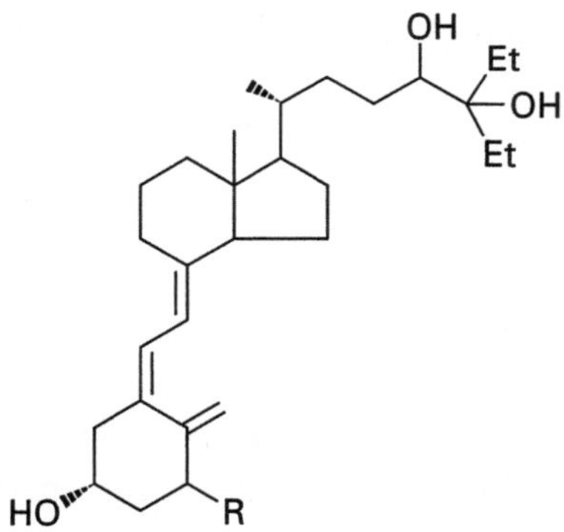

15

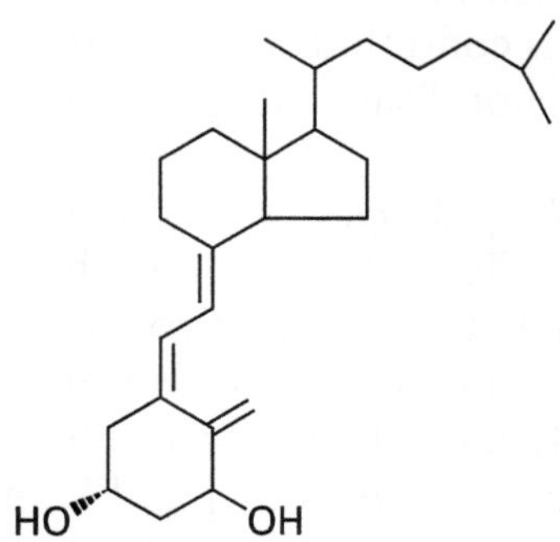

16

Fig. 5 (Continued)

1α(OH) vitamin D_3, "One-Alpha", a prodrug at low doses (0.75 μg/day) has shown a similar positive effect on bone formation as the natural vitamin D derivatives and is not associated with toxicity problems [110].

4.3 Calcitonin

Calcitonins are polypeptide hormones produced by the parafollicular or C-cells from the thyroid glands [111]. It is made up of 33 amino acids and has a mass in the range 3,500 daltons.

Calcitonin inhibits osteoclast activity and thereby prevents bone resorption. It was found [112] that calcitonin improved mineral content in the bone and slowed down loss of femoral bone in patients with high-turnover osteoporosis. Since old-age osteoporosis of type II is generally of low-turnover type, calcitonin has not been proved to be effective in such cases.

Efficacy of calcitonin in preventing bone loss in postmenopausal women has been shown by many workers [113–117]. Alternative routes of administration of calcitonin including rectal suppository and nasal spray have been investigated [118]. Intranasal administration was found to be equally effective as through intra muscular (im) injection [119, 120], and was found to have better tolerance compared to im route [121]. Recently in a one-year study, it was shown that the use of calcitonin suppository in postmenopausal women did not change the bone mineral density [122]. Use of calcitonin has been found to be helpful in patients where estrogen therapy is contraindicated [123].

A major disadvantage in the use of calcitonin is its high cost.

4.3.1 Mechanism of action

The effect of calcitonin observed in post-menopausal women is very similar to that of estrogen (E_2) treatment. A lowering of circulating calcitonin in a oophorectomized or postmenopausal state was reported [124] and estrogens were found to increase calcitonin level [125–127]. In an *in vitro* study [128] E_2 was found to enhance calcitonin production by C-cells. However, binding of calcitonin to high affinity receptors on osteoclasts was also observed [129–131], which would imply its direct action on osteoblasts. Thus, it is unclear whether the effect of E_2 in inhibiting bone resorption is mediated via increased plasma calcitonin levels.

Administration of calcitonin caused osteoclasts to move away from the bone resorption surface [132] and was also found to alter the ruffled surface structure of osteoclast which is needed for bone resorption [133]. Calcitonin also effected reduction in life span and number of osteoclasts. This could be due to inhibition of the fusion of mononuclear marrow cells which lead to osteoclast formation [134].

4.3.2 Side effects and safety

Tachyphylaxis can develop in some individuals under calcitonin treatment [135]. However, long-term administration of calcitonin in humans was found to be safe and devoid of any serious side effects [136].

4.4 Bisphosphonates

Bisphosphonates are synthetic compounds in which the P–O–P bond of pyrophosphate (**17**), a naturally occurring inhibitor of bone mineralization, has been replaced by a non-hydrolyzable P–C–P bond. These compounds have two phosphate chains of which one enables the compound to bind strongly to the hydroxyapatite crystals of the bone and the other contributes towards the biological properties and potency of the compound [137].
A number of bisphosphonates (Figure 6) showed suppression of osteoclast mediated bone resorption. Due to this anti-resorptive property, their use in the treatment of osteoporosis is indicated. Bisphosphonates generally show poor oral absorption, accounting for approximately 1–5% of the dose administered. Their elimination from the skeleton is extremely slow.

Etidronate disodium [Disodium ethane-1-hydroxy-1,1-bisphosphonate, EHDP (**18**)]:
Etidronate (**18**) is an oral preparation used for reducing bone resorption. Its continuous administration to postmenopausal osteoporotic patients at a dose of 20 mg/kg body weight per day for 6 to 12 months resulted in a 50% reduction in bone resorption and significant increase in calcium balance [138]. In a study of 66 women with postmenopausal osteoporosis a cyclic administration of **18** (400 mg/day for 2 weeks followed by 13 week gap) for 150 weeks with daily supplements of calcium and vitamin D_3 showed a significant increase in vertebral bone mineral content [139]. In another similar study a noticeable increase in the spinal bone density was observed [140].

Pamidronate disodium [Disodium (3-amino-1-hydroxypropylidene)-1,1-bisphosphonate, APD (**19**)]:
Pamidronate was found to possess osteoclastic inhibiting activity [141]. Administration of APD (150 mg/day) and calcium (1 g/day) produced a significant increase in the metacarpal cortical area and vertebral mineral density in 1 year in glucocorticoid-induced osteoporosis [142]. In animal studies **19** was found to increase bone mass in normal rats [143] and pigs [144]. It also prevents bone loss in Paget's disease [145].
Long term intermittent administration of **19** to osteoporosis patients showed an initial increase in bone density in the first two years followed by a decrease [146].

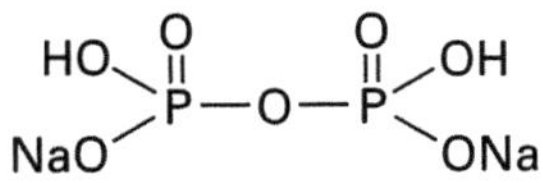

17

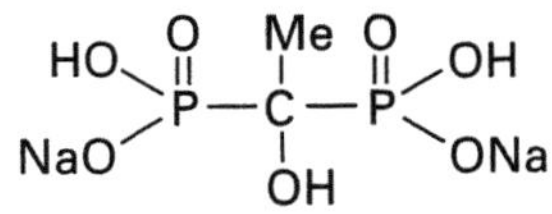

18

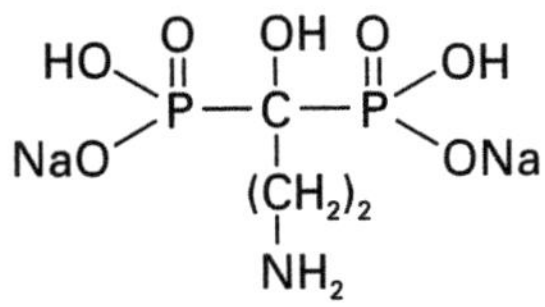

19

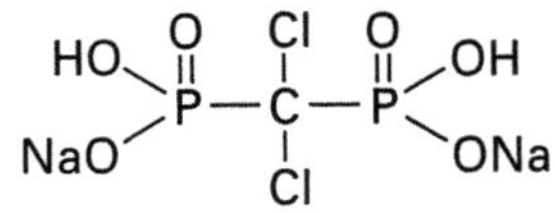

20

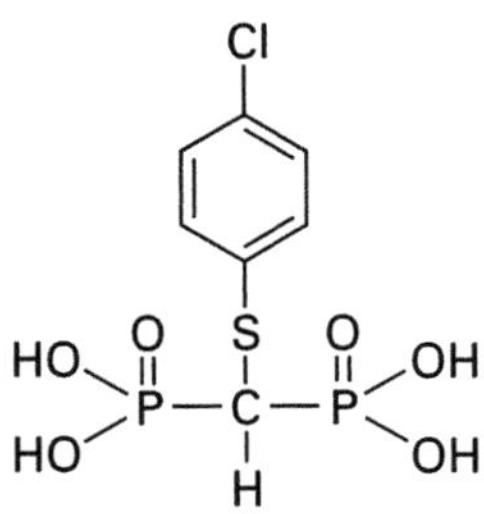

21

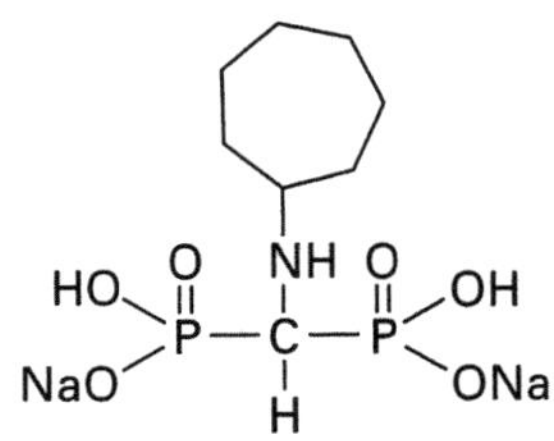

22

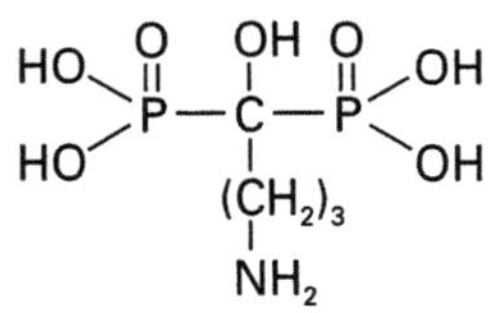

23

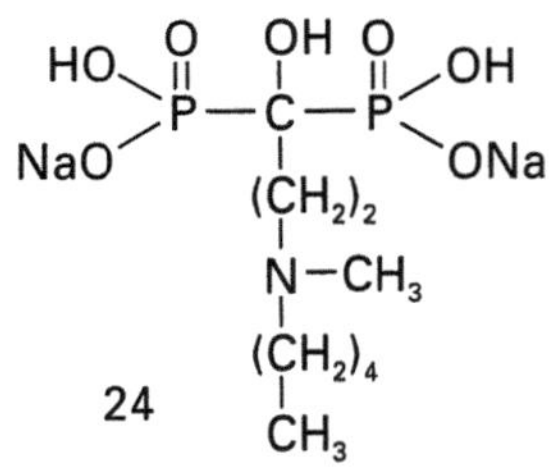

24

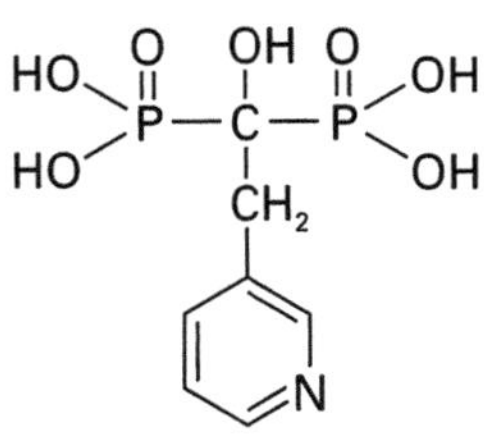

25

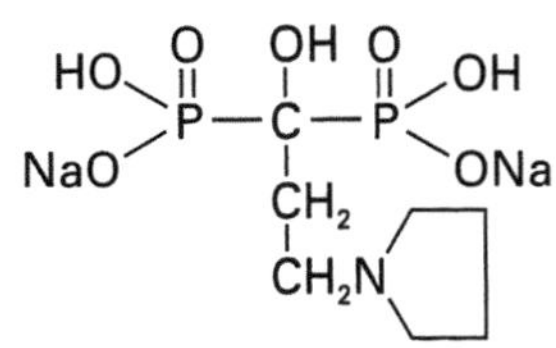

26

Fig. 6

Prolonged treatment with **19** did not show any important clinical side effect [147].

Clodronate [Dichloromethylene bisphosphonate, Cl_2 MBP (**20**)]:
In a study of 52 women with postmenopausal osteoporosis, oral administration of clodronate (**20**) 400 mg/day intermittently (once in 3 months) for one year, caused a significant increase in lumber bone density [148].

Tiludronate [(Chloro-4-phenylthiomethylene)bisphosphbonate, SR 41319 (**21**)]:
In a study conducted on 78 healthy postmenopausal women for one year, tiludronate (21) was found to check the decrease in bone mass density of the lumber spine [149]. Tiludronate has significant anti-osteoclast activity and mineralization defects were only seen at dose levels much higher than those required to decrease bone resorption [150].
More recently , a number of other bisphosphonate compounds have been shown to possess an anti-resorptive effect. YM 175 [disodium dihydrogen (cycloheptylamino) methylene-1,1-bisphosphonate (**22**)] [151], alendronate [4-amino-1-hydroxybutylidene (**23**)] [152], BM 210955 [(1-hydroxy-3-(methylpentylamino)propylidene] bisphosphonate (**24**)] [153, 154], risedronate [1-hydroxy-2-(3-pyridyl) ethylidene bisphosphonic acid (**25**)] [154], EB-1053 [(1-hydroxy-3-(1-pyrrolidinyl)propylidene] disodium bisphosphonate (**26**)] [155] are at different developmental stages. YM 175 produces an anti- resorptive effect without causing osteomalacia even at toxic doses [151].
Of the bisphosphonates mentioned above, only **18** is currently registered for the treatment of osteoporosis.
Bisphosphonates have been generally administered intermittently. This is to allow a normal period of bone formation after a short period of suppression of bone resorption leading to a positive bone balance and to minimize an adverse effect of the drug if any, on the mineralization of newly formed bones [156].

4.4.1 Mechanism of action

In *in vitro* studies bisphosphonates were found to prevent the conversion of amorphous calcium phosphate into hydroxyapatite [157, 158]. Nitrogen-containing bisphosphonates, at clinical doses, do not act through toxicity to osteoclasts or their precursors but possibly through the interference with the essential processes needed for activation of the osteoclasts [159–162]. Bisphosphonates may alter the morphology of osteoclasts, thereby inhibiting their activity [163]. YM 175 stimulates the renal production of $1,25(OH)_2$ vitamin D_3 in the serum by activating renal 25-(OH)vitamin D_3-1-hydroxylase indirectly but via some unknown factor.

4.4.2 Side effects

At high doses, all bisphosphonates may be toxic to osteoclast. Approximately 3% of the patients, during the treatment of clodronate, developed mild hypocalcemia and gastrointestinal disorders including nausea, vomitting diarrhea and epigastric pain developed in 1.8% [163]. Pamidronate has been found to cause a rise in temperature and the alteration of white cell count distribution in some patients [164]. Clodronate administration has been associated with bronchoconstriction in an aspirin-sensitive asthmatic patient [165]. Rapid bolus injection of clodronate (200 to 1500 mg/kg for 30 days could lead to acute renal failure.This type of nephrotoxicity could be avoided by slow intravenous infusion over 2 or 3 hours.

High doses of etidronate given continuously to patients with osteoporosis, induced osteomalacia [166]. Unlike pamidronate and etidronate, clodronate did not cause defective bone mineralization. Compared to **19** it showed a lower incidence of gastrointestinal problems. Clodronate appears to be more suitable than other bisphosphonates, especially in long-term therapy [163].

4.5 Estrogens and Hormone Replacement Therapy (HRT)

It is well established that estrogen deficiency is linked with the genesis of postmenopausal bone loss [167] and subsequent development of osteoporosis. Alterations in bone metabolism during the estrus cycle of rats [168] and menstrual cycle in women [169] have been reported , suggesting skeletal responsiveness to estrogen status. Thus, cessation of estrogen release upon attaining menopause or after oophorectomy results in rapid bone loss [170] which can be restored by exogenous estrogen therapy [171–174].

Use of progestins along with estrogens as hormone replacement therapy in postmenopausal women, has been found to be beneficial [175, 176] in postmenopausal osteoporosis.

A daily administration of 17β-estradiol (**27**) (2 mg) , norethisterone (**29**) (1 mg) , and calcium (500 mg) to postmenopausal women showed a significant increase in the bone mass of the spine and forearm [176].

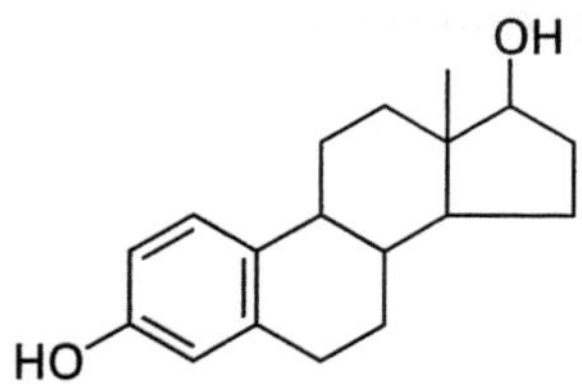

27

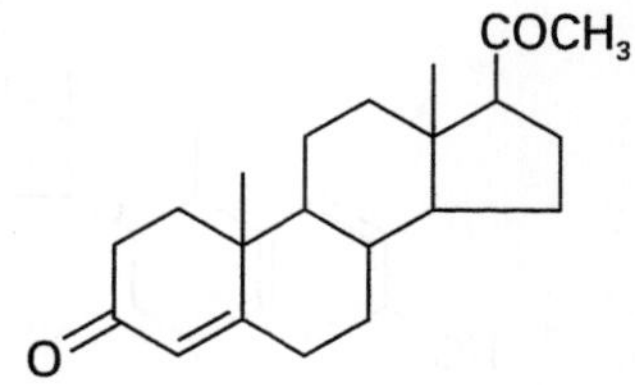

28

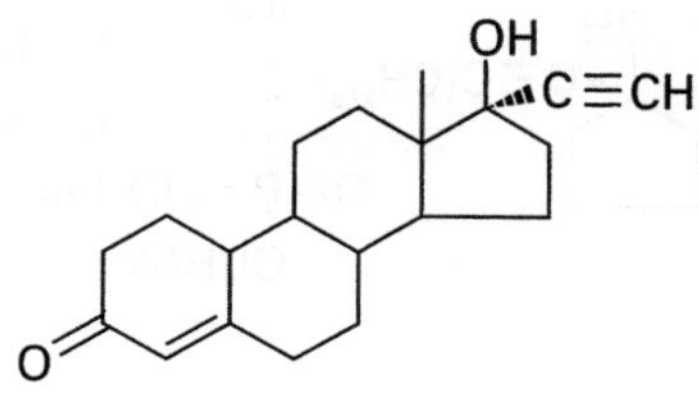

29

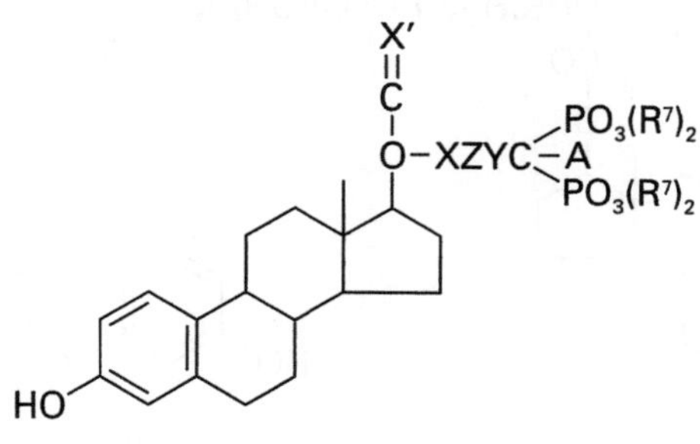

30

A=H, OH, alkylamino; R^7=H, alkyl;
X=$CR^1R^2(CR^3R^4)m$ $(CR^5R^6)n$ $(CH^2)r$;
R^1–R^6=H, Ph, cyclohexyl, alkyl,
alkenyl, (phenyl)alkenyl;
R^1R^2, R^1R^5=atoms to complete 3–6 membered rings;
X1=O,S; Y=C_{1-6} alkene; Z=CONH,NHCO

Fig. 7

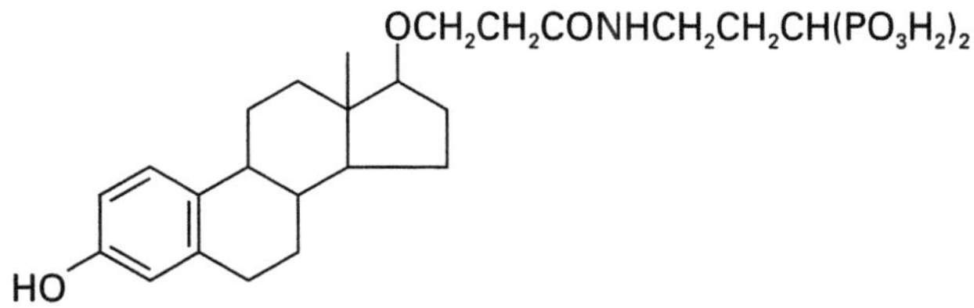

31

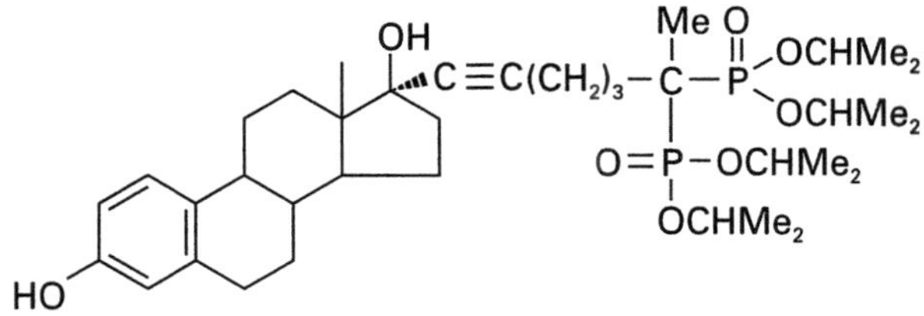

32

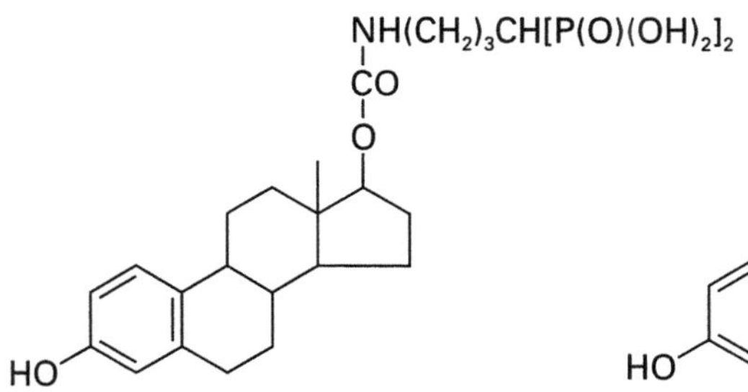

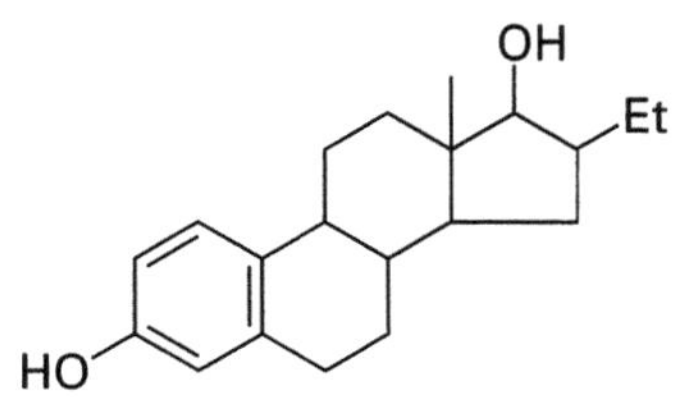

33

34

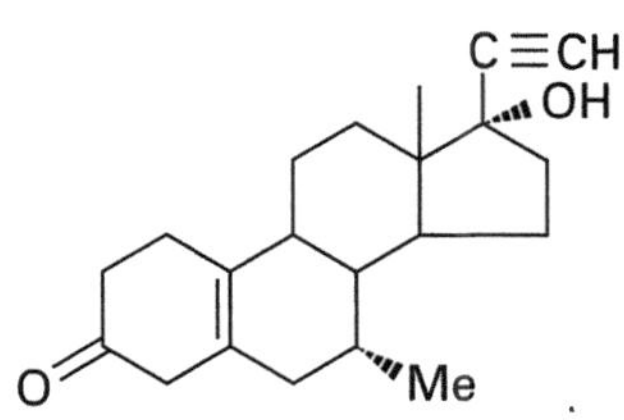

35

Fig. 7 (Continued)

Most commonly estrogens are given via oral or transdermal routes of administration. The dose of the estrogen administered appears to be critical for its effect on the skeleton. Different doses have been used for different estrogens or their combinations [177–183].

Estrogens cause depression in bone turnover primarily by decreasing bone resorption. Treatment with estrogens for some time leads to depressed bone formation [184]. Progestogens (progesterone, **28**) given alone may prevent bone loss without reducing bone formation [175, 185].

In normal menopausal patients, estrogens are generally given with progestins to protect the endometrium. Progestin is not given to those women who have undergone a hysterectomy [182].

Some estradiol diphosphate derivatives (**30–33**) which have been recently reported [186–188] for the treatment of osteoporosis are shown in Figure 7. Details for these patented compounds is not available. The 16-ethyl estradiol (**34**) [189] at 10 mg/ml inhibited 74.7% of Ca in rat embryo bone v.s. 81.0% for estradiol.

The norpregnane derivative Org OD 14 [19-norpregn-5(10)-en-20-yn-one, 17-hydroxy-7-methyl-,(7α,17α) (**35**)], with weak estrogenic, androgenic and progestational activities has been found to reduce bone resorption, without reducing serum Ca level [190–192].

4.5.1 Mechanism of action

The mechanism by which estrogen deficiency causes loss of bone is not very clear. One of the hypothesis which has been put forward is its indirect action via increase in serum calcitonin concentration [125, 193, 194]. On the other hand, estrogen receptors have been found in osteoblasts [195], several osteoblast-like cell lines [196, 197] and osteoclasts [198], which show physiological response on estrogen challenge. Also, avian osteoclasts were found to produce estrogen receptor mRNA and to exhibit estrogen dose dependent inhibition of bone resorption [198, 129]. Such findings would suggest that estrogen can directly affect bone metabolism through osteoblasts, osteoclasts or both.

Estrogen has also been found to stimulate formation of 1,25$(OH)_2$ vitamin D_3 in the kidney [199] and can reduce urinary calcium excretion in postmenopausal women [200].

4.5.2 Side effects

Estrogen therapy given to postmenopausal women has been found to increase the risk of endometrial cancer [201]. Higher incidence of hypertension, venous thrombosis and gallstones are some other side effects associated with estrogen treatment [202, 203].

4.6 Weak estrogens and anti-estrogens

Weak estrogens and anti-estrogens have an element of similarity in their molecular structure to that of potent estrogens. Generally these compounds also possess an inherent estrogenic property [204] but they may show different biological activities. Only in the recent past, some members of this class (**36–41**, Figure 8) have shown very promising activity in the treatment of postmenopausal osteoporosis and, therefore, this group of compounds deserve a separate treatment.

Ipriflavone [7-Isopropoxy-3-phenyl-4H-1-benzopyran-4-one, (**36**)]:

Ipriflavone (**36**) was found to increase the calcium concentration in the bone when administered orally to rats, sheep and chicken [205–207]. On oral administration it showed rapid absorption and was extensively metabolized [208].

Administration of **36** decreased bone remodeling and prevented bone loss in postmenopausal osteoporosis [209–212]. It also showed a beneficial effect on bone pain [213].

Ipriflavone did not show any direct estrogen-like activity [214], but when given along with low doses of estrogens, it enhanced the protective effects of estrogen on bone demineralization [215].

Ipriflavone, when administered in proper doses [110] was found to be safe and effective in preventing bone loss in acute ovarian-deficient states and in postmenopausal osteoporosis.

Clomiphene [2-[4-Chloro-1,(2-diphenyl ethenyl) phenoxy] - N,N-diethylethanamine, (**37**)]:

Clomiphene citrate (**37**) is an antiestrogen associated with significant estrogenic activity [216, 217]. Its trans isomer, enclomiphene, is predominantly antiestrogenic while the cis isomer zuclomiphene is estrogenic. It was found to prevent bone mineral loss in ovariectomized rats [218, 219] without any adverse, uterine or pituitary consequences.

Long-term administration of clomiphene to ovariectomized rats prevented osteoporosis and maintained the cortical bone thickness and total body calcium [220].

Tamoxifen [2-[4-(1,2-Diphenyl-1-butenyl) phenoxy]-N,N-dimethylethanamine, (**38**)]:

Tamoxifen (**38**) is in general a more potent antiestrogen compared to clomiphene. However, its antagonistic activity is species dependent. It behaves like a partial antagonist in rat uterus, a pure agonist in mouse and a pure antagonist in bird oviduct [221].

In birds, administration of **38** resulted in bone resorption and it prevented further development of medullary bone in estrogen-treated

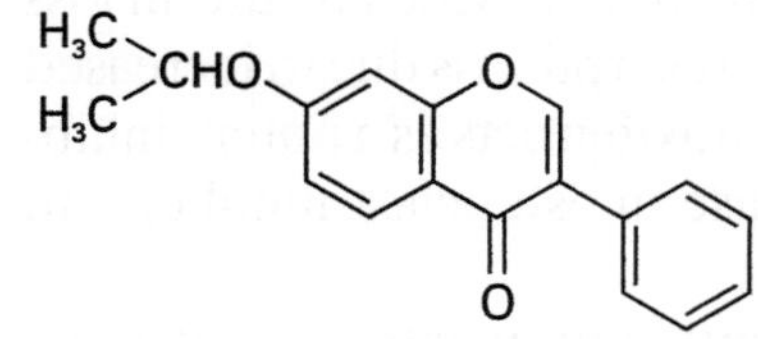

36

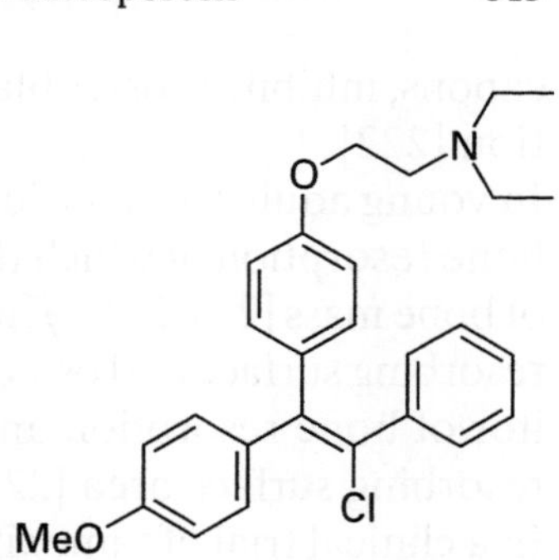

37

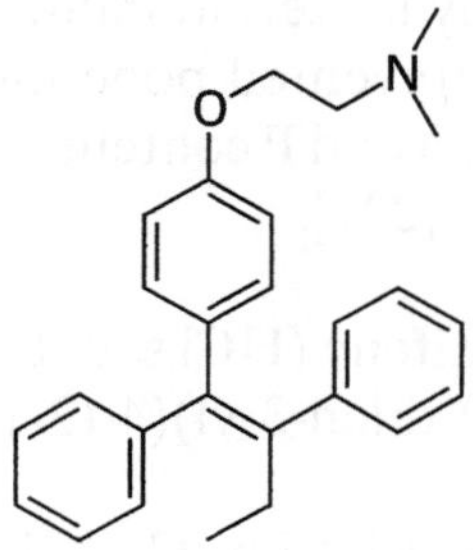

38

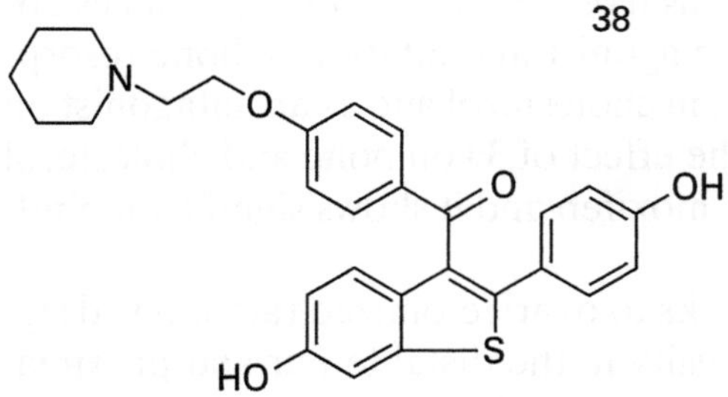

39

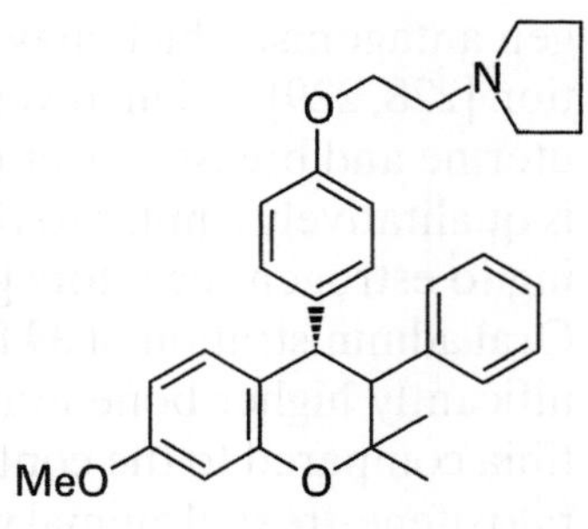

40

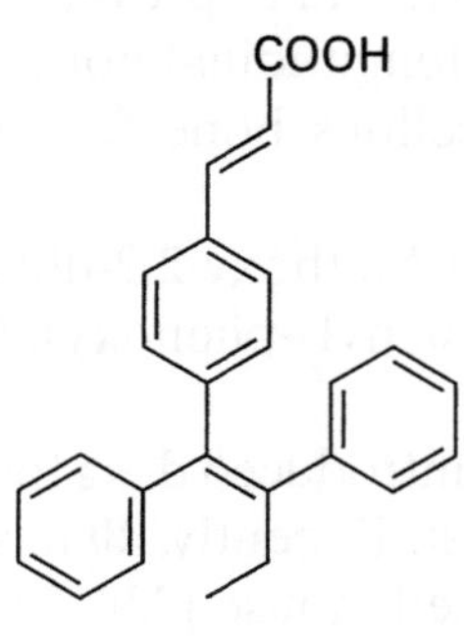

41

Fig. 8

capons, inhibiting osteoblastic function and inducing osteoclastic resorption [222].

In young adult rats, ovariectomy results in increased bone formation and bone resorption of which the latter takes precedence, which results in loss of bone mass [223, 224]. This increase in bone resorption is due to increased resorbing surface and osteoclast number. Tamoxifen acts as a potent inhibitor of bone resorption and prevents increase in osteoclast number and resorbing surface area [225].

In a clinical trial of tamoxifen alone or in combination with prednisolone in postmenopausal women with operable breast cancer, **38** was found to prevent bone loss, particularly in steroid induced patients [226].

In ovariectomized mice, **38** prevented bone loss and also any decrease either in the bone density or Ca and P content of femur. Thus it acted like a true estrogen in this species [227].

Raloxifene [LY 139481], Keoxifene (HCl·salt, LY 156758) [(6-hydroxy-2-(4-hydroxyphenyl) benzo (b) thien-3-yl)(4-(2-1-piperidyl) ethoxy) phenyl methanone (**39**)]:

Raloxifene (**39**), developed by Eli Lilly, USA, is the most studied antiestrogen for its effect in postmenopausal osteoporosis. It is a partial estrogen antagonist which may act as an agonist in inhibition of bone resorption [228, 229] and in lowering serum cholesterol and as an antagonist on uterine and breast cancer cells. The effect of **39** on bone and cholesterol is qualitatively similar to that of tamoxifen and it shows significant binding to estrogen receptors [230].

Oral administration of **39** for 5 weeks to ovariectomized rats showed significantly higher bone mineral density in the distal femur and proximal tibia compared to the control group. Serum cholesterol was lower in the raloxifene-treated animal without causing uterine hypertrophy in ovariectomized rats [231]. It was also found to prevent cancellous osteopenia as well as changes in radial and longitudinal bone growth, bone resorption and cause reduction in cancellous bone formation in ovariectomized Sprague Dawley rats [232].

Centchroman [trans-1-(2-(4-(7-Methoxy-2,2-dimethyl-3-phenyl-3,4-dihydro-2H-1-benzopyran-4-yl)-phenyl)-phenoxy)ethyl-pyrrolidine hydrochloride] (**40**)]:

Centchroman (**40**), a recently introduced drug for fertility regulation [233] is a partial estrogen antagonist. Recently, **40** has been shown to prevent bone loss in the ovariectomized mouse [234, 235]. Administration of **40** (2 x 50 μg/week) to ovariectomized mice prevented decrease in cancellous bone area of the distal femur, without causing hypertrophy.

3-[4-(1,2-Diphenylbut-1-enyl)phenyl]acrylic acid (**41**) was found to prevent loss of bone mineral density in lumber spine and the tibia in 90-day-old estrogen-deficient ovariectomized rats. Oral administration of 10 µmol/kg of **41** or tamoxifen maintained bone mineral density in rats for the duration of a 28 day-study [236].

4.6.1 Mechanism of action

The mechanism of action of antiestrogens in preventing osteoporosis is complicated and not well understood. It has been shown that ipriflavone inhibits bone resorption by directly affecting both osteoblastic growth and differentiation [237]. In *in vitro* studies, ipriflavone has been found to inhibit resorption and osteoclastogenesis [238–240]. The partial estrogen agonistic property of this class of compounds, in general, may explain their role in bone remodeling and could involve the same mechanism as is the case with estrogens. This could be particularly true for clomiphene, which is an isomeric mixture, having the cis form zuclomiphene as an estrogen. Whether the overall estrogenic property of the isomeric mixture of clomiphene is responsible for the observed bone resorption inhibitory activity is uncertain [219].

Tamoxifen has been found to act as an estrogen agonist on bone resorption [241]. The possibility of trans-tamoxifen isomerizing to the estrogenic cis-form in biophase cannot be ruled out. Tamoxifen has been found to antagonize PTH-mediated bone resorption [244]. For raloxifene it has been suggested that it may be acting as an agonist on bone cell estrogen receptors [228, 229].

Antiestrogens have the ability to bind to estrogen receptors. They may directly interact with estrogen receptors present on the osteoblast and osteoclast cells [243, 244] and may be able to distinguish between the two classes of estrogen target cells.

4.6.2 Side effects of weak estrogens and antiestrogens

There is always a possibility that the inherent estrogenicity generally associated with weak estrogens and antiestrogens may cause the side effects seen with estrogens, but in a subdued scale. However, the success of developing an antiestrogen for osteoporosis lies in a situation when the osteoporotic dose is less than the estrogenic dose as has been shown for raloxifene [245].

Tamoxifen has been shown to cause a defeminizing effect in newborn female rats without effecting masculinization. It has been found that female sexual differentiation of the brain does not proceed normally under estrogen-free conditions [246].

Tamoxifen has been found to cause a dose-related increase in the incidence of hepatocellular tumors [247].

4.7 Fluorides

Fluoride is a diet essential for normal dental and skeletal growth [248]. It is one of the most potent stimulators of bone formation in patients with osteoporosis [249, 250] and has been in use for over 30 years in the management of this disease.
Sodium fluoride (NaF) has been used in clinical studies extensively. More recently disodium monofluoro phosphate (Na_2PO_4F) has been used for the treatment of osteoporosis [251].
The use of NaF in combination with Ca and vitamin D_3 [252, 253] was found to be beneficial in improving the quality of bone formation. Calcium supplementation abolishes the increase in the bone resorption surface as seen with vitamin D_3 or NaF alone [251]. NaF in combination with Ca and estrogen for the treatment of postmenopausal osteoporosis was found to be most effective [250].

4.7.1 Mechanism of action

Fluoride directly stimulates proliferation and alkaline phosphatase activity of bone-forming cells [254]. It reduces the conversion of amorphous calcium phosphate to octacalcium phosphate and also promotes the hydrolysis of octacalcium phosphate to hydroxyapatite. At physiological concentrations, fluoride enhances the development of a more stable bone apatite. In bone apatite, hydroxyl ions are less than hydroxyapatite, resulting in open space [255] which reduces the stability of the apatite lattice. Hydrogen and fluorine being isomorphic, substitution by fluoride occurs during nucleation and growth. Fluorapatite and fluorohydroxyapatite are less soluble than hydroxyapatite and resist osteoclastically mediated bone resorption.
Physiological concentration of fluoride (2 mg/day) appears to enhance hydroxyapatite formation, therapeutic quantities promote the production of fluorapatite, increasing the stability of the mineral phase and toxic amounts of fluoride cause impairment of crystal morphology [251].
Therapeutic use of fluoride increase the number of osteoblasts. At higher doses, the osteoblasts appear less plump than normal [256, 257] and its functional capacity is impaired, resulting in woven rather than lamellar bone formation [258].

4.7.2 Side effects

A major concern in the use of NaF has been that it may lead to the production of ill-formed bones. It has also been observed that the bone mass may form at the expense of bone from another site. In particular, fluoride may increase trabecular bone while reducing cortical bone [24].
Another important side effect associated with fluoride use is gastrointestinal irritation causing nausea, vomiting, pains and diarrhea [250]. The frequency and propensity of the side effect depends on the dose of fluoride administered, its formulation and the time of administration [259]. Fewer gastrointestinal side effects are reported with sustained release or enteric-coated preparations [260, 261] and are less frequent with sodium monofluorophosphate [251]. It is less when taken with food.
Osteoarticular pain, particularly of the lower extremities, is another major side effect of fluoride use. It could be due to microfractures which develop during use [262].
Higher fracture rates have been observed in patients using fluoride [263, 264]. This could be due to improper mineralization and loss of elasticity of fluoride bones.

4.8 Parathyroid hormone

Involvement of parathyroid hormone (PTH) in osteoporosis has been mentioned above in sections 4.1.1 and 4.2.1. Further, animal studies have shown that PTH in higher concentration leads to bone resorption while in lower doses it stimulates bone formation [265]. Treatment with the hPTH (1-34), which is a segment of the intact 84 amino acid hormone, has been found to have a bone formation stimulating effect. A 100 μg daily injection of hPTH (1-34) was effective in enhancing bone turnover significantly [266].

4.8.1 Mechanism of action

In *in vitro* studies with rat bone cells and human osteoblast-like cells, PTH was found to increase production of IGF-1 and TGF-β. Both these growth factors may be responsible for the anabolic effects of PTH on bone [267].

4.8.2 Side effects

It has been found that increases in cancellous bone formation during treatment with PTH is associated with the loss of cortical bone, a problem seen with fluoride treatment [24]. This occurs because of Ca withdrawal from cortical bones for the mineralization of cancellous bone mass.

4.9 Miscellaneous compounds

A large number of compounds which do not belong to the classes mentioned earlier but show activity in the treatment of osteoporosis are also known. Detailed studies on only a few compounds are available and the rest are covered under patents with very little disclosure regarding their activity. Some of these compounds shown in Figure 9 are mentioned below to give an idea about the molecular structures which could be of interest for further exploitation in developing agents for the treatment of osteoporosis. However, the list is mainly from recent reports and is by far not an exhaustive one.

Thiazide:
Thiazide diuretics, bendroflumithiazide [3,4-dihydro-3-(phenylmethyl)-6-(trifluoromethyl)-2H-1,2,4-benzothiadiazine-7-sulfonamide 1,1-dioxide (**42**)], chlorothiazide [6-chloro-2H-1,2,4-benzothiadizine-7-sulfonamide 1,1-dioxide (**43**)], hydrochlorothiazide [6-chloro-3,4-dihydro-2H-1,2,4-benzothiadiazine-7-sulfonamide 1,1-dioxide (**44**)] [268–270] shown in Figure 9, reduce urinary calcium concentration and thereby improve calcium balance which is helpful in treating osteoporosis. Studies conducted with thiazide diuretic [268, 271, 272] showed that hypertensive men (50–80 years old) on **44** (25 mg) were found to have higher bone mineral content than those patients who had not taken thiazide or individual without hypertension.

S 12911 [3-[(3-Cyano-4-carboxymethyl-5-carboxy)-2-thienyl]-3-azapentanedioic acid, distrontium salt (**45**)]:
Strontium is a natural trace element belonging to the same group as calcium in the periodic table. When taken orally, it replaces calcium in the bone preferably in areas of active bone remodeling [273]. With increased strontium intake, its amount in the bone mineral increases [274]. At a higher level (1.5–3.0% of the dietary intake) with decrease in bone calcium it causes "strontium rickets" [275].
Strontium chloride and S 12911 (**45**) have been used for the treatment of osteoporosis. Clinical trials of strontium salt in low doses showed increased bone mass [276] in osteoporotic patients.
Studies in rats showed low doses of strontium chloride stimulated bone formation and inhibited bone resorption [277]. Dietary Sr has a marked effect on 1,25-$(OH)_2$ vitamin D_3 production [91]. In high doses it influenced the quality of bone mineral, with a decrease in size and strain of the crystals [278].

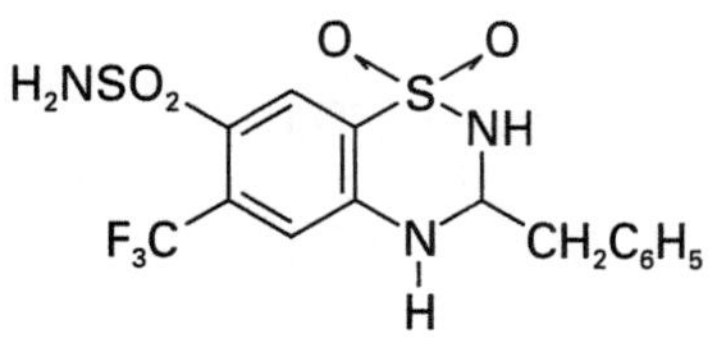

42

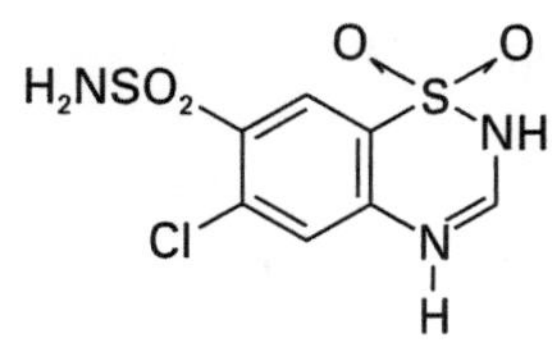

43

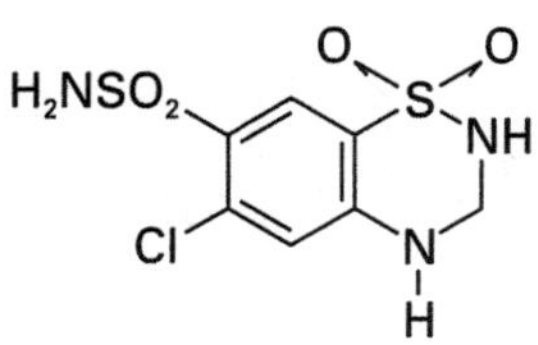

44

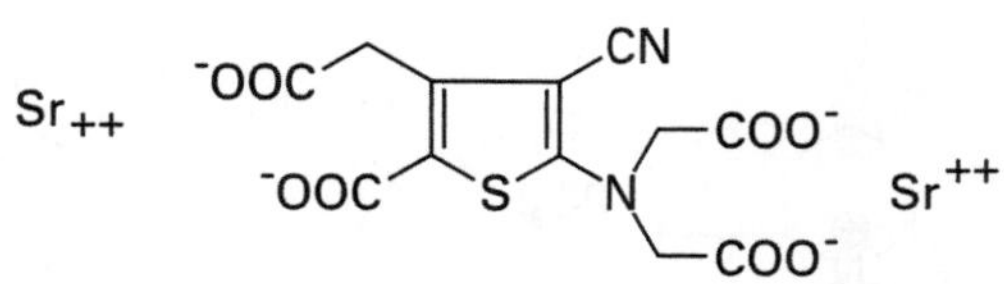

45

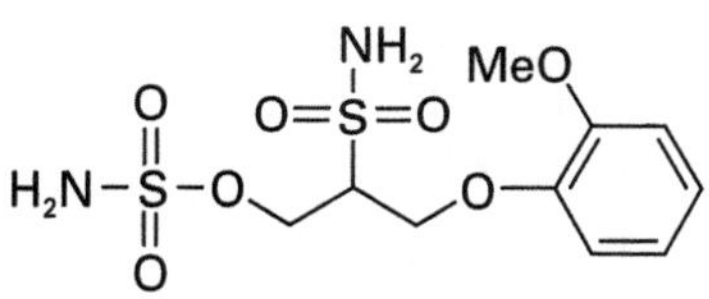

46

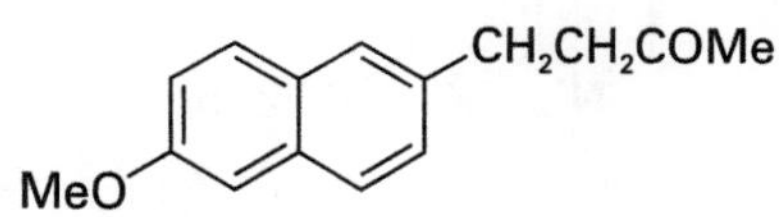

47

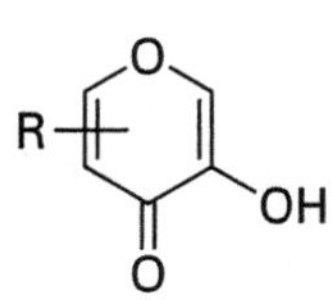

48 R=C_{1-6} hydrocarbyl

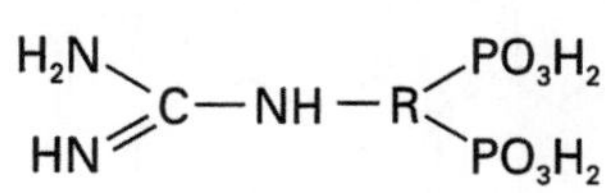

49

Fig. 9

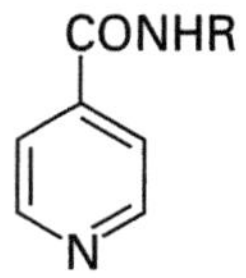

50

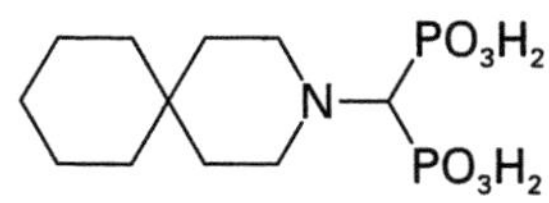

51

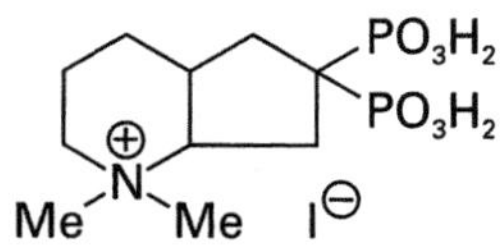

52

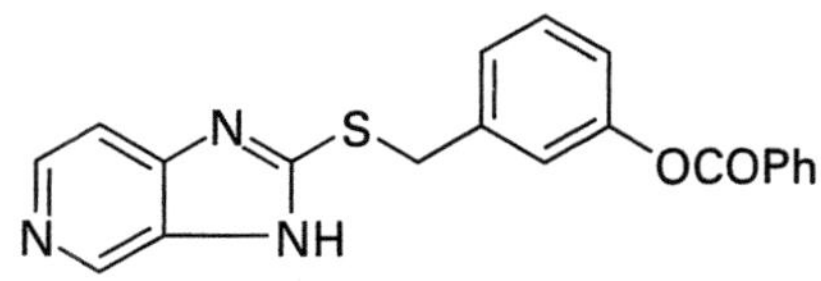

53

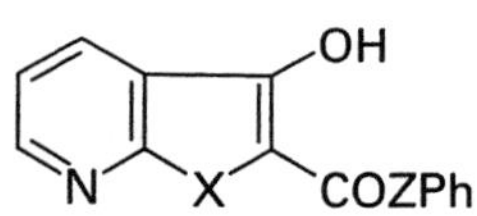

54

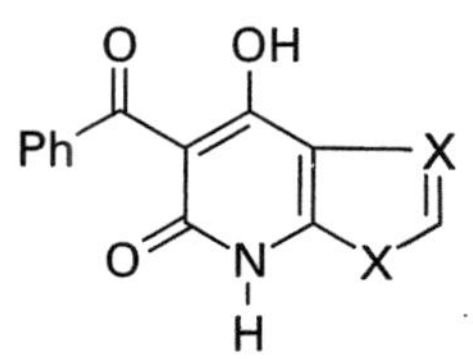

55

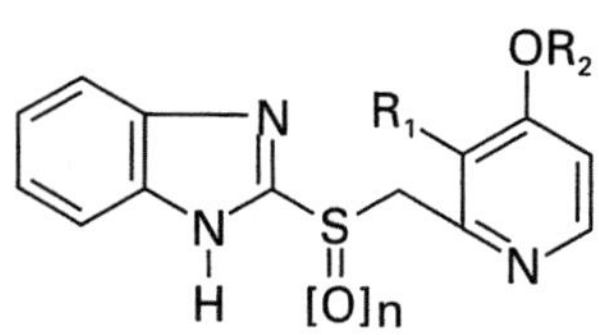

56 R_1=H, Me,
R_2=(fluorinated)$C_{1\text{-}8}$ alkyl,
n=0,1

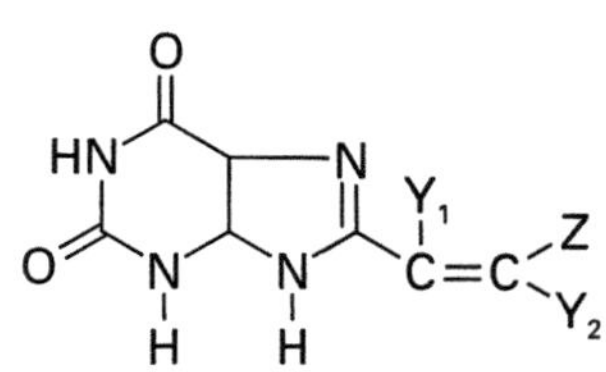

57

Fig. 9 (Continued)

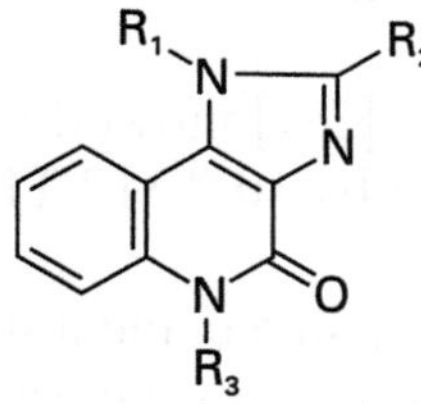

58

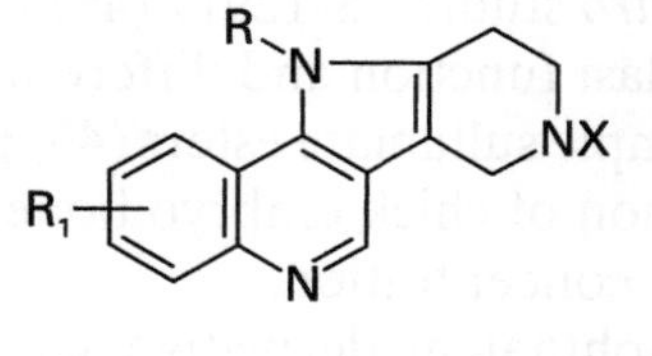

59

R=H, alkyl, Ph,
R_1=H, alkyl, Ph, OH, alkoxy, CF_3

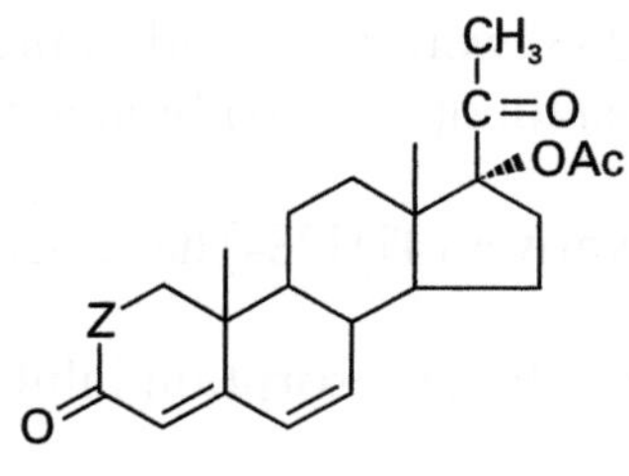

60

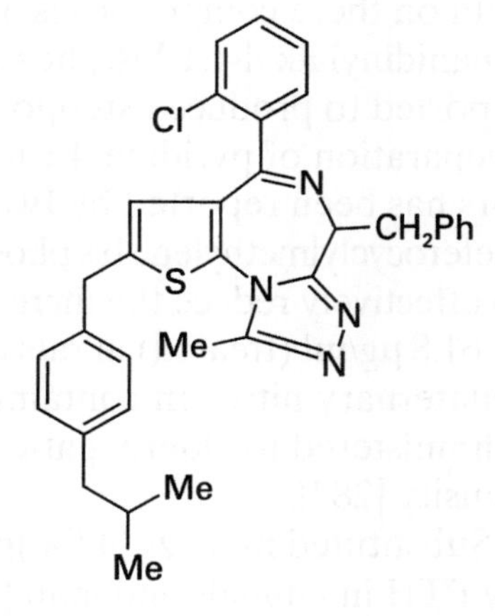

61

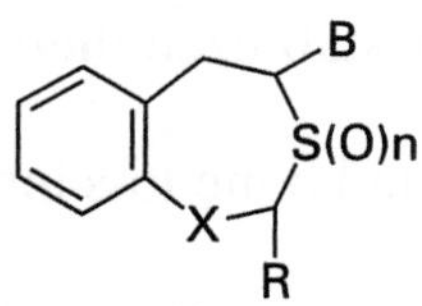

62

R=H (substituted hydrocarbyl);
B=COOH, ester or amide
X=CH(OH), CO; n=0–2

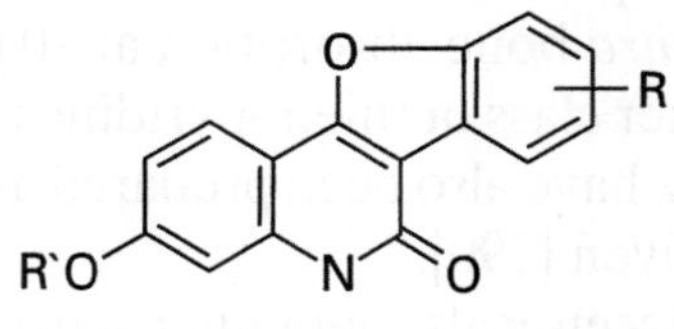

63

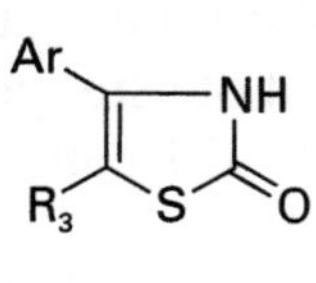

64

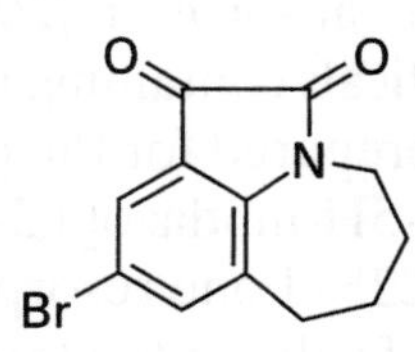

65

Fig. 9 (Continued)

In *in vitro* studies, S-12911 (**45**) was found to have an inhibitory effect on osteoclast function and differentiation [279, 280].
The simple sulfamate esters (46) prepared by Lo et al. [281] showed 100% inhibition of chick embryo bone resorption induced by 10^{-9} M PTH, at 10^{-6} M concentration.
The naphthalene derivative nambumetone (**47**) [282], in a clinical study, decreased the amount of bone resorption in patients and may have a prophylactic role in hypercalciuric patients with high bone turnover who are candidates for developing osteoporosis.
Gallium complex of 3-hydroxypyrones (**48**) [283] were prepared to prevent excessive loss of Ca from bone due to osteoporosis. No biological data on these compounds is available.
Guanidinylalkyl-1,1-bis(phosphonic acid) derivatives (**49**) [284] have been reported to produce osteoporosis effect.
Preparation of pyridine-4-carboxamides (**50**) as bone resorption inhibitors has been reported by Iwao et al. [285].
Heterocyclylmethylene bis phosphonic derivatives of structure **51** were found to effectively reduce the increase in serum Ca from 193.8 μg/ml (controls) to 61.8 μg/ml (treated) in rats at 3 x 10 mg/kg s.c. daily doses [286].
Quaternary nitrogen containing phosphonate (cis) of the type **52** when administered to elderly patients with osteoporosis, stabilized their bone density [287].
2-Substituted imidazo(4,5-c)pyridines (**53**) prevented bone loss induced by PTH in animals and man [288].
Thieno- or furopyridine derivatives (**54**) were prepared for the treatment of osteoporosis. Compound **54** (X = S, Z = O) showed 47.2% inhibition of *in vitro* bone absorption at 10 μg/ml in mice [289].
Another class of thienopyridines **55**, having substitutions on the pyridine moiety, have also been prepared as antiosteoporosis drugs. No data is however given [290].
Pharmaceuticals containing benzimidazoles of type **56** have been prepared for the treatment of osteoporosis [291]. No data on biological activity is given. Appropriately substituted xanthines of type **57** were found to inhibit (119%) bone absorption [292].
Pharmaceuticals containing imidazo[4,5-c]quinolin-4-one derivatives (**58**) have been prepared for the prevention and treatment of osteoporosis. 5-n-Butyl-1H-5H-imidazo[4,5-c]quinolin-4-one at 10^2 μM concentration showed a 122% bone resorption inhibition rate [293].
A number of substituted tetrahydropyrido [3',4';4,5] pyrrolo[3,2-c]quinolines (**59**) have been prepared. By virtue of their ability to inhibit interlukin-1 and to modify the balance between bone production and bone

resorption, some of these compounds are useful as antiinflammatory agents and for the treatment of osteoporosis [294]. 2-Oxa- or 2-azapregnane derivatives of structure **60** (A = H, lower alkanoyl; X = halo; Z = O,NR, R = H, lower alkyl) were tested on oophorectomized rats on a Ca-deficient diet and were found to increase bone ash [295].
Calcium resorption was found to decrease by 30.7% in mice, upon treatment with diazepine derivative **61** at a 20 μM concentration [296].
Bone resorption activity was observed with 1,2,4,5-tetrahydro-5-oxo-benzothiapines of type **62** (R = H, substituted hydrocarbyl; B = COOH, ester or amide, X=CH(OH), CO, n=O-2 and/or salts) [297].
Some of the recent entries include benzofuro[3,2-c]quinolinones (**63**) [298], arylthiazolones (**64**) [299–301], benzazapine derivatives (**65**) [302], shown in Figure 9. No details regarding their biological activity is available.

5 Management of osteoporosis

Along with the development of chemotherapy, the success in the management of a disease, depends on two major factors: i) Timely identification of the problem diagnosis, and ii) treatment of the disease as per requirement with appropriate drugs – disease status and therapy.
The above two factors in regard to osteoporosis are discussed below in brief.

5.1 Diagnosis of osteoporosis

Detection of onset of osteoporosis before it leads to a fracture and the extent of the disease even after the damage, helps in its prevention and treatment. In the clinical diagnosis of this disease some reduction in the bone mass may not be obvious under X-ray, but can be detected by different methods of bone density measurements and evaluation using biochemical markers discussed below.

5.1.1 Methods of measuring bone density

Measurement of bone mass provides an effective method for the identification of individuals at high risk for fracture. For this purpose, depending upon the type of bone mass measurement required, single or dual photon absorptiometry (SPA or DPA) is in use [303, 304].
A more precise and stable method for density measurement is dual energy X-ray absorptiometry (DEXA). With this device, precision measurement is obtained with the lowest radiation exposure and less scan time [305, 306].

Quantitative computed tomography (QCT) is another method for the determination of dimensional imaging and thus a "true" density measurement of cancellous bones. QCT requires more time and greater radiation exposure. It is more costly and less precise [307–310].
Measurements by radiographic absorptiometry (RA) of the metacarpals correlates well with measurements at other sites and could provide risk assessment [311].
Ultrasound is another important technique for assessing both skeletal mass and other characteristics of bone. Measurement of speed of sound through bone and the attenuation of the energy give valuable information [312]. The advantages of this method are absence of ionizing radiation and a relatively brief scanning time.

5.1.2 Biochemical markers

The rate of formation and resorption of bone can be gauged by monitoring the prominent enzymatic activity of the bone forming or resorbing cells released into the circulation during the process. These enzymatic markers for the two processes are discussed below.

Markers for bone formation

Osteocalcin:

The most efficient marker for bone formation is osteocalcin. Osteocalcin or bone Gla-protein (BGP), is a small non-collagenous protein that is predominantly synthesized by the osteoblast cells. It gets incorporated into the extracellular bone matrix but a fraction of the newly synthesized osteocalcin passes into the circulation which can be measured by radioimmunoassay technique [313].
The level of BGP increases under situations characterized by increased bone turnover such as primary and secondary hyperparathyroidism, hyperthyroidism, acromegaly, Paget's disease of bone etc. and is decreased in hypothyroidism, hypoparathyroidism and in glucocorticoid-treated patients [314, 315].
Other markers which have also found use in measuring bone formation are i) bone alkaline phosphatase [316], ii) total alkaline phosphatase [314] and iii) procollagen I extension enzyme [317].

Markers for bone resorption

Urinary pyridinium crosslink:

Pyridinoline (Pyr) and deoxypyridinoline (dPyr) are two non-reducible pyridinium cross-links present in the matured form of collagen [318] and are most efficient markers for bone resorption.

The concentration of Pyr & dPyr is very low and varies dramatically with tissue type. During bone degradation Pyr and dPyr are released from bone matrix. It has been observed that a 50–100% increase in the urinary Pyr and dPyr takes place at the time of menopause which returns to normal after estrogen therapy [319]. The release of these pyridinium cross-links in the urine can be measured by fluorimeter and HPLC methods. Recently, immunoassays have been developed to measure free urinary pyridinolins [320].
These urinary cross-links appear to be quite specific for bone turnover and do not metabolize easily. A good correlation is obtained in levels of urinary cross-link and bone turnover in osteoporosis patients [321, 322]. Other less efficient markers of bone resorptions are i) urinary hydroxyproline [323], ii) urinary hydroxylysine glycosides [324] and iii) plasma tartrate-resistant acid phosphatase [325].

6 Osteoporosis, stages and therapy

In a recent review by Ringe [325], four different clinical stages of osteoporosis have been identified and suitable therapy for such stages has been recommended. For detailed information, the reader is advised to consult the review articles and the references cited therein.
Stage O – Risk patients:
This stage refers to subjects who have not developed osteoporosis but have a higher probability of developing the disease. Such cases are to be given more preventive measures such as high calcium diet, exercise, and diet which influence enteral absorption (phosphate, oxalate, phylate), and renal loss (excess protein, NaCl, caffeine) of calcium should be minimized. HRT for women who have either primary or secondary amenorrhea has been suggested.

Stage 1 – Preclinical osteoporosis:
This is a stage when some reduction in bone mass has occurred which is not obvious in X-rays. This is usually the case in the early post-menopausal stage. The treatment is aimed at preventing further progression of the stage. For postmenopausal women, HRT treatment has been recommended [326]. Treatment with low-dose calcitonin (nasal spray) has been suggested for patients for whom estrogen therapy is contraindicated [123]. A calcium-rich diet, regular exercise, avoidance of risk factors [325], and an annual osteodensitometry check up are required for both sexes.

Stage 2 – Borderline osteoporosis:
This is an important but ambiguous stage between 1 and 3. There is an obvious reduction in the bone mass as shown by X-rays. A reduction of calcium content but no significant spinal deformity or fractures and at times general back discomfort are markers for stage 2. Controlled fluoride-calcium therapy and long-term cyclic intermittent use of etidronate has been suggested. Use of anabolic therapy has also some beneficial effect. However, its side effects are also to be taken into consideration at this age.

Stage 3 – Early manifest osteoporosis:
This stage is associated with significant loss of height or breaks in 1-3 vertebrae. It is accompanied generally by severe back pain and occasional extra-vertebral fractures. The treatment involves pain relief and prevention of further fractures by blocking accelerated bone loss. Drugs which retard some resorption such as bisphosphonates, calcitonin, estrogens, find use in the treatment. Calcitonin has the added advantage of having some analgesic effects. Use of calcitriol could be helpful. Bone-forming agents like fluoride and calcium are also helpful. However, there is no single drug which can take care of this stage effectively.
Stage 4 – Late manifest osteoporosis:
This is the latest stage in osteoporosis: multiple vertebral deformities and fractures, associated with severe, mild or no back discomfort. In these cases, a symptomatic analgesic therapy is given if desired. Oral calcium administration, physiotherapy and intermittent use of anabolic drugs has been suggested.

7 Conclusion

Development of agents for the successful treatment of osteoporosis is required to assure a person a happy, long life. A number of agents such as calcium compounds, vitamin D_3 and its derivatives, bisphosphonates, calcitonins, estrogens, antiestrogens, fluoride, PTH and a large number of miscellaneous structural prototypes have been found to be effective in the treatment of osteoporosis.
The agent needed for the therapy is chosen according to the type and clinical stage of the disease. Fluoride compounds help in bone formation but quite often it leads to the formation of bones which are not normal. PTH also shows a stimulatory effect on bone formation. Most of the other compounds interfere with the process of bone resorption. These anti-resorp-

tive agents are helpful in preventing bone loss but may affect the rate and extent of bone turnover, giving rise to weaker bones. Use of antiestrogens in hormone replacement therapy in postmenopausal women, is showing much promise. A number of candidate drugs are under advanced stages of development.

A number of growth factors, mainly present in bone, have been identified and are associated with bone remodeling. Although these have not been used for the treatment of osteoporosis due to their complexity of biological action and poor availability in pure form, they might help in the development of bone formation stimulators which would restore bone mass.

The wide variety of agents mentioned above which are involved in bone remodeling, would suggest that there may be different mechanisms involved in the manifestation of drug action. How these mechanisms are interrelated in order to produce the same effect is poorly understood. There is need for a proper structure activity relationship study for different classes of organic compounds showing bone remodeling activity in order to understand drug-receptor interaction and the mechanism of drug action.

A suitable compound to prevent osteoporosis or correct bone loss in osteoporotic patients without causing any unwanted side effects is yet to be achieved.

References

1. Bouillon, R., Burckhardt, P., Christiansen, C., Fleisch, H.A.,Fujita,T., Gennari, C., Martin, T.J., Mazzuoli, G., Melton. L.J., Ringe, J.D., Riis, P., Peck, W.A., Samsioe, G. and Shulman, L.E. (1991). Amer. J. Med. *90*, 107–110.
2. Riggs, B.L. and Melton, J. (1983). Amer. J. Med. *75*, 899–901.
3 AMA Council on Scientific Affairs: Social effects and other factors affecting health care for the elderly. (1990). Arch Intern Med. *150*, 1184–1189.
4. Cummings, S.R., Kelsey, J.C., Neviti, M.C., O'Dowd, K.J. (1985). Epidemiology Reviews 7, 178–208.
5 Mazess, R.B. (1982).Clin.Orthop.*165*, 239–252.
6 Riggs,R.L., Wahner, H.W., Dunn, W.L., Mazess, R.B., Offord, K.P., Melton, L.J.iii, (1981), J.Clin.Invest. *67*, 328–335.
7 Hamilton, J.A., Lingelbach, S., Psartridge, N.C., Martin, T.J. (1985). Endocrinology *116*, 2186–91.
8 Chambers, T.J.,Darby, J.A., Fuller, K. (1985). Cell Tissue Res. *241*, 671–5.
9 Shen, V., Rifas, L., Kohler, G., Peck, W.A. (1986). J. Bone Miner. Res. *1*, 243–9.
10 McSheehy P.M.J., Chambers, T.J. (1986). Endocrinology *119*, 1654–9.
11 Baron, R., Neff, L., Van P.T., Nefussi, J.R., Vignery, A. (1986). Am. J. Pathol. *122*, 363–78.
12 Baron, R., Neff, L., Louvard, D., Courtoy, P.J. (1985). J. Cell Biol. *101*, 2210–22.
13 Marcus, R. (1989). Hosp. Prac. *24*, 189–218.

14 Raisz, L.G. (1988). New Engl. J. Med. *318*, 818–828.
15 Parfitt, A.M., Mathews, C.H.E., Villanueva, A.R., Kleerekoper, M., Frame, B., and Rao, D.S. (1983). J.Clin. Invest. *72*, 1396–1409.
16 Erikson, E.F., Mosekilde, L., Melsen, F. (1985). Bone *6*,141–146.
17 Kaplan, F.S. (1987). Clin. Symp. *39*, 8.
18 Nordin, B.E.C. et al. (1975). Hormone Res. *3*, 131.
19 Frost, H.M. (1969). Calcit Tissue Res. *3*, 211.
20 Robbins, S.L. and Cotran, R.S. (1979). In Pathologic Basis of Diseases, W.B.Sunders Company.
21 Riggs, B.L., Melton, L.J. III (1986). New Engl. J. Med. *314*, 1676–1686.
22 Melton, L.J. III, Wahner, H.W., Richelson, L.S., O'Fallon, W.M., Riggs, B.L. (1986). Am. J. Epidemiol. *124*, 254–261.
23 Mundy, G.R. (1991). Molecular and Cellular Endocrinology *75*, C19–C25.
24 Rubin, R.D. (1991). Am. J. Med. Sciences *301*, 281–298.
25 Forero, M.S., Klein, R.F., Nissenson, R.A., Nelson, K., Heath, H.III, Arnand, C.D., Riggis, B.L. (1987). J. Bone Miner Res. *2*, 363–366.
26 Young, G., Marcus, R., Minkoff, J.R., Kim, L.Y., Segre, G.V. (1987). J. Bone Miner Res. *2*, 367–374.
27 Wilson, R., Rao, S.D., Kleerekoper, M., Parfitt, A.M. (1987). J. Bone Miner Res. *2*, Suppl.1: S19 abstract.
28 Gunness–Hey, M, Hock, J.M. (1984). Metab. Bone Dis. Relat. Res. *5*, 177–181.
29 Slovik, D.M., Rosenthal, D.I., Doppelt, S.H., Potts, J.T., Daly, M.A., Campbell, J.A., Neer, R.M. (1986). J. Bone Miner. Res. *1*, 377–381.
30 Gallagher, J.C., Jerpbak, C.M., Jee W.S.S., Johnson, K.A., DeLuca H.F., Riggs, B.L. (1982). Proc. Natl. Acad. Sci. USA *79*, 3325–3329.
31 Hurley, D.L., Tiegs, R.D., Wahner, H.W., Heath, H. III. (1987). N. Engl. J. Med. *317*, 537–41.
32 Tiegs, R.D., Body, J.J., Wahner, H.W., Barta, J., Riggs B.L., Heath H III (1985). N. Engl. J. Med. *312*, 1097–100.
33 Foresta, C., Zanatta, G.P., Busnardo, B., Scanelli, G., Scandellari, C. (1985). J. Endocrinol Invest. *8*, 377–9.
34 Raisz, L.G. (1980). Prog. Biochem. Pharmacol. *17*, 212–9.
35 Chyun, Y.S., Kream, B.E., Raisz, L.G. (1984). Endocrinology *114*, 477–80.
36 Kream, B.E., Smith, M.D., Canalis, E., Raisz, L.G. (1985). Endocrinology *116*, 296–302.
37 Hui, S.L., Epstein, S., Johnston, C.C.Jr. (1985). J. Clin. Endocrinol Metab. *60*, 74–80.
38 Heath, H III, Melton, L.J. III, Chu, C.P. (1980). N. Engl. J. Med. *303*, 567–570.
39 Auwerx, J., Bouillon, R. (1986). Q. J. Med. *60*, 737–752.
40 Coindre, J.M., David, J.P., Riviere, L., Goussot, J.F., Roger, P., Demascara Meunier, P.J. (1986). Arch. Intern. Med. *146*, 48–53.
41 Riggs, B.L., Wahner, H.W., Melton, L.J.III, Richelson, L.S., Judd, H.L., Offord, K.P. (1986). J. Clin. Invest. *77*, 1487–1491.
42 Stanley, H.L,Schmitt, B.P., Poses, R.M.,Diess,W.P. (1991). J. Am. Geriatr. Soc. *39*, 766–71.
43 Selby, P.L., Peacock, M., Barkworth, S.A., Brown, W.B., Taylor, G.A. (1985). Clin. Sci. *69*, 265–271.
44 Christiansen, C., Riis, B.J., Nilas, L., Rodbro, P., Deftos, L. (1985). Lancet *2*, 800–801.
45 Malluche, H.H., Faugere, M.C., Rush, M., Friedler, R. (1986). Endocrinology *119*, 2649–2654.

46 Klibanski, A., Greenspan, S.L. (1986). N. Engl. J. Med. *315*, 542–546.
47 Centrella, M., Canalis, E. (1985). Endocrine Rev. *6*, 544–551.
48 Canlis, E., McCarthy, T., Centrella, M. (1991). Annu. Rev. Med. *42*, 17–24.
49 Hock, J.M., Centrella, M., Canalis, E. (1988). Endocrinology *122*, 254–260.
50 Spencer, E.M., Liu, C.C., Si, E.C.C., Howard, G. A., (1991). Bone *12*, 21–26.
51 Schelechter, N.L., Russell, S.M., Spencer, E.M., Nicoll, C.S. (1986). Proc. Natl. Acad. Sci. USA *83*, 7932–4.
52 Ibbotson, K.J., Orcutt, C.M., Dsouza, S.M., Paddock, C.L., Arthur, J.A., Jankowsk, M.L., Boyce, R.W. (1992). J. Bone Mineral 7, 425–432.
53 Seydin, S.M., Thompasan, A.Y., Bentz,H., Rosen,D.M., McPherson, J.M., Conti, A., Siegal N.R., Galluppi, G.R, and Piez, K.A., (1986). J.B.C. *261*, 5693–5695.
54 Seydin, S.M., Sagarini, P.R., Rosen, D.M., Thompson, A.Y., Bentz, H., and Graycar, J.(1987). J.B.C. *262*, 1946–1949.
55 Oursler, M.J., Cortese, C., Keeting, P.E., Anderson, M.A., Bonde, S.K., Riggs, B.L., Splesberg, T.C. (1991). Endocrinology *129*, 3313–20.
56 Noda, M. and Rodan, G. (1986). Biochem. Biophysics Res. Comm. *140*, 56–65.
57 Tashjian, A.H., Voelkel, E.F., Lloyd, W., Derynck, R., Winkler, M.E. and Lerine, L. (1986). J. Clin. Invest. *78*, 1405–1409.
58 Pfeilschifter, J.P., Seyedin, S. and Mundy, G.R. (1988). J. Clin. Invest. *82*, 680–685.
59 Oreffo, R.O.C., Bonewald, L., Kukita, A.,Garrett, I.R., Seydin, S.M., Rosen, D. and Mundy G. R., (1990). Endocrinology *126*, 3069–3075.
60 Urist, M.R.,Dchange, R.J.,Finerman, G.A.M. (1983). Science *220*, 680–686.
61 Pfeilschifter, J.,Bouewald, L. and Mundy, G.R. (1990). J. Bone Miner. Res. *5*,49–58.
62 Hauschka, P.V., Mavarakos, A.E., Lafrati, M.D., Doleman, S.E. and Klagsbrun, M. (1986). J. Biol. Chem. *261*, 12665–12674.
63 Canalis, E. (1980). Metabolism *30*, 970–975.
64 Kukita, A., Bonewald, L., Rosen, D., Seyedin, S., Mundy, G.R. and Roodman, G.D. (1990). Proc. Natl. Acad. Sci. USA. *87*, 3023–3026.
65 Raisz, L.G., Kream, B.E. (1983). N. Engl. J. Med. *309*, 29–35, *309*, 83–9.
66 Gowen, M., Mundy, G.R. (1986). J. Immunol. *136*, 2478–82.
67 Seeman, E. (1993). Amer J.Med. *95*, 5A–28.
68 Girasole, G.,Jilka, R.L.,Passeri,B.S.,Boder, G.,Willams, D.C., Manolagas, S. (1992). J. Clin. Invest. *89*, 883–891.
69 Gowen, M.,Chapman, K., Littlewood, A.,Hughes, D.E., Evans, D.,Russel, R.G.G. (1990). Endocrinology *112,* 1250–55.
70 Ishimi, Y., Miyaura, C., Jin, C.H., Akatsn, T., Abe E., Nakamura, Y., Yamaguchi, Aj, Yoshike, s., Matsuda, T., Hirano, T., Kishimoto, T., and Suda, T. (1990). J. Immunol. *145*, 3297–3303.
71 Pacifici, R., Rifas, L., Teitelbaum, S., Slatopolsky, E., Mc Cracken, R., Bergfeld, M., Lee, W.F, Avioli, L.Y., and Peck, W.A. (1987). Proc. Natl. Acad. Sci. USA. *84,* 4616–4620.
72 Morris, N. (1993). Fertility and Sterility *59*, 707–725.
73 Heaney, R.P., Gallagher, J.C., Johnston, C.C., Neer, R., Parfitt, A.M., Whedon, G.D. (1982). Am. J. Clin. Nutr. *36*, Suppl. 5, 986–1013.
74 Holbrook, T.L., Barrett-Connor, E., Wingard, D.L. (1988). Lancet *2*, 1046–9.
75 Heaney, R.P. (1987). Clinical Obstet. Gynecol. *30*, 833–46.
76 Sheikh, M.S., Santa Ana, C.A., Nican, M.J., Schiller, L.R. and Fordtran, J.S. (1987). N. Engl. J. Med. *317*, 532–6.

77 Nilas, L.,Christiansen, C., Rodbro, P. (1984). Br. Med. J. *289*, 1103–06.
78 Havey, J.A., Zobitz, M.M., Pak, C.Y. (1985). J. Clin. Endo. Metab. *61*, 1223–5.
79 Gallagher, J.C., Goldgar, D. (1990). Ann. Inter. Med. *113*, 649–55.
80 Aslovia, J.F., Vaswani, A., Yeh, J.K., Ellis, K., Yasumura & Cohn S.H. (1988). Am. J. Med. *84*, 401–408.
81 Chapuy, M.C., Arlot, M.E., Duboeu, F., Brun, J., Crouzet, B., Arnaud, S., Delmas, P.D., Meunier, P.J. (1992). N. Engl. J. Med. *327*, 1637–42.
82 Reeve, J., Tellez, M., Green, J.R.,Hesp, R., Elsasser, U., Wootton, R., Hulme, P., Williamson, D., Kanis, J.A., Russell, R.G.G., Mawer, E.B., and Meunier, P.J. (1992). Acta Endocrinol. *101*, 636–40.
83 DeLuca, H.F. (1978) Arch. Intern. Med. *138*, 838–.
84 Holick, M.F., Schnoes, H.K. and DeLuca, H.F. (1971). Proc. Nat. Acad. Sci. USA 68, 803–804.
85 Omdahl, J.L., Garry, P.J., Hunsaker, L.A., Hunt, W.C., Goodwin, J.S. (1982). Am. J. Clin. Nutr. *36*, 1225–33.
86 Tsai, K.S., Heath, H. III, Kumar, R., Riggs, B.L. (1984). J. Clin. Invest. *73*, 1668–72.
87 Underwood, J.L., DeLuca, H.F. (1984). Am. J. Physiology. *246*, E 493–E 498.
88 McShechy, P.M.J., Chambers, T.J. (1987). J. Clin. Invest. *80*, 425–9.
89 Ptkovich, P.M., Wrana, J.L., Grigoriadis, A.E., Heersche, J.N.M., Sodele, J. (1987). J. Biol. Chem. *262,* 13424–8.
90 Holtrop, M.E., Cox, C. A., Clark, M.B., Holick, M.F. and Anast, C.S. (1981). Endocrinology *108*, 2293–2301.
91 Boyle, I.T., Gray, R.W. and Deluca, H.F. (1971). Proc. Nat. Acad. Sci. *68*, 2131–2134.
92 Tanaka, Y. and Deluca, H.F. (1973). Arch. Biochem. Biophys. *154*, 566–574.
93 Orwoll, E., Oviatt, S., McClung, M., Doglos, L., Sexton, G. (1990). Ann. Int. Med. *112*, 29–34.
94 Jensen, G.F., Christansen, C., Transbol I. (1982). Clin. Endocrinol. *116*, 515–524.
95 Ott, S.M. and Chesnut, C. H. III (1989). Ann. Intern. Med. *110*, 267–74.
96 Schwartzman, M.S., Franck, W.A. (1987). Am. J. Med. *82*, 224–230.
97 Christiansen, C., Rodbro, P., Christsiansen, S., Hartnack, B., Trransbol, I.B. (1978). Lancet *2*, 700–703.
98 Miyamoto, K., Murayama, E., Ochi, K., Watanabe, H., and Kubodera, N. (1993). Chem. Pharm. Bull. *41*, 1111–13.
99 Kobayashi, T., Okano, T., Tsugsanoa, N., Murano, M., Masuda, S., Takeuchi, A., Seto, K., Kishii, X. (1993). Biorg. Med. Chem. Lett. *3*, 1815–19.
100 Junqueira, L.C., Carneiro, J., Contopoulos, A.N. (1977). Basic Histology, 2nd Edition, Chapter 8, p. 134. Lange Medical Publication, Los Altos, California.
101 Tachibana, Y. (1992). Eur. Pat. Appl. E.P. 506388. Chem. Abstr. *117*, 251624k.
102 Tachibana, Y., Yokoyama, S., Tefima, T., Okmoto, Y., Hongy, T. (1993). Eur. Pat. Appl. EP 562497. Chem. Abstr. *120*,107476h.
103 Malluche, H.H., Bognar, B., Friedler, R.M., Faugere, M.C. (1991). Proc. Workshop Vitamin D 8th (Vitamin D) 537–8. Chem. Abs. *119*, 109701f (1993).
104 Deluca, H.F., Schnoes, H.K. (1993). Eur. Pat. Appl. EP 567,353. Chem. Abstr. *119*, 262541y (1993).
105 Deluca, H.F., Schnoes, H.K. (1993). Eur. Pat. Appl. EP 567,352. Chem. Abstr. *119*, 262542 z (1993).
106 Seino, Y., Ishizuka, S. (1991). Proc. Workshop Vitamin D, 8th (Vitamin D). 565–71.
107 Binderup, L. and Bramm, E. (1988). Biochem. Pharmacology *37*, 889–95.

108 Kikuchi, Y., Otomo, S., HIfguchi, S., Harada, M., Ikegawa, N. (1993). PCTR Int. Appl. WO 93,12,082. Chem. Abstr. *120*, 107471C.
109 Lancet *i*, 973–974 (1978).
110 Brandi, M.L. (1993). Am. J. Med. *95*, 5A–74S.
111 Foster, G.V., Baghdiantz, A., Kumar, M.A., Slack, E., Soliman, H.A., MacIntyre, I. (1964). Nature *202*, 1303–1305.
112 Civitelli, R., Gonnlli, S., Zacchei, F., Bigazz, S., Vattimo, A., Avioli, L., Gennari, C. (1988). J. Clin. Invest. *82*, 1268–1274.
113 MacIntyre, I., Stevenson, J., Whitehead, M., Wimalawansa, S., Banks, L., Healy, M. (1988). The Lancet *1*, 900–902.
114 Reginster, J.Y., Albert, A., Lecart, M.P., Lambilin, P., Denis, D., Deroisy, R., Fontaine, M.A., Franchimont, P. (1987) Lancet *ii*. 1481–1483.
115 Reginster, J.Y. (1993). Am. J. Med. *95* (Suppl.5A) 5A–46S.
116 Overgaard, K., Riis, B.J., Christiansen, C., Hansen, M.A. (1989). Brit. Med. J. *299*, 477–79.
117 Ribot, C., Tremollieres, F., Pouilles, J.M., Chaumet, R. (1992). J. Bone Miner. Res. *7*, (Suppl.1), 140.
118 Buclin, T., Randin, J.P., Jacquet, A.F., Azrio, M., Attinger, M., Gomej, F., Burckhardt, P. (1987). Calif. Tissue Int. *41*, 252–7.
119 Reginster, J.Y., Denis, D., Albert, A., Franchimont, P. (1987). Bone Miner. *2*, 133–40.
120 Dedeuxchaisnes, C.N., Devogela, J.P., Huaux, J.P., Dufour, J.P., Esseline, W., Engelbee, J.P., Stass, P., Hermans, P., and Debuisse, J.P. (1987). Clin. Orthop. *217*, 56–71.
121 Reginster, J.Y., Fanchimont, P. (1985). Clin. Exp. Rheumato *3*, 155–7.
122 Hermann, K.G., Brixen, A.P., Lindblad, K., Mosekilde, B.E., Ott, L.S. (1994). Calif. Tissue Int. *54*, 12–15.
123 Ringe, J.D. (1991). Arzneim-Ther. *9*, 343–7.
124 Hillyard, C.J., Stevenson, J.C., MacIntyre, I. (1978). Lancet (*1*), 961–62.
125 Stevenson, J.C., Abeyasek, G., Hillyard, C.J., Phang, K.G. Macintyre, I., Campbell, S., Lane, G., Townssend, P.T., Young, O., Whitehea, M.I. (1983). Eur. J. Clin. Invest. *13*, 481–87.
126 Brown, E.M., Gardner, D.G.,Aurbach, G.D. (1980). Endocrinology *106*, 133–138.
127 Whitcherd, M.I., Lane, G., Towsend, P.T., Abeyasekera, G., Hillyard, C.J., Stevenson, J.C. (1982). Acta. Obstet. Gynecol. Scand (Suppl). *106*, 27.
128 Greenberg, C., Kukreja, S.C., Bowser, E.N., Hargis, G.K., Henderson, W.J., Williams, G.A. (1986). Endocrinology *118*, 2594–2598.
129 Eriksen, E.F., Berg, N.J., Graham, M.L., Mann, K.G., Spelsberg, T.C., Rigg,s B.L. (1987). J. Bone Min. Res. *2* (Suppl. 1), 238.
130 Nicolson, G.C., Moseley, J.M., Sexton, P.M., Mendelsohn, F.A.O. (1986). J. Clin. Invest. *78*, 355–360.
131 Chambers, T.J., Magnus, C.J. (1982). J. Pathology. *136*, 27–29.
132 Kallio, D.M., Garant, P.R., Minkin, C. (1972). J. Ultrastructur. Res. *39*, 205–16.
133 Chambers, T.J., Dunn, C.J. (1983). Calif Tissue Int. *35*, 566–79.
134 Feldman, R.S., Krieger, N.S., and Tashjian, A.H. Jr. (1980). Endocrinology *107*, 1137–43.
135 Austin, L., Heath, H. (1981). N. Engl. J. Med. *304*, 269–278.
136 Wimalawansa, S.J. (1993). Calif Tissue Int. *53*, 90–93.
137 Fleisch, H. (1983). Bisphosphonates: mechanism of action and clinical application. In: Peck, W.A., ed., Bone and Mineral Research Annual. Amsterdam. Exerpta Medica 319–57.

138 Heaney, R.P. and Saville, P.D. (1976). Clin. Pharmacol. Ther. *20*, 593–604.
139 Storm, T., Thomsborg, G., Steiniche, T., Genant, H., Sorensen, O. (1990). N. Engl. J. Med. *322*, 1265–1271.
140 Watts, N.B., Harris, S.T., Genant, H.K., Wasnich, R., Miller, P., Jackson, R., Licata, A., Ross, P., Woodson, G., Yanover, M., Mysin, J., Kohse, L., Rao, M., Steiger, P., Richmond, B. (1990). N. Engl. J. Med. *323*, 73–79.
141 Frijlink, W.B., Velde, J.T., Bijvoet, O.L.M., Heynen, G. (1979). Lancet (*1*) 799–803.
142 Reid, I.R., King, A.R., Alexander, C.J., Ibbertson, H.K. (1988). Lancet (*1*) 1433–146.
143 Reitsma, P.H., Bijvoet, O.L.M., Potokar, M., Van der Wee-Pals L.J.A., Van Wijk-van Lennep, M.M.L. (1983). Calif. Tissue Int. *35*, 357–61.
144 de Vernejoul, M.C., Pointillart, R., Bergot, C., Bielakof, J., Morieux, C., Jeantet, A.M.L., Miravet, L. (1987). Calcif. Tissue Int. *40*, 160–65.
145 Dedeuxchaisnes, C., Nagant D., Devogelar, J.P., Esselinck, W., Depresseux, G., Rombouts-Lindemans, C., Huaux, J.P. (1983). Brit. Med. J. *286*, 1648.
146 Devogelaer, J.P., Nagant de Deuxchaisner, C. (1990). J. Bone Miner. Res. *5* (Suppl. 12), 5251.
147 Mautalen, C.A., Casco, C.A., Gonzalez, D., Ghiringhelli, G.R., Massironi, C., Fromm, G.A., Plantalech, I. (1984). Brit. Med. J. *288*, 828–29.
148 Guannine, S., D'Angelo, A., Malvasi, L., Castrignano, R., Pati, T., Troncar, R., Liberto, L., Nobile, M., Crepaldi, G. (1993). Bone *14*, 137–141.
149 Reginster, J.Y., Deroisy, R., Denis, D., Collette, J., Lecart, M.P., Sarlet, N., Ethgen, D., Franchimont, P. (1989). Lancet (*ii*) 1469–1471.
150 Charhon, S., Meunier, P., Etghen, D., Lacheretz, F., Breliere, J.C., Roncucci, R. (1985). Calif. Tissue Int. *38*, 533.
151 Nagao, Y., Ishitobi, Y., Kinoshita, H., Fukushima, S. and Kawashime, H. (1991). Biochemical Biophysical Res. Comm. *180*, 1172–1178.
152 Guy, J.A., Shea, M., Peter, C.P., Morrissey, L., Hayes, W.C. (1993). Calcif. Tissue Int. *53*, 283–288.
153 Gall,R., Bosies, E. Gen. offen. DE 3623,397 Jan 1988, Chem. Abst. *108*, p186991a.
154 Mundy, G.R. (1994). Drugs of Today *30,* 589–597.
155 Binderup E.T., Liisberg, S. (1989). PCT Int Appl WO 8909,775. 9th Oct.1989.Chem. Abstr. *112*: P 139567q.
156 Hodsman, A.B. (1989). Bone Miner *5*, 201–12.
157 Francis, M.D. (1969). Science *165*, 1264–1266.
158 Fleisch, H., Russell, R.G.G. (1969). Science *165*, 1262–1264.
159 Boonekamp, P.M., Vander Wee-Pals, L.J.A., Van Wijk-van Lennep, M.M.L., The-singh, C.W,. Bijvoet, O.L.M. (1986). Bone Mine. *1*, 27–39.
160 Hughes, D.E., MacDonald, B.R., Russell, R.G.G., Gowen, M. (1989). J. Clin. Invest. *83*, 1930–5.
161 Sahni, M., Guenther, H.L., Martin, T.J., Fleisch, H. (1993). J. Clin Invest. *91*, 2004–11.
162 Boonekamp, P.M., Lowik, C.W.G.M., van der Wee-Pals, L.J.A., van Wijk-van Lennep, M.M.L., Bijvoet, O.L.M. (1982). Bone Miner. *2*, 29–42.
163 Plosker, G.L., Goa, K.L. (1994) Drugs *47*, 945–982.
164 Bijvoet, O.L.M., Frijlink, W.B., Jie, K., Vanderti, H., Meijer, C.J.L.M., Mulder, H., Vanpaass, H.C., Reitsma, P.H., Tevelde, J., Devries, E. (1980). Arthritis Rheum. *23*, 1193–1204.
165 Rolla, G., Bucca, C., Brussino, L. (1994), Lancet, 426–27.
166 Jowsey, J., Riggs, B.L., Kelly, P.J., Hoffman, D.L., Bordier, P. (1971). J. Lab. Clin. Med. *78*, 574–584.

167 Slemenda, C., Hui, S.L., Longcope, C.,and Johnston, C.C., (1987). J. Clin. Invest. *80*, 1261–69.
168 Whitson, S.W., Dawson, L.R., Jee, W.S.S. (1978). Endocrinology *103*, 2006–2010.
169 Nielsen, H.K., Brixen, K., Bouillon, R., Mosekilde, L. (1990).J. Clin. Endocrinol. Metab. *70,* 1431–1437.
170 Horsman, A., Simpson, M., Kirby, P.A. and Nordin, B.E.C. (1977). Br. J. Radiol. *50*, 504–507.
171 Lindsay, R., Hart, D.M., Forrest, C., Baird, C. (1980). Lancet (*ii*), 1151–11533.
172 Christiansen, C., Christiansen, M.S., McNair, P., Hagen K., Estocklund, C. and Transbol, I. (1990). Eur. J. Clin. Invest. *10*, 273–279.
173 Lindsay, R., Sex steroids in the pathogenesis and prevention of osteoporosis. In Riggs, B.L., ed., Osteoporosis: Etiology, Diagnosis and Management. New York: Raven Press (1988). 333.
174 Seibel, M.J., Cosman, F., Shen, V., Gordon, S., Dempster, D.W., Ratcliff, A., Lindsay, R. (1993). J. Bone Miner. Res. *8*, 881–9.
175 Lindsay, R., Hart, D.M., Purdie, P., Ferguson, M.M., Clark, A.C., Kraszewski, A. (1978). Clin. Sci. Mol. Med. *54*, 193–5.
176 Christiansen, C., Riis, B.J. (1990). J. Clin. Endocrinol. Metab. *71*, 836–41.
177 Lindsay, R. and Hart, D.M., Clark, D.M. (1984). Obstet. Gynecol. *63*, 759–63.
178 Ettinger, B., Genant, H.K., Steiger, P., Madvig, P. (1992). Am. J. Obstet. Gynecol. *166*, 479–88.
179 Genant, H.K., Baylink, D.J., Gallagher, J.C., Harris, S.T., Steiger, P., Herber, M. (1990). Obstet. Gynecol. *76*, 579–84.
180 Lindsay, R., Tohme, J. (1990). Obset. Gynecol. *76*, 290–5.
181 Christiansen, C., Lindsay, R. (1991). Osteoporosis Int. *1*, 7–13.
182 Lindsay, R. (1993). Am. J. Med. *95* (Suppl.5A) 5A–39S.
183 Lindsay, R., Aitken, J.M., Anderson, J.B., Hart, D.M., McDonald, E.B. (1976). Lancet (*i*) 1038–40.
184 Parfitt, A.M. (1984). Calif. Tissue Int. *36*, 37–45.
185 Christiansen, C., Riis, B.J., Nilas, L., Rodbro, P., Deftos, L. (1985). Lancet *2*, 800–1.
186 Bossies, E., Esswein, A., Bauss, F., Ger Offen DE 4029,499 (1992), Chem. Abstr. *116*, 235961s.
187 Nakamura, T., Katsumata, T., Yamamoto, M. JP 05222,073 [93,222,073] (1992), Chem. Abst. *120*, 134926m.
188 Saari, W.S., Rodan, G.A., Fisher, T.E., Anderson, P.S. (1992). Chem. Abstr. *117*, 212787w.
189 Miki, T., Kumazuki, T., Yamazaki, I., Goto, G., Jpn. Kokai Tokyo Koho JP 04,145,024 (1992). Chem. Abstr. *117*, 198537f.
190 Netelnbos, J.C., Siregar-Emok, M.T.W., Schot, L.P.C., Van Ginke F.C., Lips, P., Leeuwenkamp, O.R. (1991). Maturitas *13*,137–149.
191 Geusens, P., Dequeker, J., Gielen, J., Scot, L.P.G.(1991). Maturitas *13*, 155–62.
192 Schot, L.P.C. (1989), PCT Int. Appl WO 89 09,058 Oct. 1989. Chem. Abstr. *113*, P46277a.
193 Greenberg, C., Kukreja, S.C., Bowser, E.N., Hargis, G.K., Hendersosn, W.J., Williams, G.A. (1990). Endocrinology *118*, 2594–8.
194 Gennari, C. and Agnusdei, D. (1990). J. Steroid Biochem. Mol. Biol. *37*, 451–55.
195 Turner, R.T., Bell, N.H., Gay, C.V. (1993). Poultry Sci. *72*, 728–740.
196 Benz, D.J., Haussler, M.R., Komm, B.S. (1991). J. Bone Min. Res. *6*, 531–541.
197 Eriksen, E.F., Colvard, D.S., Berg, N. J., Graham, M.L., Mann, K.G., Spelsberg, T.C., Riggs, B.L. (1988). Science *241*, 84–86.

198 Oursler, M.J., Osdoby, P., Pyfferoen, J., Riggs, B.L., Spelsberg, T.C. (1991). Proc. Natl. Acad. Sci. USA *88*, 6613–6617.
199 Castillo, L., Tanaka, Y., Deluca, H.F., Sunde, M.L. (1977). Arch. of Biochem. Biophysics. *179,* 211–217.
200 Albright, F., Smith, P.H., Richardson, A.M. (1941). JAMA *116*, 2465–74.
201 Judd, H.L., Medrum, D.R., Degtos, L.J., Henderson, B.E. (1983). Ann. Inter. Med. *98*, 195–205.
202 Wilson, P.W.F., Garrison, R.J., and Castelli, W.P. (1985). N. Engl. J. Med. *313*, 1038–43.
203 Stampfer, M.J., Willett, W.C., Coltiz, G.A. Bosner, B., Speizer, F.E. and Hennekness, C.H. (1985). N. Engl. J. Med. *313*, 1044–9.
204 Durani, S., Agarwal, A.K., Saxena, R., Setty, B.S., Gupta, R.C., Kole, P.L., Ray, S., and Anand Nitya (1979). J. Steroid Biochem. *11*, 67–76.
205 Amazaki, I., Shino, A., Shimizu, Y., Tsukuda, R., Shirakawa, Y., and Kinoshikta, M. (1986). Life Sciences *38*, 951–8.
206 Yamazaki, I., Shino, A., Tsukuda, R. (1986). J. Bone Miner. Metab. *3*, 205–10.
207 Shino, A., Matsuo, T., Tsuda, M., Yamazaki, I., Tsukuda,R., Ketazaki, T., Shiota, K., Odaka, H., Yoshida, K. (1986). Nippon Kotsu Taisha Gakkai Zasshi *3*, 177–87 (Eng.). CA, 105, 54414t.
208 Rondelli, I., Acerbi, D., Ventura, P. (1991). Int. J. Clin. Pharm. Res. *XI*, 183–92.
209 Agnusdei, D., Zacchei, F., Bigazzi, S., Zacchei, F., Bigazzi, S., Cepollar, C., Nardi, P., Montagna, M., Gennarie, C. (1989). Drugs Expt. Clin. Res. *XV*, 97–104.
210 Agnusdei, D., Camporea, A., Zacchei, F., Gennari, C., Baroni, M.C., Costi, D., Biondi, M., Passeri, A., Sbrennd, C. (1992). Curr. Ther. Res. *51*, 82–91.
211 Gambacciani, M., Spinetti, A., Cappagli, B., Taponeco, F., Felipetto, R., Parrini, D., Cappelli, N., Fioretti, P. (1993). J. Clin. Invest. *16*, 333–7.
212 Passeri, M., Biondi, M., Costi, D., Bufalino, L., Castigli, G.N., Dipeppe, C., Abate, G. (1992). Bone Mineral (suppl. 1) S57–S62.
213 Scali, G., Mansanti, P., Zurlo, A., Miola, F., Parti, M., Nardelli, A., Magnani, D., Zagathi, A. M., Kambanis, J., Bufalino, L. (1991). Curr. Ther. Res. *49*, 1004–10.
214 Melis, G.B., Paoletti, A M., Cagnacci, A., Bufalino, L., Spinetti, A., Gambacci, M., Floretti, P. (1992). J. Endocrinol. Invest. *15*, 755–61.
215 Melis, G.B., Poletti, A.M., Balducci, M.T., Bruni, Y., Becorpi, A., Otanell, S., Floretti, P. (1992). Bone Miner. *19* (Suppl. 1) S49–S56.
216 Clark, J.H. and Markaverich, B.M. (1982). Pharmac. Ther. *15*, 467–519.
217 Stewart, P.J., Stern, P.H. (1986). Endocrinology *118*, 125–.
218 Chakraborty, P.K., Brown, J.L., Ruff, C.B., Nelson, M.F. and Mitchell, A.S. (1991). J. Steroid Biochem. Molec. Biol. *40*, 725–729.
219 Jordan, V.C., Phelps, E. and Lindgreen, J.A. (1987). Brit. Cancer Res. Treatment *10*, 31–35.
220 Beall, P.T., Misra, L.K., Young, R.L., Spjut, H., J.Evans, H.J. and LeBlanc (1984). Calif. Tissue Int. *36*, 123–27.
221 Sutherland, R., Mester, J. Baulieu, E.E. (1977). Nature *267*, 434–435.
222 Kusuhara, S., Ishida, K. (1986). Jpn. J. Zootech. Sci. *57*, 726.
223 Wronski, T.J., Walsh, C.C., Ignaszewski, L.A. (1986). Bone 7, 119.
224 Turner, R.T., Vandersteenhoven, J.J., Bell, N.H. (1987). J. Bone Min. Res. *2*, 115.
225 Turner, R.T., Walkey, G.K., Hannon, K.S. and Bell, N.H. (1987). J. Bone Miner. Res. *2*, 449–456.
226 Fentiman, I.S., Saad, Z., Caleffi, M., Chaudary, M.A. and Fogelman, J. (1992). Eur. J. Cancer *28*, 684–685.

227 Broulek, P.D. (1991). Endocrine Regulation *25*, 217–219.
228 Jones, C.D., Suarez, T., Massey, E.H., Black, L.J. and Tinsley, F.C. (1979). J. Med. Chem. *22*, 962–66.
229 Black, L.J., Jones, C.D., Falcone, J.F. (1983). Life Sci. *32*, 1031–1036.
230 Jordan, V.C., Murphy, C.S. (1990). Endocrine Rev. *11*, 578–610.
231 Black, L.J., Sato, M., Rowley, E.R., Magee, D.E., Bekle, A., Williams, D.C., Culliam, G.J., Bendele, R., Kauffman, R.F., Bensch, W.R., Frolik, C.A., Termine, J.D. and Bryant, H.U. (1994). J. Clin. Invest. *93*, 63–69.
232 Evans, G., Bryant, H.U., Magee, D., and Turner, R.T., (1994). Endocrinology *134*, 2283–2288.
233 Kamboj, V.P., Ray, S., Dhawan, B.N. (1992). Drugs of Today *28*, 227–232.
234 Bain, S.D., Celino, D.L. Lantry, M., Strachan, M.I., Edwards, M.W., Piggott, I.R. and Labroo, V.M. (1993). Annual Meeting of the American Soc. for Bone & Mineral Society held on Sept. 18–21, 1993, Tampa, Florida.
235 Labroo, V.M., Creek, M., Piggott, J.R., Bothell, Bam, S.D., US Pat. No.5,280,040 dt. Jan.18, 1994.
236 Willson, T.M., Henke, B.R., Momtahen, T.M., Charijson, P.S., Batchelor, K.W., Lubahn, D.B., Moore, L.B., Oliver, B.B., Sauls, H.R., Triantafillous, J.A., Wolf, S.G., Baer P.G. (1994). J. Med. Chem. *37*, 1550–1552.
237 Benvenuti, S., Tanini,A. Frediani, U., Bianchi,S., Masi, L. Casano, R., Bufalino, L., Serio, M. and Brandi, M.L. (1991). J. Bone Mineral Res. *6*, 987–96.
238 Brandi, M.L. (1992). Bone Miner. *19* (Suppl.) S. 3–14.
239 Notoya, K., Yoshida, K., Taketomi, S., Yamazaki, I., Kumegawa, M. (1992). Calif. Tissue Int. *51* (Suppl) S3–6.
240 Albanese, C.V., Cudd, A., Argintino, L., Zambonin-Zallone, A. and MacIntyre, L. (1994). Biochemical and biophysical Res. Comm. *199*, 930–936.
241 Turner, R.T., Evans, G.L., Wakley, G.K. (1993). J. Bone Miner. Res. *8*, 359–66.
242 Orimo, H., Fujita, T., Yoshikawa, M. (1972). Endocrinol *90*, 760.
243 Komm, B.S., Terpening, C.M., Benz, D.J., Graeme, K.A., Gallegos, A., Korc, M., Greene, G.L., O'Malley, B.W., Haussler, M.R. (1988). Science *241*, 81–84.
244 Eriksen, E.F., Colvard, D.S., Berg, N.J., Graham, M.L., Spelsberg, T. C., Riggs, B.L. (1988). Science *241*, 84–86.
245 Arnett, R, Lindsay, R, Dempster, D.W.,(1986). J.Bone Mineral Res. [Suppl.1] *1*, 99 (Abstract).
246 Doehler, K.D., Hancke, J.L., Srivastava, S.S., Hofmann, C., Shryne, J.E., Gorski, R.A. (1984). Prog. Brain Res. *61* (Sex Differ. Brain) 99–117.
247 Greaves, P., Goonetilleke, R., Nunn, G., Tophan, J., Orton, T. (1993). Cancer Res. *53*, 3919–24.
248 Mertz, W. (1981). Science *213*, 1332.
249 Riggs, B.L., Hodgson, S.F., Hoffman, D.L., Kelly, P.J., Johnson, K.A., Taves, D. (1980). J. Am. Med. Assoc. *243*, 446.
250 Riggs, B.L., Seeman, E., Hodgson, S.F., Taves, D.R. and O'Fallon, W.M. (1982) N. Engl. J. Med. *306*, 446–450.
251 Kanis, J.A. (1993). Am. J. Med. *95* (Suppl. 5A) 53S.
252 Joysey, J., Riggis, B.L. Kelly, P.J., Hoffman, D.L. (1972). Am. J. Med. *53*, 43–9.
253 Chapuy, M.C., Chapuy, P., Meunier, P.J. (1987). Am. J. Clin. Nutr. *46*, 324–28.
254 Farley, J.R., Wergedale, J.E., Baylink, D.J. (1983). Science *222*, 330–32.
255 Eanes, E.D., Reddi, A.H. (1979). Metab. Bone Dis. Relt. Res. *2*, 3–10.
256 Kanis, J.A., Meunier, P.J. (1984). Q. J. Med. *53*, 145–64.

257 Chavassieux, P., Pastoure, P., Boivin, G., Chaupuy, M.C., Delmas, P.D., Milhand, G., Meunier, P.J. (1991). Osteoporosis Int. *2*, 26–33.
258 Baylink, D.J., Bernstein, D.S. (1967). Clin. Orthop. *55*, 51–85.
259 Parson, V., Mitchell, C., Eimond, A., Darby, A.J., The use of sodium fluoride and calcium suppliments and vit. D. in the treatment of axial osteoporosis. In: Dixon A. St.J., Russell, R.G.G., Stamp T.C.B. eds. Osteoporosis, a multidisciplinary problem. London Royal Soc. of Medicine academic press (1983). 259–64.
260 Deuxchaisnis, N.C., Devogdaer, J.P., Stein, F. (1990). Eur. J. Bone Miner. Res. *5* (Suppl. 2) S251.
261 Pak, C.Y.C., Sakhaee, K., Piziak, V., Peterson, R.D., Breslau, N.A., Boyd, P., Poindexter, J.R., Herzog, J., Heart-Sakhaee, A., Haynes, S., Adams-Huet, B., and Reisch, J.S., Ann. Inter. Med. *120*, 625–632.
262 John A. (1993) Amer. J. Med. *95* (Suppl.) 5A–61S.
263 Inkovaara, J., Heikinheimo, R., Jarvinen, V., Kasurinen, U., Hanhijarvi, H., Iisalo, E. (1975). Br. Med. J. *3*, 73–4.
264 Riggs, B.L., Hodgson, S.F., O'Fallon, M.W., Chao, E.Y., Wahner, H.W., Muhs, J.M., Cedel, S.L., and Melton, L.J. III. (1990). N. Eng. J. Med. *322*, 802–9.
265 Slovik, D.M., Neer, R.M., and Potts, J.T. Jr. (1981) . J. Clin. Invest. *68*, 1261–71.
266 Reeve, J., Meunier, P., Parson, J.A., Bernat, M., Bijvoet, O.L.M., Courpron, P., Edouard, C., Klenerman, L., Neer, R.M., Renier, J.C. Slovik, D., Vismans, F.J.F.E., Potts, J.T. Jr. (1980). Brit. Med. J. *280*, 1340–44.
267 Reeve, J., Hesp, R., Williamson, D., Hulme, P., Klenerman, L., Zanelli, J.M., Darby, A.J., Tregear, G.W., Parson, J.A. (1976). Lancet *1*, 1035–38.
268 Wasnich, R., Benfante, R., Katsuhiko, Y., Heilbrun, L., Voge, J. (1983). N. Eng. J. Med. *309*, 344–347.
269 Brickman, A.S., Massry, S.G., and Coburn, J.W., (1972), The J. Clin. Invest. *51*, 945–954.
270 Duarte, C.G., Winnacker, J.L., Becker, K.L. and Pace, A. (1971). *284*, 828–830.
271 Transbol, I., Christensen, M., Jensen, G., Christensen, C., McNair, P. (1982). Metabolism *31*, 383–386.
272 Lacroix, A.Z., Wienpahl, J., White, L.R.,Wallace, R.B., Scherr, P.A., George, L.K., Cornoni-Huntly, J., Ostefeld, A.M. (1990). N. Engl. J. Med. *322*, 286–290.
273 Bauer, G.C., Wendeberg, B. (1959). J. Bone Joint Surg. (B) *41*, 558–80.
274 Skoryna, S.C. (1981). Can. Med. Assoc. J. *125*, 703–12.
275 Storey, E. (1961). Aust. Ann. Med. *10*, 213–22.
276 McCaslin, F.E.Jr., Janes, J.M. (1959). Proc. Staff Meet Mayo Clin. *34*, 329–34.
277 Marie, P.J., Garba, M.T., Hatt, M., Miravet, L. (1985). Miner. Electrol. Metal. *11*, 5–13.
278 Grynpas, M.D., Marie, P.J. (1990). Bone *11*, 313–9.
279 Su, Y., Bonnet, J., Deloffre, P., Tsouderos, Y., Baron, R. (1992). Bone Miner. *17*, A 449.
280 Su, Y., Bonnet, J., Deloffre, P., Tsouderos, Y., Baron, R. (1992). J. Bone Miner. Res. *7*, A 853.
281 Lo, Y.S., Nolan, J.C., Walsh, D.A., Welstead, W.J.Jr. (1989). Eur. Pat. Appl. EP 403, 185. Chem. Abstr, *116*, 20788e.
282 Grossi, E. (1990). PCT Int. Appl.WO 9204,892. Chem. Abstr. *117*, 83452g.
283 Shah, M. (1990). PCT. Int. Appl.WO 9117,751. Chem. Abstr. *116*, 136251d.
284 Lang, H.J., Naumann, C., Carniato, D., Moura, A.M., Satoh, R., Katoh, M. (1993). Eur. Pat. Appl. EP 546,548. Chem. Abstr. *119*, 117544x.

285 Iwao, K., Yasua, O., Haruki,T., Nobuo,K., Akio, I., Joji, N., Hiroyuki, I., Katsushi, G. (1994). Eur. Pat. Apple. EP. 578,419, Chem. Abstr. *120*, 244689u.

286 Ohishi, Y., Tamura, M., Hayashida, M., Ikegami, S., Itiyama, Y., Awa, T., Ichikawa, T., Nomiyama, K., Handa, K.M., Mimura, M. (1992). Eur. Pat. Appl. EP 498,424. Chem. Abstr. *117*, 212723x.

287 Ebetino, F.H., Kass, S.M., Francis, M.D. PCT Int. Appl. WO 9324, 499 (1993). Chem. Abstr. *120*, 245509x.

288 Santilli, A.A., Andrews, S.M., Strike, D.P., US 5,288,871 (1994). Chem. Abstr. *120*, 245109s.

289 Ohe, T., Akagi, T., Chiba, K., Amano, Y. PCT Int. Appl.WO 9203,427 (1992). Chem. Abstr. 3 *117*, 69849 k.

290 Suzuki, F., Miwa, Y., Hayashi, H., Kuroda, T., Ohmon, K., Nakazima, H. Eur. Pat. Appl. EP 505,058 (1992). Chem. Abstr. *117*, 251343t.

291 Soda, T., Kubo, K., Tsuda, M., Jpn Kokai Takkyo Koho JP 01,203,325 (1992). Chem. Abstr. *112*, 104881 k.

292 Suzuki, F., Shimada J., Ishii, A., Nanaka, H., Kosaka, N., Ichikawa, S. PCT Int. Appl. WO 920,6976 (1992). Chem. Abstr. *117*, 90312 q.

293 Suzuki, F., Kuroda, T., Ishii, A., Kosaka, N. Jpn Kokai Takkyo Koho JP 03,291,226 (1991). Chem. Abstr. *116*, 228260j.

294 Skotnicki, J.S., Kearney, R.M., US 5,281,608 (1994). Chem. Abstr. *120*, 270359f.

295 Takahashi, H., Saito, T. Jpn. Kokai Takkyo Koho JP 0454,195 (1992). Chem. Abstr. *117*, 76475 p.

296 Tahara, T., Moriwaki, M., Chiba, K., Manobe, S., Shindo, M., Nakagawa, T., Nakamura, T. PCT Int. Appl.WO 9307,129 (1991). Chem. Abstr. *120*, 270 466 P.

297 Sohada, T., Xamazahi, I., Eur. Pat. Appl. EP 460,488 (1991). Chem. Abstr. *116*, 151599S.

298 Kamijo, T., Ujue, S., Tsutsumi, N., Tsubaki, A., Jpn Kokai Takkyo Koho JP 02,142,792 (1988). Chem. Abstr. *113*, 172001u.

299 Isomura, Y., Sakamoto, S., Yoshida, M., Abe, T., Jpn Kokai Takkyo Koho JP 63,112,573. (1988). Chem. Abstr. *109*, 170418d.

300 Isomura, Y., Sakamolo, S., Yoshida, M., Abe, T., Jpn Kopkai Tokkyo Koho JP 63,112,572. (1988) Chem. Abstr. *109*, P110423s.

301 Isomura, Y., Sakamoto, S., Yoshida, M., Abe, T., Jpn Kokai Tokkyo Koho JP 63,112,574 (1988). Chem. Abstr. *109*, 110424t.

302 Miyashita, M., Kohno, Y., Kojima, E., Saito, K. PCT Int Appl. W09100,273 (1991). Chem. Abstr. *114*, P 185308v.

303 Slemenda, C.W., Hui, S.L., Longeope, C., Wellman, H. and Johnston, C.C.Jr. (1990). Ann. Internal. Med. *112*, 96–101.

304 Stevenson, J.C., Lees, B., Devenport, M., Cust, M.P., Ganger, K.F. (1989). Br. Med. J. *298*, 924–8.

305 Faulkner, K.G., Gluer, C.C., Palermo, L., Black, D., Genant, H.K., Cumming, S.R. (1992). J. Bone Miner. Res. *7* (Suppl.I) 98.

306 Johnston, C.C. Jr., Simenda, C.W. (1993). The Amer. J. Med. *95*, 5A–55.

307 Kalender, W.A., Rienmull, R., Seissler, W., Behr, J., Welke, M., Fichte, N. (1990). Radiology *175*, 265–68.

308 Sandor, T., Felsenberg, D., Kalenda, W.A., Clain, A., Brown, E. (1992). Calif Tissue Int. *50*, 502–6.

309 Smith, D.A.S., Hosie, C.J., Deacon, A.D., Hamblen, D.L. (1990). Br. J. Radiol. *63*, 776–82.

310 Genant, H.K., Ettinger, B., Harris, S.T., Block, J.E., Steiger, P. Quantitative computed tomography in assessment of osteoporosis. In: Riggs, B.L., Melton, L.J.III, eds. Osteoporis. Actiology, Diagnosis and Management. New York. Raven Press 1988). 221–50.
311 Cosman, F., Herrington, B., Himmelstein, S., Lindsay, R. (1991). Osteoporosis Int., *2*, 343–8.
312 Herney, R.P., Avioli, L.V., Chestnut, C.H. 3d, Lappe, J., Recker, R.R., Brandenburger, G.H. (1989). JAMMA *261*, 2986–90.
313 Price, P.A., Parthemore, J.G., Deftos, L.J. (1983). J. Clin. Invest. *71*, 1316–21.
314 Delmas, P.D. (1993). The Amer. J. Med. *95*, 5A–16S.
315 Delmas, P.D., Demiaux, B., Malaval, L., Chapuy, M. C., Edouard, C., and Meunier, P.J. (1986). J. Clin. Invest. *77*, 985–91.
316 Posen, S., Cornish, C., Kleerekoper, M. (1977). Alkaline phosphatase and metabolic bone disorders. In: Metabolic bone diseases. LV Avioli and S.M.Krane eds. Academic Press Inc. NY 941–181.
317 Ebeling, P.R., Peterson, J.M., Riggis, B.L. (1992). *7*, 1243–1250.
318 Eyre, D.R. (1987). Enzymology *144*, 115–39.
319 Uebelhart, D., Schlemmer, A., Johansen, J., Gineyts, E., Christiansen, C., Delmas, P.D. (1991). J. Clin. Endocrinol. Metab. *72*, 367–7.
320 Seyedin, S., Zuk, R., Kung, V., Daniloff, Y., Shepard, K. (1993). J. Bone Miner. Res. *8*, 635–42.
321 Eastell, R., Hampton, L., Colwell, A. Urinary collagen crosslinksare highly correlated with radio isotopic measurements of bone resorption. In: C.Christiansen and K.Overgaard eds. Proceedings of the Third International Symposium on osteoporosis. Osteopress, Aalberg, Denmark (1990). 469–70.
322 Delmas, P.D., Schlemmer, A., Grineyts, E., Riis, B., Christiansen, C. (1991). J. Bone. Miner. Res. *6*, 639–44.
323 Podenphant, J., Larsen, N.E., Christiansen, C. (1984). Clin. Chim. Acta *142*, 145–8.
324 Krane, S.M., Kantrowitz, F.G., Byrne, M., Pinnel, S.R., Singer, F.R. (1977). J. Clin. Invest. *59*, 819–27.
325 Ringe, J.D. (1994). Drugs of Today *30*, 25–32.
326 Schneider, H.P.G., Doren, M., Langzeitige Osteogen-Gestagen Substitution. In: Osteoporose. Pathogenese, Diagnostik und Therapiemöglichkeiten. Ringe J.D. (ed) Walter de Gruyter. Berlin 1991.

Index Vol. 45

The references of the Subject Index are given in the language of the respective contribution.
Die Stichworte des Sachregisters sind in der jeweiligen Sprache der einzelnen Beiträge aufgeführt.
Les termes repris dans la Table des Matières sont donnés selon la langue dans laquelle l'ouvrage est écrit.

Index of titles
Verzeichnis der Titel
Index des titres
Vol. 1–45 (1959–1995)

Author and paper index
Autoren- und Artikelindex
Index des auteurs et des articles
Vol. 1–45 (1959–1995)

Agents and Actions Supplements

Further titles in this series:

P.M. Brooks / R.O. Day, *University of New South Wales, Sydney, Australia /* **G.G. Graham,** *University of New South Wales, Kensington, Australia /* **K.M. Williams,** *University of New South Wales, Sydney, Australia (Eds)*

Variability in Response to Anti-Rheumatic Drugs

1993. 240 pages. Hardcover.
ISBN 3-7643-2869-X (AAS 44)

T.T. Hansel, *Sandoz Pharma Ltd., Basel, Switzerland /* **J. Morley,** *Muhmed Ltd., London, UK (Eds)*

New Drugs in Allergy and Asthma

1993. 320 pages. Hardcover.
ISBN 3-7643-2870-3 (AAS 43)

J.C. Cheronis, *Cortech, Inc., Denver, CO, USA /* **R.E. Repine,** *University of Colorado, Denver, CO, USA (Eds)*

Proteases, Protease Inhibitors and Protease-Derived Peptides

Importance in Human Pathophysiology and Therapeutics

1993. 248 pages. Hardcover.
ISBN 3-7643-2868-1 (AAS 42)

M.H. Schöni, *Alpine Kinderklinik, Davos, Switzerland /* **R. Kraemer,** *Inselspital, Bern, Switzerland (Eds)*

Update on Childhood Asthma

1993. 222 pages. Hardcover.
ISBN 3-7643-2867-3 (AAS 40)

W.B. van den Berg / P.M. van der Kraan / P.L.E.M. van Lent, *Dept. of Rheumatology, University Hospital, Nijmegen, The Netherlands (Eds)*

Joint Destruction in Arthritis and Osteoarthritis

1993. 276 pages. Hardcover.
ISBN 3-7643-2773-1 (AAS 39)

N.R. Ackerman / R. J. Bonney / A.F. Welton *(Eds)*

Progress in Inflammation Research and Therapy

1991. XVI + 192 pages. Hardcover.
ISBN 3-7643-2529-1 (AAS 35)

M.J. Parnham / M.A. Bray / W.B. van den Berg *(Eds)*

Drugs in Inflammation

1991. 264 pages. Hardcover.
ISBN 3-7643-2504-6 (AAS 32)

MIX
Papier aus verantwortungsvollen Quellen
Paper from responsible sources
FSC® C105338

If you have any concerns about our products,
you can contact us on
ProductSafety@springernature.com

In case Publisher is established outside the EU,
the EU authorized representative is:
Springer Nature Customer Service Center GmbH
Europaplatz 3, 69115 Heidelberg, Germany

Printed by Libri Plureos GmbH
in Hamburg, Germany